Ocular Radiation Risk Assessment in Populations Exposed to Environmental Radiation Contamination

NATO ASI Series

Advanced Science Institute Series

A Series presenting the results of activities sponsored by the NATO Science Committee, which aims at the dissemination of advanced scientific and technological knowledge, with a view to strengthening links between scientific communities.

The Series is published by an international board of publishers in conjunction with the NATO Scientific Affairs Division

A Life Sciences **B Physics**	Plenum Publishing Corporation London and New York
C Mathematical and Physical Sciences **D Behavioural and Social Sciences** **E Applied Sciences**	Kluwer Academic Publishers Dordrecht, Boston and London
F Computer and Systems Sciences **G Ecological Sciences** **H Cell Biology** **I Global Environment Change**	Springer-Verlag Berlin, Heidelberg, New York, London, Paris and Tokyo

PARTNERSHIP SUB-SERIES

1. Disarmament Technologies	Kluwer Academic Publishers
2. Environment	Springer-Verlag / Kluwer Academic Publishers
3. High Technology	Kluwer Academic Publishers
4. Science and Technology Policy	Kluwer Academic Publishers
5. Computer Networking	Kluwer Academic Publishers

The Partnership Sub-Series incorporates activities undertaken in collaboration with NATO's Cooperation Partners, the countries of the CIS and Central and Eastern Europe, in Priority Areas of concern to those countries.

NATO-PCO-DATA BASE

The electronic index to the NATO ASI Series provides full bibliographical references (with keywords and/or abstracts) to about 50,000 contributions from international scientists published in all sections of the NATO ASI Series. Access to the NATO-PCO-DATA BASE is possible via a CD-ROM "NATO Science and Technology Disk" with user-friendly retrieval software in English, French, and German (©WTV GmbH and DATAWARE Technologies, Inc. 1989). The CD-ROM contains the AGARD Aerospace Database.

The CD-ROM can be ordered through any member of the Board of Publishers or through NATO-PCO, Overijse, Belgium.

2. Environmental – Vol. 50

Ocular Radiation Risk Assessment in Populations Exposed to Environmental Radiation Contamination

edited by

A. K. Junk

Eye Radiation & Environmental Research Laboratory,
Columbia University,
New York, U.S.A.

Y. Kundiev

Institute of Occupational Health,
Academy of Medical Sciences of Ukraine,
Kiev, Ukraine

P. Vitte

Institute of Occupational Health,
Academy of Medical Sciences of Ukraine,
Kiev, Ukraine

and

B. V. Worgul

Eye Radiation & Environmental Research Laboratory,
Columbia University,
New York, U.S.A.

Kluwer Academic Publishers

Dordrecht / Boston / London

Published in cooperation with NATO Scientific Affairs Division

Proceedings of the NATO Advanced Research Workshop on
Ocular Radiation Risk Assessment in Populations Exposed to
Environmental Radiation Contamination
Kiev, Ukraine
29 July - 1 August 1997

A C.I.P. Catalogue record for this book is available from the Library of Congress.

ISBN 0-7923-5310-2

Published by Kluwer Academic Publishers,
P.O. Box 17, 3300 AA Dordrecht, The Netherlands.

Sold and distributed in North, Central and South America
by Kluwer Academic Publishers,
101 Philip Drive, Norwell, MA 02061, U.S.A.

In all other countries, sold and distributed
by Kluwer Academic Publishers,
P.O. Box 322, 3300 AH Dordrecht, The Netherlands.

Printed on acid-free paper

Printed in the Netherlands

TABLE OF CONTENTS

2. Dosimetry

PREFACE

In former Sowjet Union countries there are currently underway or being planned, several major ocular follow-up studies of populations exposed to radiation from reactor accidents, contamination from nuclear weapons manufacturing or fall-out from nuclear testing. The importance of such studies lies in their potential to provide the data necessary to:

1) help define the true extent of the impact of environmental contamination in affected regions
2) allow for a better appreciation of the degree of morbidity arising from such contamination
3) establish acceptable standards for ocular risk guidelines,
4) develop the necessary database to allow cataract to meet its potential in retrospective dose reconstruction,
5) assess the contribution of environmental radiation exposure to the incidence of senile cataract development in populations at large.

Given the complexity of such studies, the potential confounders, and the myriad of possible methods of assessment, it is in the interest of the global scientific and medical communities to, insofar as possible, standardize methodologies and agree upon minimum criteria to make inter-study comparisons possible. With this in mind the NATO Advanced Research Workshop (ARW) on "Ocular Radiation Risk Assessment in Populations Exposed to Environmental Radiation Contamination", 29 July - 1 August 1997 - Puscha Ozyorna, Kiev, Ukraine, was organized to establish minimum and standardized criteria for the acquisition, archiving, evaluating, and dissemination of data on the ocular risk of populations to environmental radiation exposure.

The approach was to have major lectures on each of the three primary components of population studies; ophthalmology, epidemiology and dosimetry. It was agreed upon from the outset that the strength and utility of any study would be determined by the weakest component and that any effort should focus on maximizing the validity of each. The ARW resulted in a series of recommendations, which are the first codification of the manner in which such studies should be executed.

Because of its relative non-ambiguity and the fact that agencies historically have conditioned their risk assessments on the induction of cataract, study design necessarily focused on cataract onset. There were readily agreed upon basic points that should be considered in the design and conduct of an eye study. They are detailed in the final chapter of this volume and are summarized below.

As regards the ophthalmological aspects careful coordination with the epidemiological component must be implemented from the outset in order to agree on such things as the best way to handle confounders and/or one and two-eyed data acquisition. Qualified ophthalmologists must be used as primary examiners. Mydriatrics must always be used to maximize posterior lens visualization. A study should not even be considered if the subjects eyes cannot be dilated. Ophthalmoscopy can be employed as part of the overall eye examination but the lens status **must** be assessed using a slit-lamp. Standardized recording forms and the training to properly use them are critical.

Central estimates of dose and estimates of uncertainty should be provided for *absorbed dose* for each type of radiation of significantly different linear energy transfer (LET), such as alpha particles, beta-gamma radiation, and neutrons; information as specific as possible should be provided on the nature of the irradiation experienced by the studied population. Adequate dosimetry support is understood to have the following requirements; assistance in the cohort-selection phase to ensure that proposed members of the cohort have a reasonable probability of having a "knowable" dose with as little uncertainty as possible. Ultimate provision of a dose to the eye lens that includes both beta and gamma components with as small an amount of uncertainty as possible. The uncertainty requirements are not specified, but a goal should be to have individual doses with an uncertainty factor of three or less. An uncertainty factor of two or less would be highly desirable.

Dosimetrists and epidemiologists should be involved early in joint discussions of possible studies so that even approximate estimates of dose can be used to examine whether a postulated epidemiologic study would have enough power to detect, in a statistically significant way, the effect to be studied. Significant dosimetric support should continue over the life of any epidemiologic study of potentially significant value (or investment). For case-control or cohort studies, doses and associated uncertainties should be determined for each individual in the study. A cohort study is the preferred study type whenever it is feasible. In planning a study it is vital to determine the sample size required to yield adequate statistical power; otherwise the study is unlikely to produce meaningful results. The sample of subjects must be systematically drawn from a defined population, ***not*** just a "convenience sample" or whoever volunteers. It is essential that a cohort study be designed so that subjects at all dose levels receive ocular examinations with the same frequency and thoroughness and the examiners should be blinded to the dose status of the subjects.

The Ukrainian-American Chernobyl Ocular Study (UACOS) was used and was discussed as a concrete example of the conduct of an epidemiologic study of ocular risk.

The committee is most grateful to the North Atlantic Treaty Organization for the exceptional support provided for this meeting and for the production of this monograph. It also acknowledges substantial support provided by Columbia University, New York, NY and the Edward S. Harkness Eye Institute at Columbia

University, New York, NY, as well as the Ministry of Public Health, Kiev, Ukraine and the Institute of Occupational Health (IOH), Academy of Medical Sciences, Kiev, Ukraine. The Editors would like to thank L. R. Anspaugh, J. Doorish, N. Kleiman, J. Koniarek and A. Wegener for taking the time to review papers contained in this volume. We thank Julissa Diaz for her invaluable help in compiling and finalising these proceedings.

Anna K. Junk
Yuri I. Kundiev
Peter Vitte
Basil V. Worgul

ORGANIZATION OF THE NATO ADVANCED RESEARCH WORKSHOP ON OCULAR RADIATION RISK ASSESSMENT IN POPULATIONS EXPOSED TO ENVIRONMENTAL RADIATION CONTAMINATION, KIEV, JULY 1997

Program Committee

Co-Directors	B. V. Worgul	Columbia University, ERERL, New York, USA
	Y. I. Kundiev	Institute of Occupational Health, Kiev, Ukraine
Members	A. M. Kellerer	GSF, Inst. of Radiobiology, Neuherberg, Germany
	I. Liktarev	Inst. Radiation Protection, Kiev, Ukraine
	N. Sergienko	Center of Eye Microsurgery, Kiev, Ukraine
	A. Wegener	Univ. Bonn, Inst. of Exp. Ophthalmol., Germany

Organizing Committee

Co-Chairmen	A. Vozinaov	Pres. Acad. Med. Sci., Kiev, Ukraine
	A. Serdyuk	Minister Pub. Health, Kiev, Ukraine
Members	Y. I. Kundiev	Institute of Occupational Health, Kiev, Ukraine
	A. Romanenko	Dir. Sci. Ctr. Rad. Med., Kiev, Ukraine
	V. Torbin	Ministry Chernobyl Prob., Ukraine
	B. V. Worgul	ERERL, Columbia University, New York, USA
Scientific Secr.	P. M. Vitte	Institute of Occupational Health, Kiev, Ukraine

Session Chairmen

L. R. Anspaugh	University of Utah, Salt Lake City, USA
M. Bausz	Semmelweis Medical School, Budapest, Hungary
W. P. Chang	Yang Ming University, Taipei, Taiwan
V. Chumak	Radiation Protection Institute, Kiev, Ukraine
S. P. Denyer	University of Brighton, Brighton, UK
A. K. Junk	Ludwig-Maximilians Univ., Munich, Germany
T. Kodama	Ehime University, Ehime, Japan
Y. I. Kundiev	Academy of Med. Sciences, Kiev, Ukraine
V. Kruchkov	State Research Center, Moscow, Russia
I. Lichtarev	Radiation Protection Institute, Kiev, Ukraine
C. Medvedovsky	Columbia University, New York, USA
G. Parkhomenko	Eye Microsurgery Center, Kiev, Ukraine
N. Sergienko	Medical Acad. Postgrad. Education, Kiev, Ukraine

R. Shore	New York University, New York, USA
P. M. Vitte	Academy of Med. Sciences, Kiev, Ukraine
B. V. Worgul	Columbia University, New York, USA

Speakers

A. Abdullina	Inst. of Oncology & Radiol., Bishkek, Kyrgyzstan
L. R. Anspaugh	University of Utah, Salt Lake City, USA
C. Baumstark-Khan	DLR, Inst. of Aerospace Med., Cologne, Germany
M. Bausz	Semmelweis Medical School, Budapest, Hungary
V. G. Bebeshko	Ukrainian Sci. Ctr. Rad. Med., Kiev, Ukraine
W. P. Chang	Yang Ming University, Taipei, Taiwan
M. W. Charles	University of Birmingham, Birmingham, UK
V. V. Chumak	Radiation Protection Institute, Kiev, Ukraine
S. P. Denyer	University of Brighton, Brighton, UK
A. I. Deyev	Russian State Medical University, Moscow, Russia
A. Eglite	Medical Academy of Latvia, Riga, Latvia
I. Galstyan	State Research Center, Moscow, Russia
P. Fedirko	Ukrainian Sci. Ctr. Rad. Med., Kiev, Ukraine
M. Froemel	Ludwig-Maximilians Univ., Munich, Germany
A. K. Junk	Ludwig-Maximilians Univ., Munich, Germany
T. Kodama	Ehime University, Ehime, Japan
V. Kruchkov	State Research Center, Moscow, Russia
Y. I. Kundiev	Institute of Occupational Health, Kiev, Ukraine
I. Kuras	Vice Prime Minister Acad, Kiev, Ukraine
I. Lichtarev	Radiation Protection Institute, Kiev, Ukraine
I. M. Logay	Filatov Inst. of Eye Diseases, Odessa, Ukraine
A. S. Madekin	Grodno State Medical Institute, Grodno, Belarus
T. N. Mikhailina	Biophysic Institute, Ozyorsk, Russia
C. Medvedovsky	Columbia University, New York, USA
A. Ruban	Eye Microsurgery Center, Kiev, Ukraine
V. I. Serduchenko	Filatov Inst. of Eye Diseases, Odessa, Ukraine
A. Serdyuk	Minister of Public Health
N. Sergienko	Medical Acad. Postgrad. Education, Kiev, Ukraine
R. Shore	New York University, New York, USA
S. Sosnovsky	Military Medical Academy, St. Petersburg, Russia
J. R. Trevithick	University of Western Ontario, London, Canada
N. M. Umovist	National Medical University, Kiev, Ukraine
P. M. Vitte	Institute of Occupational Health, Kiev, Ukraine
E. Voice	University of Essex, Colchester, UK
A. Vozianov	President of Academy of Medical Sciences
B. V. Worgul	Columbia University, ERERL, New York, USA
Y.N. Zabulonov	Human Ecology Institute, Kiev, Ukraine

LIST OF PARTICIPANTS OF THE NATO ADVANCED RESEARCH WORKSHOP ON OCULAR RADIATION RISK ASSESSMENT IN POPULATIONS EXPOSED TO ENVIRONMENTAL RADIATION CONTAMINATION

A. Abdullina	Kyrgyz Republican Registry of Radiation Victims, Inst. of Oncology & Radiology, 92 Akhunbaev St., Bishkek 720064, Kyrgyzstan
L. R. Anspaugh	Univ. of Utah, Inst. of Radiobiology, Building 585, 40 North 2030 East Front, Salt Lake City, Utah 84112-5860, USA
T. M. Avakian	Yerevan Physics Institute, Alichanian Brosst 2, Yerevan, 375036, Armenia
C. Baumstark-Khan	DLR, Inst. of Aerospace Med., Radiobiological Unit, Linder Höhe, D-51147 Cologne, Germany
M. Bausz	Semmelweis Medical School, Dept. of Ophthalmology, Tomo U. 25-29, H-1083 Budapest, Hungary
V. G. Bebeshko	Ukrainian Sci. Ctr. Rad. Med., 53 Melnikova St., 252004 Kiev, Ukraine
N. Bushuyeva	Filatov Inst. of Eye Diseases and Tissue Therapy, 49/51 Boulevard Francais, 270061 Odessa, Ukraine
W. P. Chang	Yang Ming University Medical School, Institute of Public Health, 155, Section 2, Lih-non Street, Taipei, Taiwan
M. W. Charles	University of Birmingham, School of Physics and Space Research, Edgbaston, Birmingham B15 2TT, UK
V. Chumak	External Dosimetry, Ukrainian Radiation Protection Institute, 53 Melnikova St., 252004 Kiev, Ukraine
V. Danilichev	Military Medical Academy, 6 Lebedeva St., St. Petersburg 9, Russia
S. P. Denyer	Biomaterials Research Group, University of Brighton, Cockcroft Building, Lewes Road, Moulsecomb, Brighton BN2 4GJ, UK
A. I. Deyev	Russian State Medical University, 115-1-200, Profsouznaya St., Moscow 117647, Russia
A. Eglite	Institute of Occupational and Environmental Health, Medical Academy of Latvia, Dzirciema 16, Riga LV 1007, Latvia
P. Fedirko	Ukrainian Sci. Ctr. Rad. Med., 53 Melnikova St., 252004 Kiev, Ukraine
B. Fountos	US DOE, Office of International Health Programs, EH-63/270 CC 19901 Germantown Road, Germantown, Maryland 20874-1290, USA

M. Froemel	Radiobiological Institute, Ludwig-Maximilians University, Schillerstr. 42, D-80336 Munich, Germany
I. Galstyan	State Research Center, Institute of Biophysics, 46 Zhivopisnaya St., Moscow 123183, Russia
T. Kodama	Dept. of Ophthalmology, Ehime University, School of Medicine, Shigenobu, Ehime 791-02, Japan
V. Kruchkov	State Research Center, Institute of Biophysics, 46 Zhivopisnaya St., Moscow 123183, Russia
Y. I. Kundiev	Institute of Occupational Health, Academy of Med. Sciences, 75 Saksagansky St., 252033 Kiev 33, Ukraine
I. Kuras	Vice Prime Minister Acad, Kiev, Ukraine
A. K. Junk	Dept. of Ophthalmology and Institute of Radiobiology, Ludwig-Maximilians University, Mathildenstr. 8, D-80336 Munich, Germany
I. Liktarev	External Dosimetry, Ukrainian Radiation Protection Institute, 53 Melnikova St., 252004 Kiev, Ukraine
V. Lishenko	Filatov Inst. of Eye Diseases and Tissue Therapy, 49/51 Boulevard Francais, 270061 Odessa, Ukraine
I. M. Logay	Filatov Inst. of Eye Diseases and Tissue Therapy, 49/51 Boulevard Francais, 270061 Odessa, Ukraine
A. S. Madekin	Grodno State Medical Institute, Ul. Gorkogo 80, Grodno 230015, Republic of Belarus
I. Masnyk	National Cancer Institute, Radiation Effects Branch, 6130 Executive Blvd., Suite 530, Rockville, Maryland 20852, USA
C. Medvedovsky	Columbia University, Eye Radiation and Environmental Research Laboratory, 630 W 168th St., New York, New York 10032, USA
S. Melnoz	Institute of Radiation Medicine, Minsk, Belarus
T. N. Mikhailina	Biophysic Institute, CMSI-71, 19 Ozyorsk Shosse, Ozyorsk, Chelyabinsk-65, Russia
S. Mikhalovsky	Biomaterials Research Group, University of Brighton, Cockcroft Building, Lewes Road, Moulsecomb, Brighton BN2 4GJ, UK
U. Muller Eberhard	Cornell University, Ithaca, New York 14853, USA
G. Ozola	Institute of Occupational and Environmental Health, Medical Academy of Latvia, Dzirciema 16, Riga LV 1007, Latvia
A. Ruban	Eye Microsurgery Center, 3 Avenue Komarova, Kiev 252000, Ukraine
V. I. Serduchenko	Filatov Inst. of Eye Diseases and Tissue Therapy, 49/51 Boulevard Francais, 270061 Odessa, Ukraine
A. Serdyuk	Minister of Public Health, Kiev, Ukraine

N. Sergienko	Kiev Medical Academy of Postgraduate Education, 9 Dorogojitskaya St., 252033 Kiev 33, Ukraine
V. Shevchenko	Vavilov Institute of General Genetics, Russian Academy of Sciences, 3 Gubkin St., GSP-1, Moscow 117809, Russia
R. Shore	New York University, Dept. of Environmental Medicine, 341 E 25th St., New York, New York 10010, USA
S. Sosnovsky	Military Medical Academy, 6 Lebedeva St., St. Petersburg 9, Russia
J. R. Trevithick	University of Western Ontario, Dept. of Biochemistry, London, Ontario, N6A-5C1, Canada
N. M. Umovist	National Medical University, Kiev, Ukraine
M. Vinogradova	Biophysic Institute, CMSI-71, 19 Ozyorsk Shosse, Ozyorsk, Chelyabinsk-65, Russia
P. M. Vitte	Institute of Occupational Health, Academy of Med. Sciences, 75 Saksagansky St., 252033 Kiev 33, Ukraine
E. Voice	University of Essex, Dept. of Biological and Chemical Sciences, John Tabor Laboratories, Colchester CO4 3SQ, UK
A. Vozianov	President of Academy of Medical Sciences, Kiev, Ukraine
B. V. Worgul	Columbia University, Eye Radiation and Environmental Research Laboratory, 630 W 168th St., New York, New York 10032, USA
Y.N. Zabulonov	Human Ecology Institute, Kiev, Ukraine

THE UKRAINIAN/AMERICAN CHERNOBYL OCULAR STUDY

B.V. WORGUL[1], Y.I. KUNDIEV[2], V.V. CHUMAK[3], A. RUBAN[4], G. PARKHOMENKO[4], P. VITTE[3], N.M. SERGIENKO[4], R. SHORE[5], I.A. LIKHTAREV[6], C. MEDVEDOVSKY[1], AND A.K. JUNK[1]

[1]The Eye Radiation & Environmental Research Laboratory, Columbia University, New York, NY, USA, [2]Kiev Research Institute for Occupational Health, Ukraine, [3]Ukrainian Scientific Center for Radiation Medicine, Kiev, Ukraine, [4]Eye Microsurgery Center, Ukraine, [5]Dept. Epidemiology, New York University, USA., [6]Radiation Protection Institute, Kiev, Ukraine.

1. Abstract

The Ukrainian/American Chernobyl Ocular Study (UACOS) Group has been established to provide an infrastructure to monitor the effects of radiation on ocular tissues, with particular emphasis on the lens. This consortium has been focusing on the subset of the over 250,000 individuals who were assigned clean up and maintenance duties after the accident, the so-called "Liquidators". The planned 30 year study has three main thrusts; (1) an extensive cohort study of cataract incidence in relation to dose and other factors, (2) a quantitative, longitudinal, non-subjective assessment utilizing Scheimpflug image acquisition and, finally (3) the establishment of a tissue repository for capsulotomy fragments or "tags" to be made available for investigational use. The last arm of the effort currently involves calibration of the micronucleus test in lens epithelia against known doses of radiation. The studies, which are overseen in Ukraine by the Ministry of Health and The National Academy of Sciences, and in the United States by several agencies (see acknowledgements), are organized in conjunction with six centers throughout Ukraine and three institutes in Kiev.

The longitudinal Scheimpflug slit-imaging of the eyes now in its third year, has, to date, enrolled over 360 patients ranging in age from 26 to 60 (ATE) with doses spanning 7.6 to 2500 mGy. Analyses of light-scatter from the lenses as a function of dose and/or age reveal that, if the entire lens is considered, age has a more potent negative effect on transparency than does dose. However, when corrected for age (and, more importantly, the lenticular region being considered), a trend towards a dose-dependent loss of posterior subcapsular (PSC) transparency becomes apparent. It is critical to note that, characteristically, radiation cataracts first appear in the PSC region of the lens.

A. K. Junk et al. (eds.),
Ocular Radiation Risk Assessment in Populations Exposed to Environmental Radiation Contamination, 1–12.

2. Introduction

The lens, by virtue of its primary radiopathy, cataract, and its amenability to ready, non-invasive assessment, has held out the promise of being a valuable bio-indicator for radiation exposure. The first effort at true calibration of this potential monitoring technique was done by Merriam & Focht in 1957 [1] using a limited population of radiotherapy patients. Although relatively few low dose exposures were available (the total population numbered under 300) that work, suggested a threshold for cataract of 2 Gy. The most recent ophthalmic reevaluation of the Hiroshima database using DS86 criteria proposed a minimum cataractogenic dose of about 1.4 Sv based on a two-threshold model [2]. However more recent reanalyses by the same group suggested a greater concordance with a non-threshold model [3, also see 4]. A recent study of an American population (Beaver Dam, Wisconsin) [5] indicates a higher prevalence of posterior subcapsular (PSC) cataracts in patients who had received C-T scans, suggesting that doses on the order of 100 to 300 mGy are cataractogenic. Characteristically, PSC cataracts are the initial opacities which appear following exposure [see 6]. A recent report on ocular changes in children from exposed regions around Chernobyl indicate a higher than normal incidence of PSC changes [7]. While the precise dose range cannot be ascribed to the exposed children it is very unlikely that it exceeded a few hundred mSv with a high probability that most of the children were exposed to a fraction of that. These data are consonant with experimental evidence [8] suggesting the absence of a threshold for cataracts and therefore that the cataractogenic response to radiation is purely stochastic.

As regards cataract in the Chernobyl Liquidator population, there is no question that, for at least the higher dose groups, sufficient time has elapsed to allow opacities to begin to develop. The problem is that while radiation cataracts develop in a characteristic fashion, the changes are not pathognomonic. The clinical picture requires consideration of onset time, progression, and a robust personal history to account for potential confounders. Therefore, it is important for future assessment that a non-subjective, permanent record be made of a subgroup developing lens changes. Because the subjects are available, ready to study, and the post-accident interval is such that radiogenic cataracts are appearing, ophthalmological follow-up on the Liquidator population is timely and important.

The Liquidators represent the most dosimetrically definable of the Chernobyl exposed population. Also, because the exposure was occupationally related, the health status of the Liquidators is monitored, thus, as a group, they are highly suitable for longitudinal analyses. The situation provides an unparalleled opportunity not only to consider risk issues, but modalities for monitoring populations at risk as well as to test existing theories of radiation action on normal tissues in general, and the eye in particular.

The issues surrounding risk have generated a singular sense of urgency regarding radiation effects on the eye. The ocular radiation protection standards formulated by national and international committees are all predicated on the assumption that there exists a high dose threshold for radiation cataract development.

If, as the evidence is increasingly suggesting, this supposition is incorrect, the standards set for radiation workers as well as the population at large may not be appropriate. Clearly, in order to adequately protect those populations at risk of radiation exposure this question must be resolved.

The Chernobyl Liquidator population provides, by its size, dose distribution and accessibility, the first real opportunity to address the question of whether or not radiation cataracts are deterministic or stochastic. For the same reasons, it can also supply the data necessary to allow radiation cataract to achieve its full potential as a "biological dosimeter" for assessing populations at risk and reducing uncertainties in retrospective dose reconstruction.

The joint investigations under the aegis of the Ukrainian American Chernobyl Ocular Study (UACOS) utilize state-of-the-art methodologies and technologies to assess damage to the lenses of individuals exposed to radiation resulting from the Chernobyl Reactor Number Four accident. The data which are being generated are meant not only to document the ocular health of the exposed population, but to derive therefrom a greater resolution of our understanding of the cataractogenic effects of radiation exposure in human populations, and maximize its potential for application in retrospective dosimetry. The project also includes a tissue rescue program (repository) for bioindicator calibration and future cytological reference.

The efforts focus on dose, time dependent ocular radiation effects, in the Liquidator population and include, although are not limited to, the following:

1. A cohort epidemiological study (with a nested case control subset) of cataract onset and progression using standardized subjective parameters.
2. Quantitative analyses of radiation cataract development and progression in humans employing new technologies for a longitudinal non-subjective evaluation of lens transparency.
3. The establishment of a program for the acquisition, archiving and analyses of lens epithelial tissue removed during routine cataract extraction procedures.

   Thorough ocular examinations as well as an epidemiological evaluation of exposure accompany these studies to other agents to establish potentially confounding factors which may influence the outcomes. Ultimately, the UACOS aims at achieving the following objectives:

   1. To obtain a reliable evaluation of the risk of cataract development in a critical population involved in the Chernobyl accident.
   2. To non-subjectively measure and quantify human radiation cataract development as a function of dose and establish a reference database which can be used to retrospectively assess radiation exposure in individuals.
   3. Calibrate the micronucleus assay in the lens as a potential retrospective dosimetric bioindicator for evaluating populations at risk and establish a repository of tissue for future reference.

3. STUDY GOAL 1

To obtain reliable evaluations of the risk of cataract development in a critical population involved in the Chernobyl accident.

3.1. BACKGROUND

Various studies of radiation effects on the eye have established that the initial lesion caused by ionizing radiation is a posterior subcapsular (PSC) cataract [see 6]. In terms of "spontaneous" cataracts attributable to other causes, PSCs are relatively infrequent, constituting only 15-20% of the total number of cataracts [10]. The relatively low background rate of occurrence makes it easier to statistically detect an excess risk.

Radiation cataract was the first late effect of radiation to be documented among the Japanese A-bomb survivors [11]. The current epidemiological database on radiogenic cataracts is relatively small and is marked by methodological limitations, some of which may have led to a questionable characterization of the risk function. For instance, in the aforementioned classic study by Merriam & Focht [1] which reported a threshold dose of 2000 mGy, only 33 patients with lens doses below 2000 mGy were examined for cataracts. The statistical power for detecting a modest sized risk with this small number of patients would be extremely low. The value of 2000 mGy has nevertheless been commonly used by various radioprotection groups (ICRP, NCRP, UNSCEAR, BEIR) as an assumed threshold value for acute exposure, with even higher threshold values assumed for fractionated exposures.

In a recent reanalysis [2] of a 17-year collation of data on PSCs among 2,124 subjects in the Japanese A-bomb study, the authors applied both non-threshold models that were linear or linear-quadratic in dose and models that contained dose thresholds. They found a slightly better fit from a dose threshold model (with an estimated threshold of 700 mGy for gamma radiation and 70 mGy for neutrons) than from the non-threshold models. However the difference between the goodness-of-fits was small and far from statistical significance, and, in fact, the non-threshold linear-quadratic model provided an adequate fit ($p = 0.18$) to the data. It is of interest that there was a suggestive elevation of risk in their lowest dose group of 10-990 mGy, such that the relative risk was 2.1 ($p = 0.08$, 95% confidence interval 0.8-5.8) according to our calculations. It is also noteworthy that this, the largest epidemiologic study of radiogenic cataracts, had significant limitations in that it was based on only 792 persons and 15 recorded PSCs in the dose range 10-990 mGy. Furthermore the data were collected by various investigators making it likely that the ophthalmologic examinations were probably of variable sensitivity and quality (e.g., the most recent examinations were performed without pupil dilation) [13]. The most recent report, which found a better fit for a non-threshold linear dose-response function than for a threshold function, is difficult to interpret because it lumped together significant and very minor lens changes [3].

At the other extreme from those who regard 2000 mGy as the threshold dose, a study [5] recently related PSC prevalence to anamnestic reports of diagnostic radiation. It reported that PSC was related to a history of C-T Scans (RR = 1.45, 95%

confidence interval 1.08-1.95) and was suggestively related to diagnostic procedures to the head (RR = 1.27, 95% CI 0.96-1.66). However, these data should be interpreted cautiously, since the diagnostic radiation history was based on self-reports which are subject to recall bias.

Several studies have reported an inverse association between radiation dose and time to cataract presentation [1], [2], [14]. This implies that there should be a long-term follow-up in a study that attempts to assess radiation risk of PSCs at low doses. This is one of the reasons that we anticipate a 15-year study (i.e., with total follow-up for about 25 years after exposure), with the potential to extend the study to 25 years (total follow-up = 35 years) if later it appears warranted. Some [13], but not all [1], [15], studies have also reported that the sensitivity of the lens to cataract induction is inversely associated with age at radiation exposure. This will be investigated as part of the UACOS program.

A variety of other risk factors for cataracts have been reported. These include diabetes, diastolic hypertension and hypertensive drugs [16] phenothiazines and other major tranquilizers [17], hypocalcemia, corticosteriods [18,19], ultraviolet radiation exposure [20], cigarette smoking [21], [22] and alcohol consumption [23], [24]. These factors need to be investigated as hypotheses in their own right - because some of the evidence is marginal or inconsistent – as well as potential confounder variables in analyzing radiation effects.

Intake of several nutrients may lower cataract risk: carotenoids, vitamin A [25] and vitamin C [19], [26] - although not all studies have been positive for these nutrients [18], [26]. The dietary factors merit further investigation, and the present population may provide an especially good opportunity to do so because the range of vitamin intakes is likely to be greater than in studies in the United States.

Biennial ophthalmologic examinations are about to be initiated among a cohort of 12,000 Liquidators to document PSC cataracts and other opacities of the lens. This task will center on the application of conventional slit lamp biomicroscopy in seven centers which serve the medical needs of 90% of the surviving Liquidators (see Figs. 1 & 2). When complete, this study will be the largest study ever conducted of radiation-induced lens opacities in a population with measured doses. It will constitute a dose range similar to the Japanese A-bomb ocular studies but will include 4-5 times the number of subjects [2], [13].

The study includes those Liquidators for whom real-time dose measurements had been confirmed by retrospective dosimetry and who are available for long-term follow-up. Certified ophthalmologists from each of the centers have been trained in Kiev to conduct the examinations. The routine data acquisitions are to be monitored by occasional on-site visits. In addition, the centers are expected to refer cases to the Institute of Occupational Health in Kiev for potential inclusion to the non-subjective quantitation analyses pool (Study 2). The referred cases will provide additional opportunities to verify compliance to the standardized criteria required by the study.

The approach of the study is to utilize unequivocal minimum criteria for cataract onset in order to minimize inter-observer variation during data acquisition. Therefore, the effort focuses on the incidence of cataract onset and not progression.

3.2. ORGANIZATIONAL STRUCTURE

The study is currently underway and data acquisition has begun. The protocol is designed to be compatible with existing arrangements between the Ukrainian ocular preventative disease programs at the Ministry of Health. The examinations are conducted at seven centers: Kiev, Kharkiv, Dnipropetrovsk, Donetsk, Zaporizhya, Kirovograd and Poltava (2 additional centers in Slavutich and Rivno are in the process of being certified for inclusion.

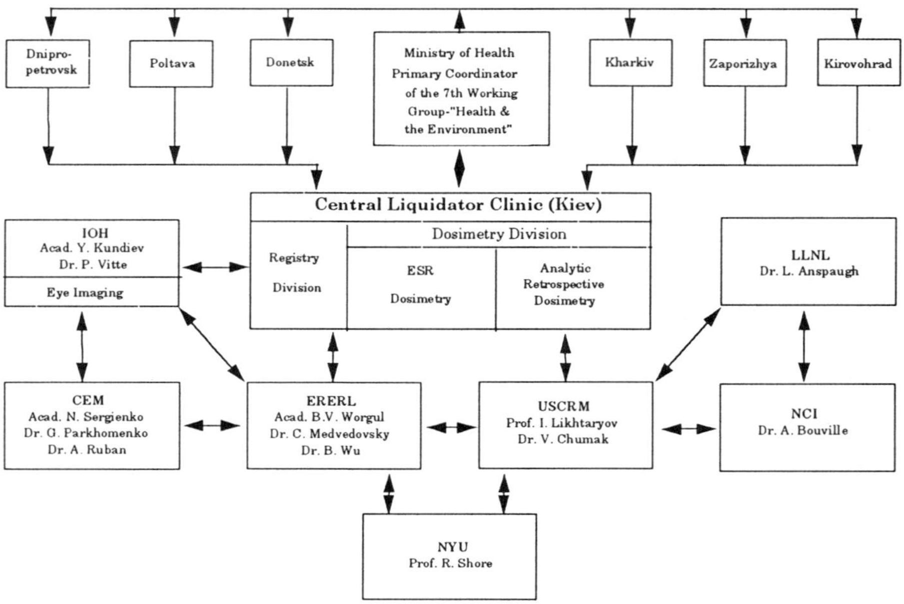

Figure 1. A flow-chart illustrating the relationships between the various components of the UACOS. Academician Yuri Kundiev and Academician Basil V. Worgul are Program Directors for the Ukraine and the United States respectively. IOH = Institute for Occupational Health (Ukraine); CEM = Center for Eye Microsurgery (Ukraine); USCRM = Ukrainian Scientific Center for Radiation Medicine (Ukraine); ERERL = Eye Radiation and Environmental Research Laboratory (US); LLNL = Lawrence Livermore National Laboratory (US); NCI = National Cancer Institute (US); NYU = New York University (US).

As shown in the flowchart (Fig. 1) Academician Yuri Kundiev, Director of the Institute of Occupational Health (IOH), provides for the overall directorial and administrative needs of the Ukrainian side of the program. Also he, together with Dr. Peter Vitte of the same institute, conduct the diet, habit and occupational background surveys. They work in close collaboration with Dr. Roy Shore of New York University on the epidemiological issues confronting the program. Professor Ilia Likhtarev and Dr. Vadim Chumak of the Ukrainian Scientific Center for Radiation Medicine (USCRM) coordinate the dosimetric aspects. Academician Nikolai Sergienko director of the Center for Eye Microsurgery (CEM) and staff members Drs. Giorgi Parkhomenko and Andre Ruban are responsible for the ophthalmological aspects of the study. Academician Basil V. Worgul director of the Eye Radiation and

Environmental Research Laboratory (ERERL) of Columbia University co-ordinates the study with Acad. Kundiev. He, Dr. Cecily Medvedovsky and Dr. Anna K. Junk are responsible for overall data analyses and logistics.

4. STUDY GOAL 2

To non-subjectively measure and quantify human radiation cataract development as a function of dose and establish a reference database which can be used to retrospectively assess radiation exposure in individuals.

4.1. BACKGROUND

The Chernobyl accident provides an unparalleled opportunity to generate an image library of human radiation cataract development amenable to non-subjective, quantitative assessment, longitudinal intra- interpatient comparative analyses, and retrospective re-evaluation. In addition to the historically subjective nature of cataract scoring, the well-known inverse relationship between time of onset (latent period) of cataractogenic expression and dose has been a major impediment to risk assessment. In fact, it is likely that the entire concept of cataract as being a deterministic effect is the direct result of the limitations imposed by the dose dependent latent period i.e. the time between exposure and the appearance of cataract. A longitudinal, long-term, study of a dosimetrically well defined population, using state-of-the-art Scheimpflug Slit Imaging, should provide the data necessary to permit extrapolation of risk as a function of dose across age groups and remaining time at risk (life span). In addition, because the instrumentation provides digitally based images stored on long-lived optical media, the application of the technique promises the establishment of an image library which can serve a reference for future reanalysis and comparison. The use of the method also serves as the ideal means to validate on a sampling basis subjective follow-up studies, such as those in Study 1.

The ongoing longitudinal study focuses on those Liquidators whose doses have been well defined or have a high probability of being determined with low uncertainty. The labor and time intensive nature of the data acquisition places an upper limit on the number of patients which can be imaged in a given period. While currently over 360 subjects are enrolled, it is anticipated that approximately 500 individuals distributed across all age subgroups will be monitored long-term using the technique.

In addition to its non-subjective nature, the methodology provides for a continuously incremental, quantitative determination of the loss of transparency over time. By generating a large number of cataract vs. time curves against dose, the aim is to establish a series of standardized data sets. Ultimately it is believed that the slopes (rates) of cataract progression will reflect the dose received at a given age. These data then can be used to retrospectively assess dose under the appropriate conditions. Such a capability does not currently exist using the subjective non-linear scoring methodologies typically employed [see 4 for a full discussion of the modalities].

4.2. ORGANIZATIONAL STRUCTURE

The equipment - a modified Zeiss Scheimpflug Imaging System and an Oxford Retroillumination Camera necessary for the quantitation are located and operated in a special Ophthalmology suite of the Institute for Occupational Health in Kiev (see Organizational Chart). The individuals selected for long term follow-up are to be a subset of the cohort/case control study (Study 1) and are selected based on the confidence in the doses received, age, and cataract status. Additional cases which arise in the remote centers but are of interest and are relevant to this subproject will be referred to the Kiev clinic for evaluation and possible inclusion. The lenses of the patients will be documented at 24-30 month intervals.

The study involves several technologies which have the capability of producing a raw image database as well as non-subjective quantitative assessment of the images themselves. Copies of the images are provided to the American counterparts for corroborative analyses and cross-indexing. Eventually the raw and analyzed images will be made available to the scientific community via the Internet. It should be noted that the use of the instrumentation also provides the basis for technological and methodological improvements in human cataract assessment [27]

4.3. CURRENT STATUS

Now in its third year, over 300 Liquidators have been processed for the first time and the group is being subjected to a second round. Meanwhile, additional subjects are being added to the cohort. Although the strengths of the technique reside in its intra-individual monitoring capability, comparing results across the population has yielded unanticipated preliminary results.

Analyses from the posterior cortex (the region expected to show the earliest and most severe radiogenic changes) as a function of dose across all ages (Fig. 2a) for those of the cohort for which we have completed confirmatory dosimetry reveals no evidence of a relationship. Using the rationale that the early post-exposure (7-9 years) age-related changes predominate over any possible radiation induced opacification we divided the Liquidators into those >50, 40-50, and <40 years of age (Fig. 2b, 2c, and 2d respectively). Clearly, the younger group reveals a positive correlation with dose while the oldest individuals do not.

The data are not to be interpreted that the older individuals have been spared radiogenic changes but that those accompanying the aging process mask any such alterations. This is confirmed by the fact that the middle age group, while showing a positive correlation with dose, is less manifest despite an overall higher mean scatter. Obviously, there are many ways, more elegant than simple regressions, to analyze the currently available data. However, inasmuch as the data is still in the acquisition phase and there is a large collaborative effort by several laboratories (the ERERL in New York, the Institute for Experimental Ophthalmology in Bonn, and at the GSF in Munich) to develop more sophisticated algorithms for evaluating the images, the preliminary results are purposefully presented in their barest forms.

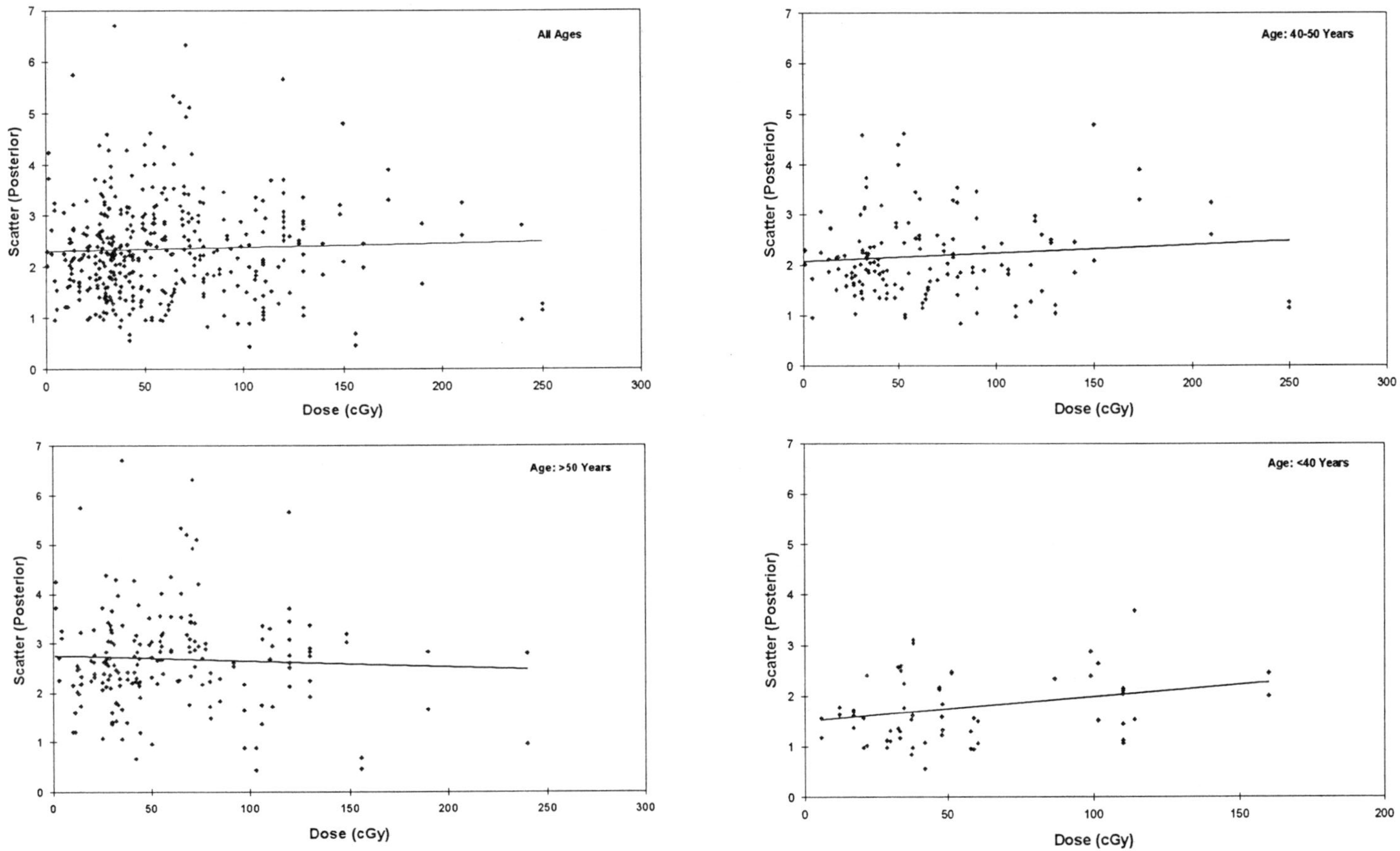

Figure 2. A plot of the light scatter from the posterior cortex of lenses from Liquidators exposed to a variety of doses. The ages shown were at the time of examination (7-9 years post-exposure). (2a) All ages. (2b) Older than 50 years of age. (2c) Ages 40 to 50 years. (2d) Younger than 40 years of age.

5. STUDY GOAL 3

Establish a repository of tissue for immediate analyses and future reference. The effort will focus on calibrating the micronucleus assay in the lens as a potential retrospective dosimetric bioindicator for evaluating populations at risk.

5.1 BACKGROUND

There exists a critical need to institute a program to acquire, reposit and analyze lens material retrieved during routine cataract operations from individuals whose history includes exposure to radiation from the Chernobyl incident. When a cataract is removed during a modern extracapsular cataract extraction (ECCE) procedure, a small piece of lens epithelium, called "tag", is removed. This tag, typically discarded, contains a monolayer of 20,000 to 90,000 undifferentiated cells which, by virtue of their anatomical location, have remained in place for most, if not all, of the post-natal life of the person from whom it comes. Thus, irrespective of the basis for the opacity that occasioned its removal, the tag can provide invaluable data on earlier damage caused by exogenous agents.

The ERERL has developed the means, and was the first to assess human tags for cytogenetic damage using the micronuclei (MN) assay. Unlike the transient nature of induced MNs characteristic of more commonly used human tissues, e.g. peripheral lymphocytes, the unique biology of the lens guarantees that MNs which are produced by agents such as ionizing radiation, are potentially retained for decades if not lifetimes [28)] Experimental studies [29]-[31]show that, as has been demonstrated for the blood and marrow, lenticular MNs are useful bioindicators of exposure to radiation. In the case of humans the tag MN assay has the added advantage of extreme longevity.

It should be emphasized that the MN assay is only one of the quantitative parameters that can be derived from the tags. Cell density, cell size, and DNA content can and should be catalogued. Furthermore, the methodology for studying tags using DNA Fluorescence In Situ Hybridization (FISH) on these cells is being perfected. Thus, the tags can serve as a resource for studying fundamental aspects of radiation injury to human tissues and cells in vivo.

In any case it is absolutely essential that the wholesale loss of this precious resource from the Chernobyl Liquidator population be prevented. Once acquired and after the MN assay is calibrated using those cases where the doses are well defined it can then be used to estimate exposure levels which are less certain. However, an urgent priority must be to ensure that every effort is made to recover each and every tag as it becomes available, and provide for their proper handling and storage for eventual assessment.

5.2 ORGANIZATIONAL STRUCTURE

As cataract extractions become necessary for those whose history includes the

Chernobyl experience, every effort will be made to recover lens epithelial tissue (tags) to be archived and eventually analyzed. The tissues will be recovered irrespective of whether or not the cataracts from which they were derived were radiogenic in origin. The effort is integrated into the medical follow-up and can program to the Ministry of Health. The American counterpart is responsible for processing and repositing the analyzed material.

The procedures are overseen by the CEM and processing of the tissues is being conducted at the ERERL.

5.3. CURRENT STATUS

The calibration study is scheduled to begin in June of 1998. Appropriate subjects are currently in the process of being identified.

Acknowledgements

The authors would like to acknowledge the support of the Ministry of Health and the National Academy of Sciences of Ukraine, the United States Department of Energy (DOE DE-FG01-95EH89658), the National Institutes of Health (ES009484), the Defense Nuclear Agency (DNA 001-92-C-0137) and Research to Prevent Blindness Inc

Details of the studies underway are available on the World Wide Web (HTTP://cpmcnet.columbia.edu/dept/eye/rad). Inquiries can also be forwarded to Professor Basil V. Worgul, <bvwl@columbia.edu>.

References

1. Merriam, G.R..Jr. and Focht, E. (1957) A clinical study of radiation cataracts and the relationship to dose, *Am. J. Roentgenol. Radium Ther. Nucl. Med.* 77,5, 759-785.
2. Otake, M. and Schull, W.J. (1990) Radiation related posterior lenticular opacities in Hiroshima and Nagasaki atomic bomb survivors based on the DS86 dosimetry system,, *Radiat Res* **121,** 3-13.
3. Otake, M., Finch, S.C., Choshi, K., Takaku, I., Mishima, H. and Takase T. (1992) Radiation related ophthalmological changes and aging among Hiroshima and Nagasaki A-bomb survivors: a reanalysis, *Radiat Res* **131**, 315-324.
4. Worgul, B.V., Kundiev, Y., Likhtarev, I., Sergienko, N., Wegener, A. and Medvedovsky, C..P. (1996) Use of subjective and nonsubjective methodologies to evaluate lens radiation damage in exposed populations - an overview, *Radiat. Environ. Biophys.* **35**, 137-144.
5. Klein B.E.K., Klein I., Linton K.L.P. and Franke T. (1993) Diagnostic X-ray exposure and lens opacities: The Beaver Dam eye study, *Am J Public Health* **83**, 588-590.
6. Merriam, G.R.Jr. and Worgul, B.V. (1983) Experimental radiation cataract - its clinical relevance. *Bull. N.Y. Acad. Med.* **59**,:372-392.
7. Day, R.., Gorin, M.B., and Eller, A.W. (1992) Prevalence of Lens Changes in Children Residing around Chernobyl, *Health Phys* **68**, 632 –642.
8. Worgul, B.V., Brenner, D.J., Medvedovsky, C., Merriam, G.R.Jr., and Huang, Y. (1993) Accelerated heavy particles and the lens VII: the cataractogenic potential of 450 MeV/amu iron ions. *Inv.Ophthal. Vis. Sci.* **34**, 184-193.
9. Sperduto, R.D. and Hiller, R. (1984) The prevalence of nuclear, cortical and posterior subcapsular lens opacities in a general population sample, *Ophthal.* **91**, 815-818.

10. Cogan, D.G., Martin, S. and Kimura, S. (1949) Atomic bomb cataracts, *Science* **110**, 654-655.
11. Choshi, K., Takaku, I., Mishima, H., Takase, T., Nerlishi, S., Finch, S. and Otake, M. (1983) Ophthalmologic changes related to radiation exposure and age in Adult Health Study sample, Hiroshima and Nagasaki, *Radiat. Res.* **96**, 560-579.
12. Merriam, G.R., Szechter, A. and Focht, E. (1972) The effects of ionizing radiations on the eye, *Front Radiat. Ther. Oncol.* **6**, 346-385.
13. Otake, M. and Schull, W.J. (1982) The relationship of gamma and neutron radiation to posterior lenticular opacities among atomic bomb survivors in Hiroshima and Nagasaki, *Radiat. Res.* **92**,:574-595.
14. Bellows, J.G. and Bellows, R.J. (1975) Presenile and senile cataract - the aging lens: clinical considerations, in J.G. Bellows (ed.), *Cataract and Abnormalities of the Lens*, Grune and Stratton, New York, pp. 303-313, 1975.
15. Isaac, N., Walker, A., Jick, H. and Gorman, M. (1991) Exposure to phenothiazine drugs and risk of cataract, *Arch. Ophthalmol.* **109**, 256-260.
16. Italian-American Cataract Study Group (1991) Risk factors for age related cortical, nuclear, and posterior subcapsular cataracts, *Am. J. Epidemiol.* **133**, 541-553.
17. Jacques, P. and Chylack, L. (1991) Epidemiologic evidence of a role for the antioxidant vitamins and carotenoids in cataract prevention, *Am. J. Clin. Nutr.* **53**, 352-355.
18. Leske, M., Chylack, L. and Wu, S. (1991) The lens opacities case-control study. Risk factors for cataract, *Arch. Ophthalmol.* **109**, 244-251.
19. Christen, W.G., Munson, J.E., Seddon, J.M., Glynn, R.J., Buring, J.E., Rosner, B. and Hennekens, C.H. (1992) A prospective study of cigarette smoking and risk of cataract in men., *JAMA* **268**,:989-993.
20. Klein, B.E.K., Klein, R., Linton, K.L.P. and Franke, T. (1993) Cigarette smoking and lens opacities: Beaver Dam eye study, *Am. J. Prev. Med.* 9, 27-30.
21. Munoz, B., Tajchman, U., Bochow, T. and West, S. (1993) Alcohol use and risk of posterior subcapsular cataracts, *Arch. Ophthal.* **111**, 110-112.
22. Ritter, L., Klein, B., Klein, R. and Mares-Perlman, J. (1993) Alcohol use and lens opacities in the Beaver Dam Eye Study, *Arch. Ophthalmol.* **111**, 113-117.
23. Hankinson, S., Stampfer, M., Seddon, J., Colditz, G., Rosner, B., Speizer, F. and Willett, W. (1992) Nutrient intake and cataract extraction in women: a prospective study, *Br. Med. J.* **305**, 335-339.
24. Hiller, R., Sperduto, R. and Ederer, F. (1983) Epidemiologic associations with cataract in the 1971-1972 National Health and Nutrition Examination Survey, *Am. J. Epidemiol.* **118**, 239-249.
25. Worgul, B.V., David, J., Odrich, S., Merriam, G.R.Jr., Medvedovsky, C., Merriam, J.C., Trokel, S.L. and Geard, C.R. (1991) Evidence of genotoxic damage in human cataractous lenses, *Mutagenesis* **6**, 6, 495-499.
26. Odrich, S., Medvedovsky C., Merriam, G.R.Jr., and Worgul, B.V. (1988) Micronucleation in the lens epithelium following in vivo exposure to physical and chemical mutagens. *Lens Res.* **5**, 203-216.
27. Worgul, B.V., Medvedovsky, C., Powers-Risius, P. and Alpen E. (1989) Accelerated heavy ions and the lens IV. Biomicroscopic and cytopathological analyses of the lenses of mice irradiated with 600 MeV/amu ^{56}Fe ions. *Rad. Res.* **120**, 280-293.
28. Tao, F., Medvedovsky, C., David, J., Broglio, T., Powers-Risius, P., Alpen, E.L. and Worgul, B.V. (1993) Accelerated heavy ions and the lens. IX The late effect of LET and dose on cellular parameters in the murine lens, *Int. J. Radiat. Biol.* **64**, 1, 103-111.

CATARACTOUS CHANGES RELATED TO RADIATION AND AGING AMONG THE ATOMIC BOMB SURVIVORS IN HIROSHIMA

T.KODAMA[1], Y.OHASHI[1], K.CHOSHI[2], H.K.MISHIMA[2]
[1] *Department of Ophthalmology, Ehime University School of Medicine, Shigenobu, Ehime 791-0259 Japan*
[2] *Department of Ophthalmology, Hiroshima University School of Medicine, Kasumi, Minami-ku, Hiroshima 734-0037 Japan*

1. Introduction

Damage to the lens epithelial cells is a well-recognized phenomenon after exposure to ionizing radiation. The explosion of the atomic bomb obviously proved the hazard of ionizing radiation. In fact, a high frequency of cataract has been observed in atomic bomb survivors in Hiroshima and Nagasaki, first reported by Cogan et al. in 1949 [1]. Lens opacities after exposure to ionizing radiation usually appear after the relatively long latent period. Although the effect of age on the development of radiation cataract has been well recognized in experimental animals [2][3], there are few data available for human radiation cataract [4][5][6]. The purpose of the present study is to evaluate the late effects of radiation upon cataractogenesis among atomic bomb survivors in Hiroshima. Part of data in this article are based on the publication reported by Choshi et al. [4].

2. Subjects and Methods

The present study consists of three series of surveys which were made in 1955, 1957-1961 and 1978-1980 to understand the long-term effects of ionizing radiation on the lens. The first investigation in 1955 was to consider the relationship for the prevalence of posterior subcapsular opacities and epilation. Posterior subcapsular opacities were found in 52 out of 80 cases. The second investigation was done in 1957-1961. Younger persons who were in the uteri at the time of the atomic bomb explosion and whose mothers received 1.0 Gy or more were selected for this study. The third investigation was done in 1978-1980. People examined in this study were selected from those in the Adult Health Study (1978-1980) who were exposed to 1.0 Gy or more in Hiroshima (1.0 Gy+ group). Control group was selected from outpatients in Hiroshima on the basis of simple random stratified sampling by age and sex. Ophthalmological examinations were performed regularly at the time of Adult Health Study. These studies were done in collaboration with the Adult Health Study Program

A. K. Junk et al. (eds.),
Ocular Radiation Risk Assessment in Populations Exposed to Environmental Radiation Contamination, 13–19.

of the Atomic Bomb Casualty Commission and Radiation Effects Research Foundation.

For the histological study of atomic bomb cataract, a lens extracted from a Japanese man aged 41 with doughnut-shaped opacities was fixed in 10% formalin and embedded in paraffin. Thin sections were made and stained with hematoxylin and eosin.

3. Results

Figure 1 shows the classification of typical atomic bomb cataracts by severity and the pathological manifestation of doughnut-shaped opacities in the posterior subcapsular region. A characteristic feature of atomic bomb cataract was an initial axial opacity which appeared as a dot located at the posterior pole (Fig. 1-A). This punctate opacities developed to small granules and vacuoles (Fig. 1-B) and progressed to a doughnut-shaped appearance (Fig. 1-C). The histological findings of atomic bomb cataract extracted from a Japanese man aged 41 showed balloon-cell formation beneath the posterior capsule and subadjacent amorphous debris in Figure 1-D.

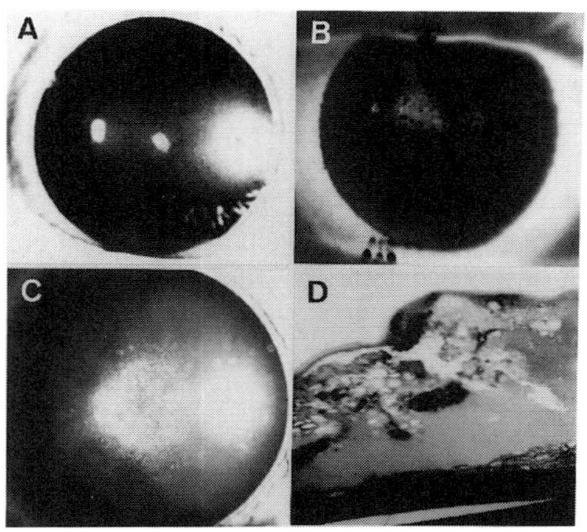

Figure 1. Clinical and pathological characteristics of atomic bomb cataract; (A) Punctate posterior subcapsular opacities; (B) Small posterior subcapsular granular opacities; (C) Large posterior subcapsular plaque opacities; (D) Lens from 41 year old male with doughnut shaped opacities: balloon-cell formation beneath the posterior capsule (x 200), hematoxylin and eosin

Figure 2 shows a high correlation between posterior subcapsular changes and epilation. The incidence of posterior subcapsular opacities increased as the degree of hair loss became worse. Figure 3 and Figure 4 show the relationship between the radiation dose and either posterior subcapsular changes (331 cases) or axial opacities (350 cases), respectively. A closer correlation was found between prevalence of cataract and radiation doses (100 rad are equivalent to 1 Gy).

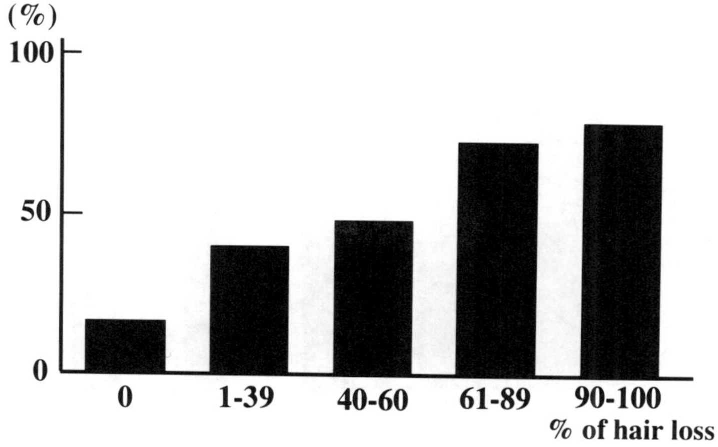

Figure 2. Relationship between epilation and posterior subcapsular opacities

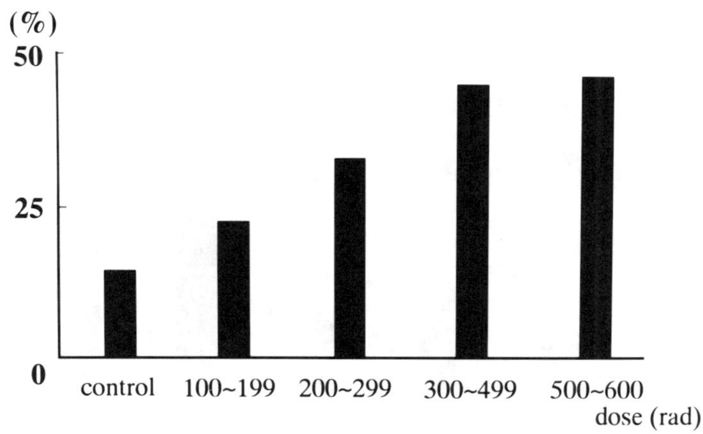

Figure 3. Prevalence of posterior subcapsular opacities in relation to dose

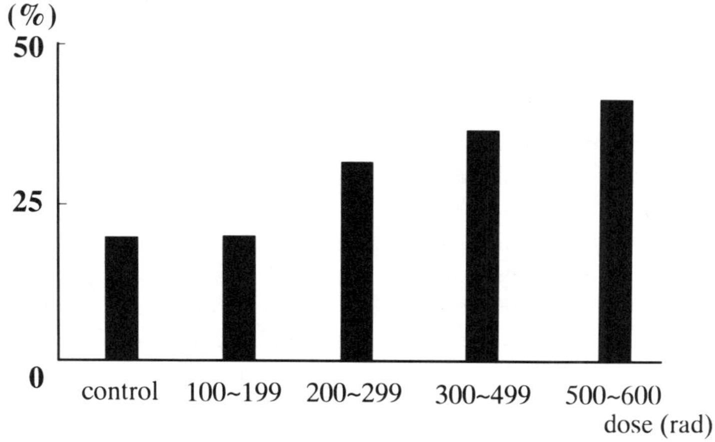

Figure 4. Prevalence of axial opacities in relation to dose

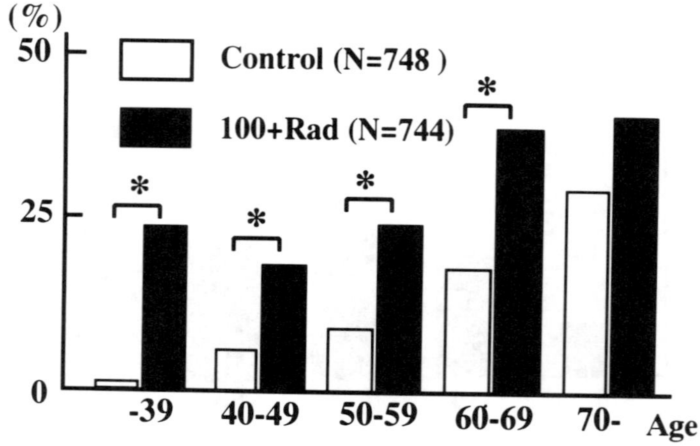

Figure 5. Prevalence of posterior subcapusular opacities in control group and 1.0 Gy+ group (*P<0.001)

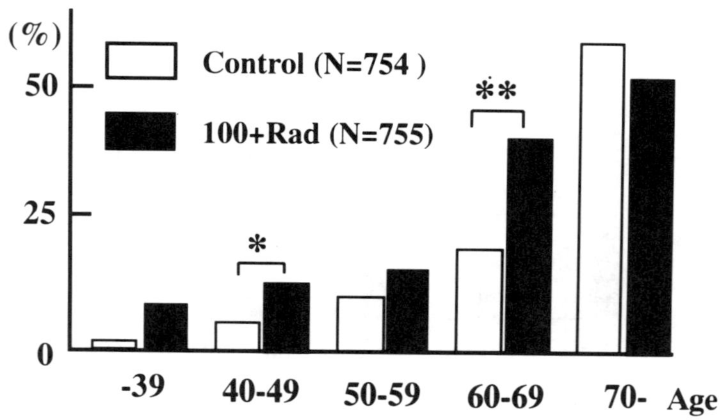

Figure 6. Prevalence of axial opacities in control group and 1.0 Gy+ group (* P<0.05; ** P<0.001)

Figure 5 shows the prevalence of posterior subcapsular change in the control and 1.0 Gy+ group. Incidence of cataract of the 1.0 Gy+ group was always higher than that of the control group. The highly significant excess was observed for all groups other than 70+ age (P<0.001). The most remarkable risk of cataract was for the group under 40. The prevalence of persons who had axial opacities in the control and 1.0 Gy+ groups is given in Figure 6. In both groups, the prevalence of axial opacities increased with age. There is an increasing tendency in the 1.0 Gy+ group for all age groups less than 70. The risk of cataract in the 1.0 Gy+ group was significantly greater than that in the control both in the 40 to 49-year-old and in the 60 to 69-year-old age groups. No sex differences for all ages was observed in the control and 1.0 Gy+ groups (data not shown). The occurrence rate was also examined for cortical and nuclear cataract. There was no remarkable difference in the prevalence of those lesions between the control and 1.0 Gy+ group (data not shown).

TABLE 1. The relationship between the distance form hypocenter and the incidence of cataract in utero group

Distance from hypocenter (km)	Subjects	Radiation cataract (%)
0 ~ 1.0	18	0
1.0 ~ 1.2	20	2 (11.1)
1.2 ~ 1.4	18	2 (11.1)
1.4 ~ 1.6	50	1 (2.0)
1.6 ~ 1.8	30	0
1.8 ~ 2.0	38	2 (5.3)
2.0 ~ 3.0	56	1 (1.8)
Total	230	8 (3.5)

Children exposed to ionizing radiation in uteri were examined in order to evaluate the radiation-induced damage to the fetal lens (Table 1). Cataractous changes were present in only eight (3.5%) of 230 cases. Interestingly there was no radiation cataract in this group when exposed within 1.0 km from the hypocenter.

4. Discussion

The most frequent manifestation of lens opacities related to radiation and aging was the occurrence of axial opacities in the posterior subcapsular region. Miller et al. reported that clinical manifestations of atomic bomb cataract in Hiroshima and Nagasaki were axial opacities, visible by ophthalmoscopy, as shown in Figure 1-A, and polychromatic sheen visible by slit lamp biomicroscopy [7][8][9]. The polychromatic sheen is defined as a minimal radiation effect of iridescent changes located in the posterior capsule and can not be photographed [8][9]. As shown in figure 1 D, the histological appearance of atomic bomb cataract consists of balloon cell formation in the posterior subcapsular region. Balloon cells seem to represent swollen equatorial cells after their migration beneath the capsule towards the posterior pole. This morphological alteration is not an unusual manifestation of degenerative processes [10][11].

Figures 3 and 4 show a close correlation of cataract and calculated radiation doses. Interestingly, the incidence of posterior subcapsular opacities was closely correlated with the degree of hair loss [12][13]. Cells in growing hair follicles divide rapidly and are damaged by relatively small doses of radiation. The resulting interference with hair growth leads to loss of hair [14]. Therefore degree of epilation was adopted as an index of radiation dose.

Axial opacities and posterior subcapsular changes suggest a stronger aging effect in persons exposed early rather than late in life. The most significant excess risk of posterior subcapsular opacities was observed in the age group of 40 years or less. Lenses in this group whose individuals were 15 years or less at the time of explosion were most sensitive to radiation. This result suggests a relatively stronger aging effect for survivors exposed early rather than late in life. In general, the younger the age of irradiation, the shorter the latent period. Since rapidly dividing cells appear to be the most susceptible to ionizing radiation damage, development of cataract may depend on the repairing ability of the lens, radiation dose and age. This implies that lenses of the young individuals are more radiosensitive than those of older people.

The fetal lens might be expected to be the most susceptible to radiation and show the shortest latent period. Unexpectedly, the incidence of radiation-induced cataract in children exposed in the uteri was too small. Table 1 shows that only eight of 230 cases (3.5 %) revealed cataractous changes, although the younger lens is much more susceptible to ionizing radiation than the older one. The absorbed dose of a fetus in the uterus varied not only with the distance from the hypocenter, but also with the orientation of the fetus to the atomic bomb explosion. Moreover, it was dependent on the stage of pregnancy at the time of explosion. The effect of age on the development of radiation cataract in mice lenses was studied by Gajewski et al. [3]. Their results showed that the mice lenses were not equally radiosensitive at different ages. On the contrary, Merriam and Szechter reported that young lenses were not more sensitive to X-ray in the rat radiation cataract [2]. A more complex relationship among radiation dose, age and cataractogenesis will continue to be an important subject of radiation biology.

5. Summary

Lens opacities after exposure to ionizing radiation usually appear after latent period. People examined in this study were selected from the atomic bomb survivors who were exposed to 1.0 Gy or more. A control group was selected from the outpatient department. They were living out of Hiroshima at the time of the bombing. A highly significant risk for axial opacities and posterior subcapsular changes was observed in all age groups other than 70+ . The most significant excess risk of posterior subcapsular opacities was found in the age group of less than 15 years at the time of atomic bomb explosion. On the contrary, the incidence of radiation-induced cataract in children exposed in uteri was only eight of 230 cases (3.5 %), although the younger lens is much more susceptible to the exposure of ionizing radiation. These data are believed to be important in understanding radiation-induced cataract and aging. Their synergetic effects might influence the late effects of the atomic bomb on radiation cataract.

6. References

1. Cogan, G., Martin, S.F., and Kimura, S.J. (1949) Atomic bomb cataracts. Science **110**, 654- 655.
2. Merriam, G.R.Jr., and Szechter, A. (1975) The relative radiosensitivity of rat lenses as a function of age. Radiat.Res. 62,488-497.
3. Gajewski, A.K., Majewska, K., Slowikowska, M.G., Chomiczewski, K. and Kulig, A. (1977) Types and rate of cataract development in mice irradiated at different ages. Radiat. Res. **71**, 471-480.
4. Choshi, K., Takaku, I., Mishima, H., Takase, T., Neriishi, S., Finch, S.C. and Otake, M. (1983) Ophthalmic changes related to radiation exposure and age in adult health study sample, Hiroshima and Nagasaki. Radiat. Res. **96**, 560-579.

5. Otake, M. and Schull, W.J. (1982) The relationship of gamma and neutron radiation to posterior opacities among atomic bomb survivors in Hiroshima and Nagasaki. Radiat. Res. **92**, 574-595.
6. Otake, M., Finch, S.C., Choshi, K., Takaku, I., Mishima, H. and Takase, T. (1992) Radiation-related ophthalmological changes and aging among Hiroshima and Nagasaki A- bomb survivors :A reanalysis. Radiat. Res. **131**, 315-324.
7. Cogan, G. and Dreisler, K.K. (1953) Minimal amount of X-ray exposure causing lens opacities in the human eye. Arch. Ophthalmol. **50**, 30-34.
8. Miller, R.J., Fujino, T. and Nefzger, M.D. (1967) Lens findings in atomic bomb survivors. A review of major ophthalmic surveys at the atomic bomb casualty commission(1949-1962). Arch. Ophthalmol. **78**, 697-704.
9. Nefzger, M.D., Miller, R.J. and Fujino, T. (1969) Eye findings in atomic bomb survivors of Hiroshima and Nagasaki:1963-1964 Amer.J.Epidemiol. **89**, 129-138.
10. Kimura, S.J. and Ikui, H. (1951) Atomic-bomb radiation cataract. Case report with histopathologic study. Amer. J. Ophthalmol. **34**,811-816.
11. Cogan, D.J., Donaldoson, D.D. and Reese, A.B. (1952)Clinical and pathological characteristics of radiation cataract. Arch. Ophthalmol.**47**, 55-70.
12. Sinskey, R.M.K., Slowikowska, M.G., Chomiczewski, K. and Kulig, A. (1977) Types and rate of cataract development in mice irradiated at different ages. Radiat. Res. **71**, 471- 480.
13. Neriishi, K., Wong, F.L., Nakashima, E., Otake, M., Kodama, K. and Choshi, K. (1995) Relationship between cataracts and epilation in atomic bomb survivors. Radiat. Res. **144**, 107-113.
14. Patt, H.M. and Quastler, H. (1963) Radiation effects on cell renewal and related systems. Physiol. Rev. **43**, 357-396.

QUANTIFICATION OF LENS OPACITIES WITH DIGITAL SCHEIMPFLUG IMAGING

M. FROEMEL[1], P. EGNER[1], H.ROOS[2], A.M. KELLERER[1,2]
[1]GSF, National Research Center for Environment and Health, Institute of Radiobiology, Ingolstaedter Landstrasse 1, D-85764 Neuherberg, Germany
[2]University of Munich, Radiobiological Institute, Schillerstrasse 42, D- 80336 Munich, Germany

1. Abstract

Scheimpflug imaging of the human ocular lens is optimally suited for quantification of lens opacities if connected with digital image processing. For application in cataract studies a TOPCON SL-45 B Scheimpflug slitlamp has, therefore, been upgraded by substituting the conventional camera with an electronic camera and an electronic image storing system. The output signals are digitized by an image processing board and are stored on optical disks. To account for variations of the flash light, the intensity is monitored by a light sensitive detector, and appropriate correction factors are applied to the opacity values of the digitized image. To guarantee long-term stability of the instrument a recalibration procedure has been developed. We have analysed the geometric image distortions, and computer algorithms have been developed and applied successfully, to correct them. For quantification of lens opacities light attentuation within the lens needs to be taken into account. A tentative correction has been derived to consider this influence.

2. Materials and Methods

2.1. THE ELECTRONIC SCHEIMPFLUG SYSTEM

With Scheimpflug photography [5], it is possible to obtain a sharp image of a plane section through the human ocular lens. Therefore, Scheimpflug imaging, especially if connected with digital image processing, is optimally suited for quantification of lens opacities. In view of the need to assess lens opacifications as a late effect of exposure to ionizing radiation, we have developed an electronic Scheimpflug system. This instrumentation is based on a commercially available *Topcon SL-45 B* Scheimpflug camera. The main modification is the substitution of the conventional camera with an electronic camera and an electronic image storing system. The image of the ocular

A. K. Junk et al. (eds.),
Ocular Radiation Risk Assessment in Populations Exposed to Environmental Radiation Contamination, 21–26.

lens is recorded by a CCD-camera (*Sony*) and the output signals are continuously digitized by an image processing board (*Leutron*) which is installed in a personal computer. The image and the patient's data are written on a write-once optical disk for permanent storage.

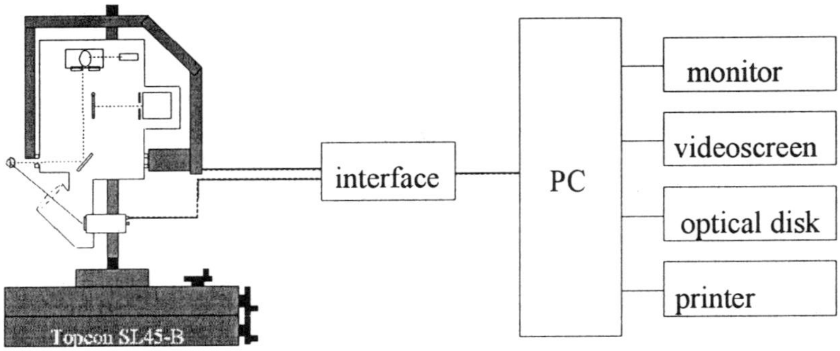

Figure 1: Electronic Scheimpflug system equipped with digital image recording and processing

2.2 MEASUREMENT OF OPACITIES

Quantitative evaluations of lens opacities from Scheimpflug images suffer from several constraints which are inherent in the technique:

- geometric image distortions
- distortion of local intensities due to geometric distortions
- intensity distortions caused by the fact that the imaging lenses do not accept the same fraction of scattered light from different positions in the lens

With digital image processing it has become possible to overcome these constraints. We have developed computer algorithms and have applied them successfully to eliminate these influences [2]. However, in addition to the above factors, the measured local opacities are affected by attentuation of light within the lens.

In the Scheimpflug technique a plane section of the lens is illuminated by a slitlamp. The light scattered in the lens is utilized for imaging of the illuminated plane (*Figure 2*). Due to light absorption and scattering posterior parts of the lens are illuminated with less intensity than anterior parts. In addition, the degree of attentuation of light emerging from the lens depends on its pathlength within the lens.

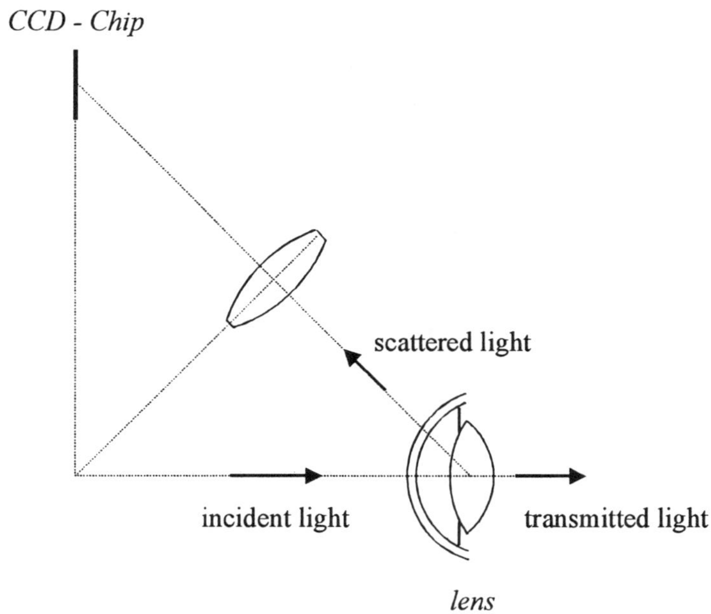

Figure 2: Schematic diagram of the Scheimpflug imaging technique. Light scattered in the lens is measured to determine local opacities.

To account for these effects a tentative correction has been developed. The calculation assumes that light intensity decreases exponentially in the lens. The age- and wavelength-dependent 'attentuation coefficients' are chosen in such a way that the transmission criteria of Pokorny et al. [4] are met. For scattering of light, Rayleigh scattering with its λ^{-4} wavelength dependence is assumed. The calculation is performed for a 45° Scheimpflug geometry. As an example the relative intensity of light from the posterior capsule is given in *Figure 3*, as it is seen by the camera. The intensity depends on the wavelength and - apart from individual variations - on the patient's age.

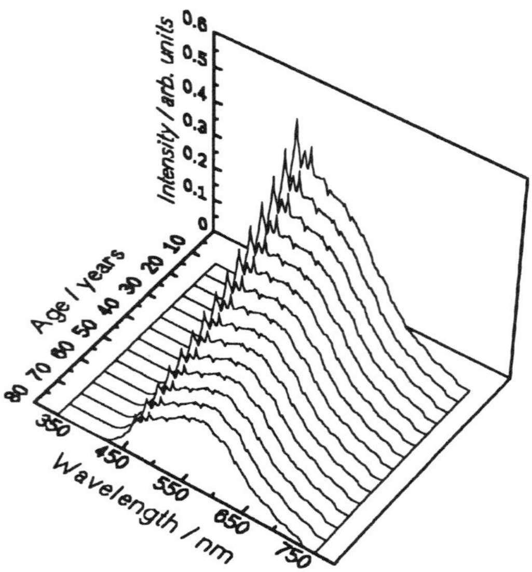

Figure 3: Intensity, to the detector, of light emerging from the posterior capsule in its dependence on wavelength and on patient's age.

3. Results

In *Figure 4* spectra of *Figure 3* are integrated to show the distribution of wavelengths. In the case of the posterior capsule the measured opacity values are reduced by 47% for a 20 year old person. For a 60 year old person the values are reduced by 64%.

In *Figure 5* factors are given to account for light attentuation within the lens. The factors are averaged over the main anatomical substructures of the lens (anterior capsule, anterior cortex, nucleus, posterior cortex and posterior capsule). The factors increase with age and are higher for the posterior parts of the lens than for the anterior parts.

For precise quantification of lens opacities all the influences above mentioned need to be taken into account. In epidemiological studies, where a group of exposed persons is compared to a control group, the determination of absolute values is less essential, provided, the measurements in both groups are performed with the same instrumentation. However, precise quantification is required to faciliate inter-comparisons between the results of different groups if they use different instrumentations.

Through the various steps of correction Scheimpflug imaging has become a more powerful tool for the quantification of lenticular opacities.

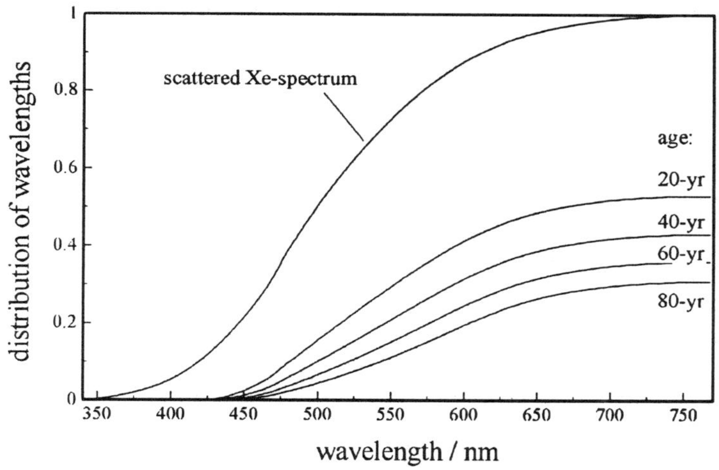

Figure 4: Distribution of wavelengths of light scattered from the posterior capsule. The lines refer to different ages. For comparison, the corresponding line for the Xe-flashlight is inserted.

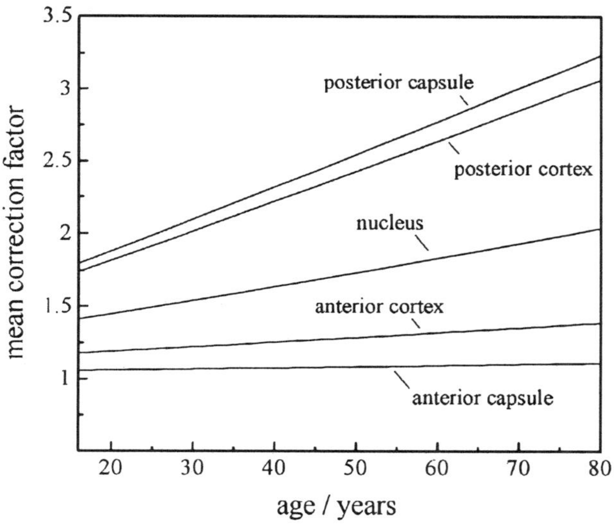

Figure 5: Factor to account for the attentuation of light within the lens. The factor is given in its dependence on age for the main anatomical substructures.

4. References

1. Boettner, E.A. and Wolter, J.R. (1962) Transmission of the ocular media, *Investigative Ophtalmology* **1**, 776-783
2. Egner, P., Roos, H. and Kellerer A.M. (1995) Applicability and technical features of an Electronic Scheimpflug System for Cataract Studies, *International Forum on Advanced Techniques in Lens & Cataract Research, Kanazawa, Japan*
3. Froemel, M., Junk, A., Roos, H. and Kellerer A.M. (1997) A Control Group for radiation induced Lens Opacities using an Electronic Scheimpflug System, *NATO book series*
4. Pokorny, J., Smith, V.C. and Lutze M. (1987) Aging of the Human Lens, *Applied Optics* **26**, 1437-1440
5. Scheimpflug, T. (1906) Der Photoperspektrograph und seine Anwendung, *Photogr. Korr.* **43**, 516

A CONTROL GROUP FOR RADIATION INDUCED LENS OPACITIES USING AN ELECTRONIC SCHEIMPFLUG SYSTEM

M. FROEMEL[1], A. JUNK[2], H.ROOS[2], A.M. KELLERER[1,2]
[1]*GSF, National Research Center for Environment and Health, Institute of Radiobiology, Ingolstaedter Landstrasse 1,D-85764 Neuherberg, Germany*
[2]*University of Munich, Radiobiological Institute, Schillerstrasse 42, D-80336 Munich, Germany*

1. Abstract

Opacification of the ocular lens is an important late effect of exposure to ionizing radiation. To assess minor opacifications and to quantify the results, the Scheimpflug technique needs to be applied. To compare the degree of opacifications in the radiation exposed cohorts with normal levels, measurements in a reference group are required to determine average degrees of lens opacifications due to aging. With our electronic Scheimpflug system we started to establish such a reference group by examining a cohort of 395 persons with the Scheimpflug technique. The age span of the group covers 67 years, from age 14 to age 81. Increasing opacity with increasing age is found for all anatomical substructures, except the posterior capsule. As this appears to be caused by the influence of reduced illumination of the posterior lens segments due to light absorption in the anterior segments, tentative correction factors have been derived to account for this artefact. The corrected opacity values show an increase with age for all substructures, including the posterior capsule.

2. Materials and Methods

2.1. THE ELECTRONIC SCHEIMPFLUG SYSTEM

Opacification of the lens of the eye is one of the radiation effects that may be important even at relatively low doses. Several cohorts of radiation exposed persons have been examined qualitatively in the past. However, it has been difficult to quantify the results and, in particular, to assess quantitatively slight opacifications or the evolution of opacifications. The conventional slit lamp technique is not optimally suited for such investigations and, therefore, the Scheimpflug technique needs to be

A. K. Junk et al. (eds.),
Ocular Radiation Risk Assessment in Populations Exposed to Environmental Radiation Contamination, 27–32.

applied. With this technique it is possible to obtain sharp images of plane sections through the ocular lens. By analysing these pictures, quantitative density values of different points within the lens can be measured.

Our electronic Scheimpflug system is based on a *Topcon SL-45 B* Scheimpflug camera equipped with a CCD-camera and an electronic image storing system. the flash light intensity of the camera is detected with a photoelectric cell to ensure correct scaling of the observed opacity values. For calibration of the instrument and to guarantee long-term stability, a sphere of opaque glass is used as a 'reference eye'. In each series of examinations, an image of the glass sphere is taken and the opacities of this image are used as reference density.

2.2 ANALYSIS OF SCHEIMPFLUG IMAGES

In epidemiological studies of radiation induced lens opacities not all the details are relevant that are visible on a Scheimpflug image. Therefore, mean values of the opacities are determined for the main anatomical substructures of the lens which are anterior capsule, anterior cortex, nucleus, posterior cortex, posterior capsule and whole lens. This division is adapted to the 'LOCS II + LOCS III' and 'New Grading System for Cataracts' which are commonly used for the classification of cataracts.

2.3. REFERENCE GROUP

With the electronic Scheimpflug system we started to establish a reference group for lens opacifications by examining a cohort of 395 persons with the Scheimpflug technique. Two different groups are part of the cohort: 307 male German Air Force employees were examined during the regular, annual health check up. These persons included jet pilots and ground personnel. This is a selected group, but the advantage of this cohort is the reliable documentation of the health status during the past and that these people will be available for several years for repeated examinations. As there are no women and no persons older than 55 years in this group, the control cohort had to be completed. We have therefore added 88 patients of the Eye Clinic with minor refractive errors, excluding patients who were referred to the clinic because of lens opacities. The age span covers 67 years, from age 14 to age 81. The sum distribution of ages for the reference group is shown in *Figure 1*.

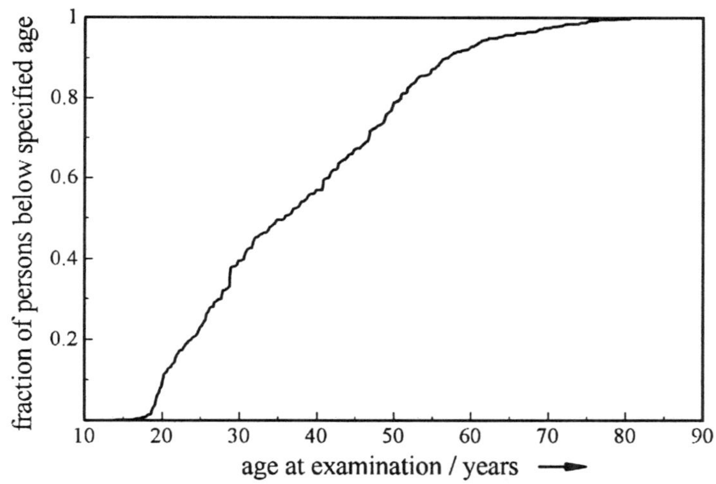

Figure 1: Sum distribution of ages for the reference group

3. Results

Figure 2 shows the mean opacity values of the control group for the different anatomical substructures and for the whole lens in their dependence on the patient's age at examination. From each person 5 images, at different angular orientations of the camera, were taken of each eye. There were no significant differences between the left and the right eye, so the data were averaged. The points represent, therefore, averaged opacities for individual persons. To increase the readability, the diagrams in *Figure 3* show the opacity averages within age at examination intervals of 4 years.

4. Discussion

Increasing opacity with increasing age is found for all substructures, except the posterior capsule. For the posterior capsule, a reversed age trend is seen, but it appears to be caused by the influence of reduced illumination of the posterior lens segments due to light absorption in the anterior segments. To account for this artefact, tentative correction factors have been derived under the assumption that light attentuation in the ocular lens is predominantly due to absorption [2]. For the correction procedure, the spectrum of the Topcon Xe-flashlight is rescaled with age- and wavelength-dependent absorption coefficients deduced from the lens transmission data of Pokorny et al. [4]. For simplicity, we have assumed Rayleigh scattering. The mean reduction of light due to absorption in the lens was found to be 47% for a 20 year old person and 64% for a 60 year old person in the case of the posterior capsule.

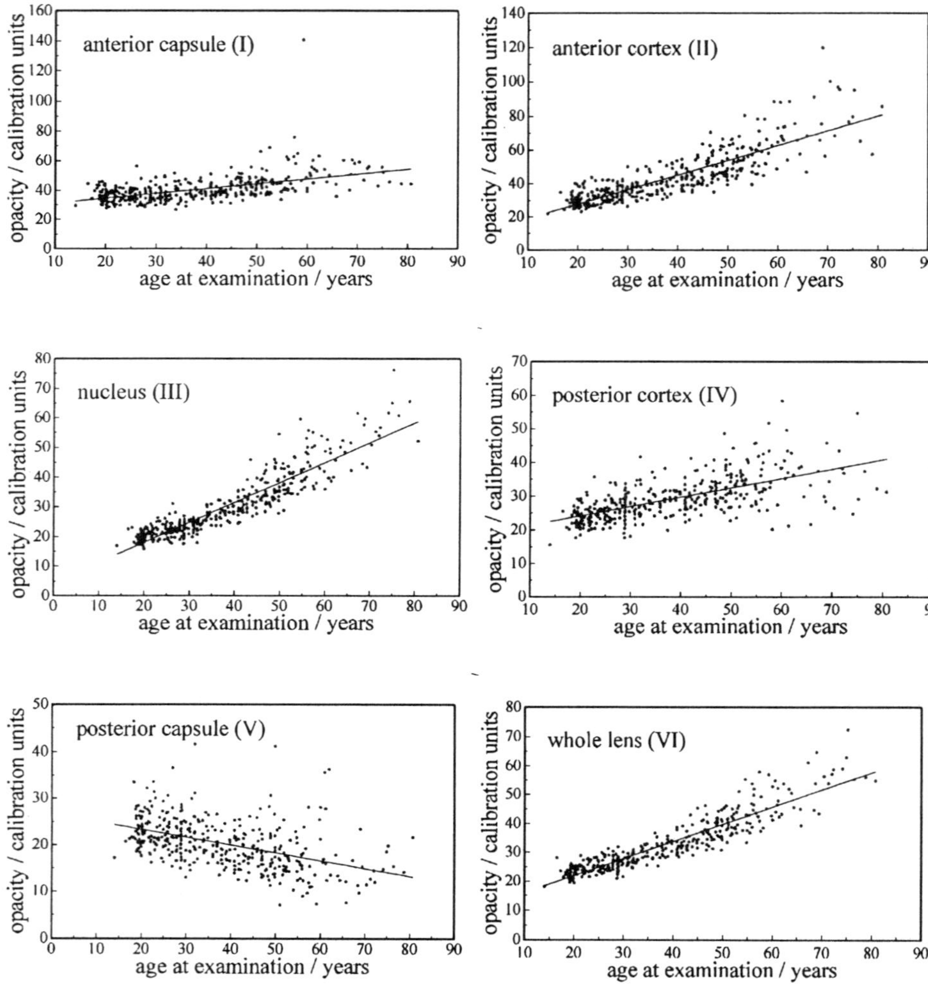

Figure 2: mean opacity values vs. age at examination for the control group. The solid lines refer to linear quadratic regression.

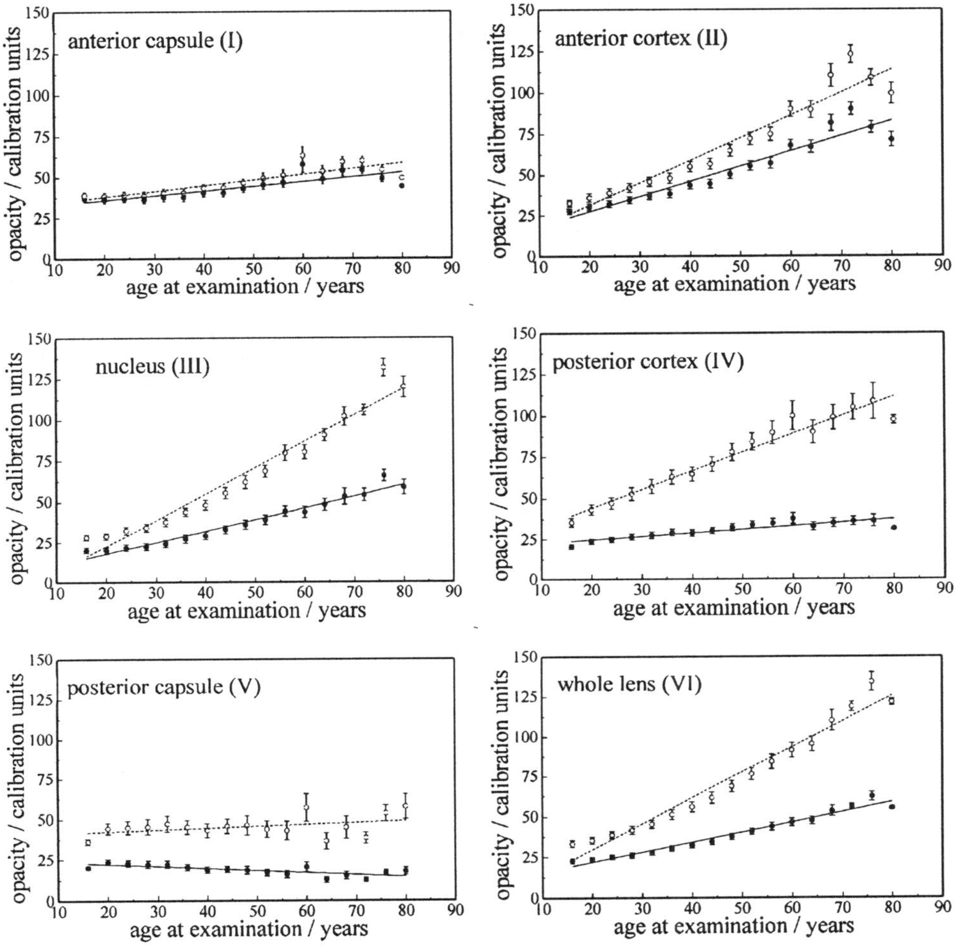

Figure 3: mean opacity values vs. age at examination for the control group before (black dots) and after (white dots) correction. The lines refer to linear quadratic regression. The values are averaged over an age at examination interval of 4 years, the error bars are standard deviations.

The correction factors have been applied to the mean opacity values of the reference group. The modification is most evident in the posterior structures. The corrected mean opacity values, inserted as white dots in *Figure 3*, show an increase with age for all substructures, including the posterior capsule. The age specific increases of the values for nucleus and posterior cortex are substantially steeper than the increases of the uncorrected values. The correction should be improved further. In particular, corneal scattering, a more realistic straylight mechanism and the relation between absorption and scatter will have to be taken into account. One limitation of the present correction is also that it does not account for the shadow of the pupil due to insufficient dilatation. Although cases with poor dilatation were excluded, a suitable correction would further increase the slopes of the dependencies in the present data.

Concerning the reference group, there is still a lack of persons older than 65 years and of younger women. Further examinations at the Munich Eye Clinic are under way.

5. References

1. Egner, P., Roos, H. and Kellerer A.M. (1995) Applicability and technical features of an Electronic Scheimpflug System for Cataract Studies, *International Forum on Advanced Techniques in Lens & Cataract Research, Kanazawa, Japan*
2. Froemel, M., Egner, P., Roos, H. and Kellerer A.M. (1997) Quantification of Lens Opacities with Digital Scheimpflug Imaging, *NATO book series*
3. Mellerio, J. (1970) Light Absorption and Scatter in the Human Lens, *Vision Research* **11**, 129-141
4. Pokorny, J., Smith, V.C. and Lutze M. (1987) Aging of the Human Lens, *Applied Optics* **26**, 1437-1440
5. Sample P. A., Quirante J. S. and Weinreb R. N. (1991) Age-related Changes in the Human Lens, *Acta Ophtalmologica* **69**, 310-314
6. Scheimpflug, T. (1906) Der Photoperspektrograph und seine Anwendung, *Photogr. Korr.* **43**, 516

POSTERIOR SUBCAPSULAR CATARACT AND DRY EYE SYNDROME AFTER RADIATION EXPOSURE BY THE CHERNOBYL ACCIDENT

A.K. JUNK[1,2], P. EGNER[2], B. SWENSSON[1], R.U. PETER[3], F.H. STEFANI[1], A.M. KELLERER[2]
Ludwig-Maximilians-University Munich, Germany, [1]Department of Ophthalmology, [2]Radiobiological Institute, [3]Department of Dermatology; present address: (Chairman) Department of Dermatology, University of Ulm, Germany

1. Summary

During the nuclear accident of Chernobyl in April 1986 numerous reactor workers and fire fighters were exposed to large doses of ionizing radiation. In addition to high ambient γ-ray exposures, these men suffered from a very inhomogenous contamination with fission products on their wet and insufficiently protective clothing, and a resulting severe exposure of the skin, predominantly with β-rays.
16 Chernobyl clean-up workers and 4 persons exposed during nuclear accidents at other nuclear installations were repeatedly examined between September 1991 and September 1996. The radiation exposures ranged from 0.35 to 9 Gy, according to data notified by GUS authorities. They were, in their general trend, confirmed by the determination of chromosome aberrations. The medical therapeutic measures were focused on orthopedic prosthetics and the treatment of chronic radiation dermatitis. Ophthalmological examinations included biomicroscopy of the anterior and ophthalmoscopy of the posterior eye segments. Quantitative assessment of ocular radiation damage, especially to the lens and the documentation of subsequent development of cataract was achieved by application of an electronic Scheimpflug camera system (Topcon SL-45, modified) that included image analysis for quantification of lens opacities.
2 patients had already undergone cataract extraction at first presentation, posterior subcapsular lens opacities were seen in 6 patients, 1 patient presented dense corticonuclear cataracts and pseudoexfoliation-like changes. 4 patients had chronic dry eye syndrome (reduced tear production in Schirmer test). Retinal radiation damages were not detected. No ocular radiation injuries were detected in 9 patients.
Posterior subcapsular cataracts were found to be the predominant consequence of ocular radiation exposure in our patients. There is, at this point, no distinct correlation of ocular findings with the distribution and level of chronic cutaneous radiation damage or with the whole body doses.

A. K. Junk et al. (eds.),
Ocular Radiation Risk Assessment in Populations Exposed to Environmental Radiation Contamination, 33–42.

2. Keywords

radiation, radiation cataract, posterior subcapsular opacity, dry eye syndrome, cutaneous radiation syndrome, basal cell carcinoma, Scheimpflug-photography

3. Introduction

In April 1986 several hundred persons were - reactor personnel or fire fighters in the first phase of the Chernobyl nuclear power plant accident or subsequently members of the rescue and clean-up teams - exposed to high doses of ionizing radiation. Apart from high ambient γ-ray doses, they were inhomogenously contaminated predominantly with β-ray emitting fission products. Among more than 200 men, selected for immediate hospital treatment, 19 patients received bone marrow transplantation [1], 115 developed acute radiation disease of varying severity with lethal outcome for 28 victims [6]. Characteristic symptoms were caused by radiation and /or thermal damage to skin and eye, to haemopoietic tissues and gastrointestinal tract. The consequences of the combined injuries are not yet fully understood. Long-term follow-up of affected patients is necessary to provide continued individual medical care. In addition, experience gained in the follow-up will be valuable in the future, for appropriate treatment and for predicting the course of acute or chronic radiation disease, in particular if signs and symptoms can be related to radiation dose received.

In this study we compare dermatological and ophthalmological findings obtained between September 1991 and September 1996 from 16 victims of the Chernobyl accident and 4 victims of radiation accidents in a nuclear research institute at Moscow with doses assigned by GUS authorities and partially assessed by the analysis of chromosomal aberrations in peripheral blood lymphocytes [5].

4. Materials and methods

CASE REPORTS

For all 20 male patients a history of acute radiation syndrome is reported, first treatment ensued at Hospital No. 6, Moscow. All patients were being treated for symptoms of the delayed stage of cutaneous radiation syndrome with skin involvement of about 4% to 50 % of the body surface, primarily on the lower legs and distal parts of the arms but also on other regions, including face and neck. Total body exposure - according to the assessment by GUS authorities - ranged from 0.35 to 9.0 Gy in the Chernobyl victims. Individual case reports are presented in brief (assigned doses are given in brackets):

(1) DA31 worked at the reactor during the night of the accident, was transferred to hospital on day 1, died of late bone marrow complications in 1995 [5.5 Gy].

(2) PP50 worked within the power plant at 40 m distance from the reactor core during the night of the accident. Carried severely contaminated colleague on his shoulders out of the endangered area and was irradiated for 10 minutes; walked through shallow contaminated water for 20 minutes, was transferred to hospital on day 1, received bone marrow transplantation [5.8 Gy].

(3) SW59 worked outside the power plant at about 500 m distance from the reactor, his entire body was covered with dust and ashes, transferred to hospital on day 1 [5.4 Gy].

(4) KA45 was a visiting engineer on an inspection trip during the night of the accident. Stayed for 3 - 4 hours at about 50 m distance from the reactor and waited for 1 hour outside for transport to hospital [5.7 Gy].

(5) KN46 worked as a consulting engineer with the liquidation teams from week 1 until 9 months after the accident. Wore a protective suit, which left the hands and the nape of the neck free. Contamination with radioactive water on day 1, developed a prolactinoma [1.5 Gy].

(6) NA42 worked as a technician at the reactor during the night of the accident. Exposed during cleaning procedures for over 6 hours, contaminated with radioactive water for over 1 hour. Changed clothes and showered after 7 hours, treated for 2 years in Hospital No. 6, received bone marrow transplantation, amputation of left lower leg due to non healing ulcers [6.5 Gy].

(7) IA61 worked at the reactor during the night of the accident at a distance of about 50 -70 m from the explosion. Spent about 40 minutes in the contaminated area, washed and changed clothes 1 hour later, transferred to hospital 24 hours after the accident, received multiple skin transplantations [4.0 Gy].

(8) RG58 worked in block IV at the time of the accident at a distance of 30 - 40 m from the reactor, with hands severely contaminated and wet clothes, remained in the contaminated area for about 1 hour, changed clothes and showered after 2 hours, multiple skin transplantation and amputation of left finger V (2.5 Gy].

(9) TA61 worked in block IV at a distance of 100 m from the reactor, severely contaminated through sitting on contaminated pipes, changed clothes for the first time 3.5 hours after the accident. Transferred to hospital on day 1 after the accident, received bone marrow transplantation, excision of a verruca vulgaris gigantea, cataract extraction both eyes [9.0 Gy].

(10) BI13 worked as a watchman walking at about 150 m distance around the reactor during the night of the accident until 8 a.m., chronic ulcerations on the affected legs [5.0 Gy].

(11) GO60 worked at the reactor during the night of the accident for 1.5 hours, contaminated by radioactive water, exposed for about 10 minutes at 150 m distance from the reactor [4.5 Gy].

(12) KA64 arrived at the reactor site 1 week after the accident and worked as a liquidator for several months [0.35 Gy].

(13) TA64 worked as a watchman during the night of the accident, stayed close to the reactor for 1 day and 2 nights and was covered with graphite dust, lost hair and nails at day 20, received bone marrow transplantation [5.0 Gy].

(14) CV38 lived 2 km from the power plant and arrived to work on the morning after the accident, worked for 1 h at 400 m distance from the reactor, received bone marrow transplantation [no dose assignment by GUS authorities].

(15) CA34 worked as a member of the liquidator teams, protected on the body by lead but hands and feet unprotected [1.0 Gy and 2.0 Gy].

(16) BA40 was employed as engineer at the power plant, worked on day 2 from 7 a.m. until 5.30 p.m. at reactor block IV, transferred in the night of day 2 to hospital for acute radiation syndrome [1.3 Gy].

(17) FW33 had radiation accident (neutron- and γ-radiation) at nuclear research institute in Moscow 1971, wore protective clothing on lower extremities and received higher doses on upper body, multiple basal cell carcinomas and parotid tumor [4.4 Gy].

(18) MD39 engineer, involved in nuclear accident with FW33 in 1971. Patient stood elevated in 2 m distance with his back towards accident source, received higher doses on lower extremities, 1973 amputation of both lower limbs, 2 basal cell carcinomas at the back [3.8 Gy].

(19) KW40 worked as technician in nuclear plant, 1975 accident with radioactive isotopes, dose unknown, amputation of both forearms, cataract extraction on both eyes, radiotherapy for larynx carcinoma [no dose assignment by GUS authorities].

(20) KO42 had radiation accident at nuclear research institute in Moscow 1979, involving right upper extremity with very high doses [50 - 100 Gy]. Worked from month 3 to 6 after the Chernobyl accident as liquidator. In 1988 and 1991 employed as engineer in Chernobyl [no dose assignment by GUS authorities].

The patients were presented repeatedly to the university hospitals of Munich from September 1991 till September 1996. They had routine examination and treatment for chronic cutaneous radiation syndrome and secondary malignancies. Orthopedic prostheses were provided where necessary.
Ophthalmological examination included best corrected visual acuity, Schirmer test, Jones test and break-up-time for diagnosis of dry eye syndrome, applanation tonometry, biomicroscopy of the anterior eye and funduscopy. An electronic Scheimpflug camera system based on a Topcon SL-45, was employed for quantitative assessment of radiation cataracts. Scheimpflug images were taken in several defined planes through the optic axis of the eye and were processed by integration analysis of 5 anatomically defined lens regions and the whole lens, thus obtaining comparable opacity scores - subsequently termed scores in terms of calibration units - for each area [2,3].

5. Results

5.1. DERMATOLOGICAL

15 Chernobyl victims suffered from severe chronic cutaneous radiation damage of the exposed skin, presenting with dermal sclerosis, epidermal atrophy, disseminated homogeneously colored dark-brown macules, telangiectasias, subcutaneous fibrosis and disseminated keratosis, partially leading to chronic radiation ulcer and necrosis. Predominantly affected areas included the lower extremities (walking through contaminated water), buttocks (sitting on contaminated objects) and the upper part of the body (contamination by wet clothing), unprotected hands and faces. Patient KA46 presented only very distinct telangiectasias on the nape of the neck [4]. 1 patient (DA31) died of late bone marrow complications.

The two patients, who were involved in the same accident (neutron and γ-radiation) at a nuclear research institute in Moscow, FW33 and MD39, developed multiple basal cell carcinomas at the sites of chronic cutaneous radiation damage.

5.2. OPHTHALMOLOGICAL

Posterior subcapsular opacities of different magnitude were documented in four of the Chernobyl victims (GO60, KA45, NA42, PP50).

Figure 1a. right eye

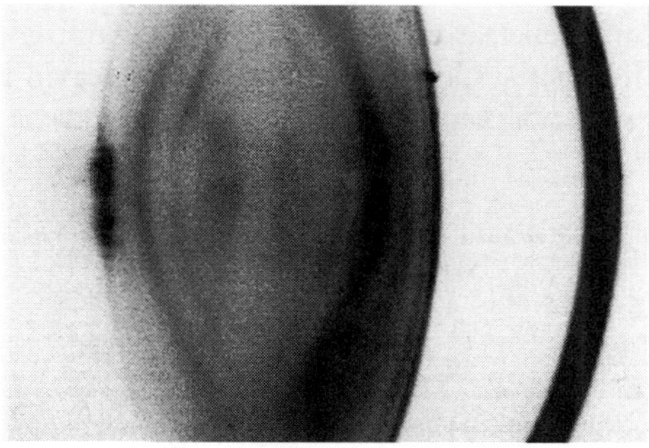

Figure 1b. left eye

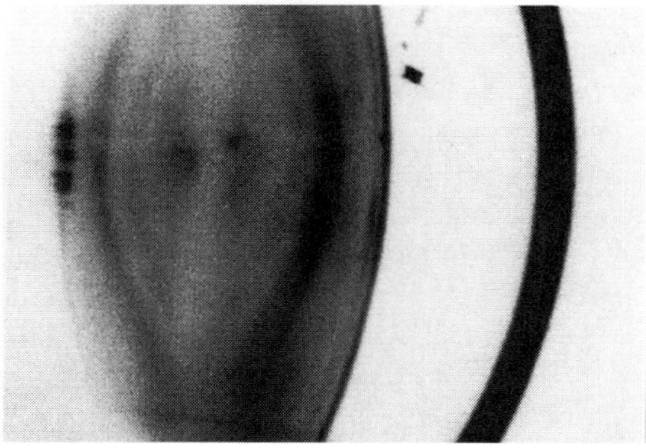

Figure 1a,b. Scheimpflug images of right (1a) and left (1b) anterior eye segment (NA42), note the differing amont of posterior subcapsular opacity

TA61 had cataract extraction before first presentation. BI13 presented dense corticonuclear cataracts and pseudoexfoliation-like changes; etiological conclusions to differentiate between age related changes and secondary alterations due to thermal and radiation injury, remain speculative in this patient.

Dry eye syndrome was found in three (KA45, SW59, TA64) Chernobyl victims, DA31 reported three episodes of amaurosis fugax - in retrospection a possible early sign of his bone marrow complication, IA61 complained of pruritus on both eyes and repeated conjunctival bleeding.

Among the group of men exposed at the nuclear research institute in Moscow, posterior subcapsular cataracts were documented in two (FW33, MD39) patients, KW40 had cataract extraction before first presentation, secondary glaucoma, treated by iridectomy, and remained with dry eye syndrome.
The remaining patients presented normal age related lens opacities and no signs of radiation damage to the eye (BA40, CA34, CV38, DA31, IA61, KN46, KA64, RG58, and KO42). Radiation retinopathy was not detected in any of our patients.
Densitometric evaluation of Scheimpflug images in the anatomical lens regions of anterior capsule (I), anterior cortex (II), nucleus (III), and whole lens (VI) revealed normal values within the standard deviation of an age matched normal collective. An exception were the 2 patients with cataract extraction prior to their examination and BI13 with dense corticonuclear cataract; they were arbitrarily assigned to the top of the opacity scale. It is not surprising that opacities increased in the posterior cortex (IV) and on the posterior capsule (V), the typical regions for manifestation of radiation cataract.

Figure 2a-e. Densitometric evaluation of Scheimpflug images in the anatomical lens regions in comparison to normal age related distribution

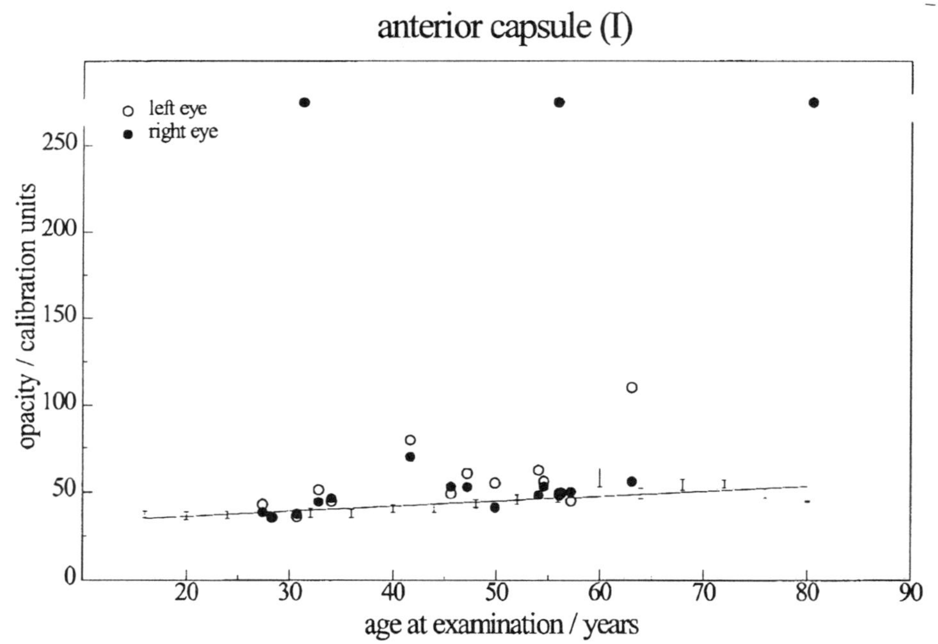

Figure 2a. anterior capsule (I)

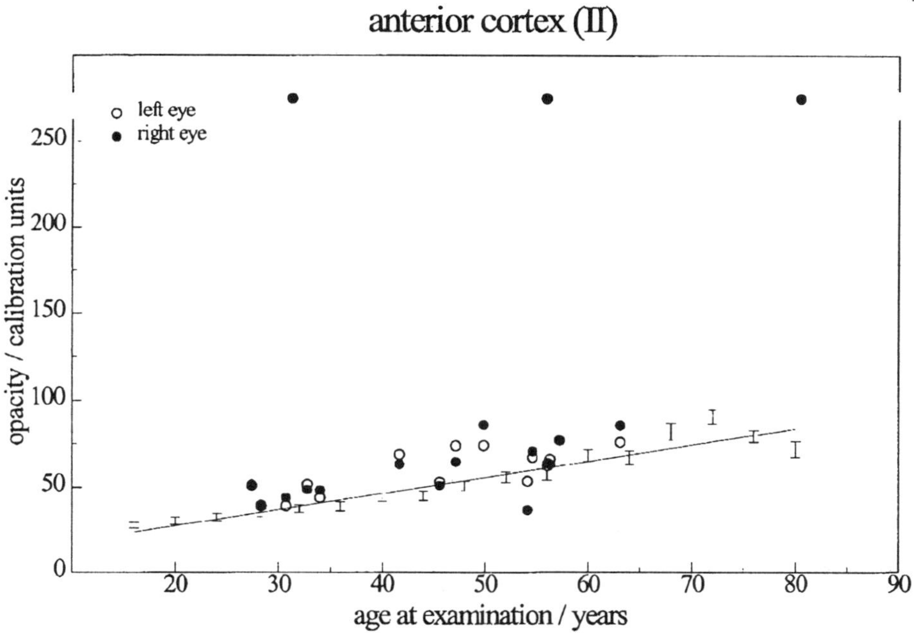

Figure 2 b. anterior cortex (II)

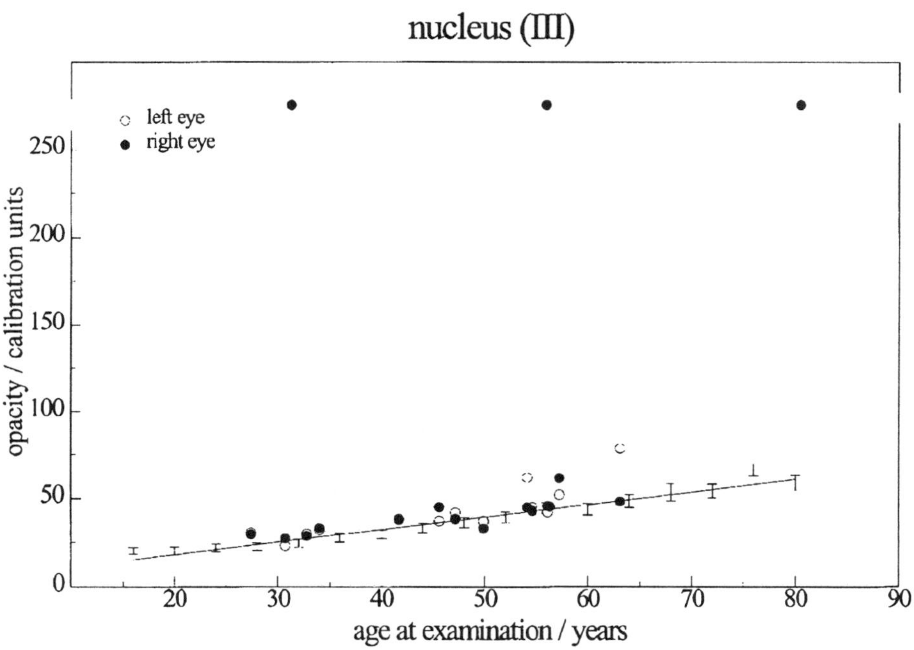

Figure 2 c. nucleus (III)

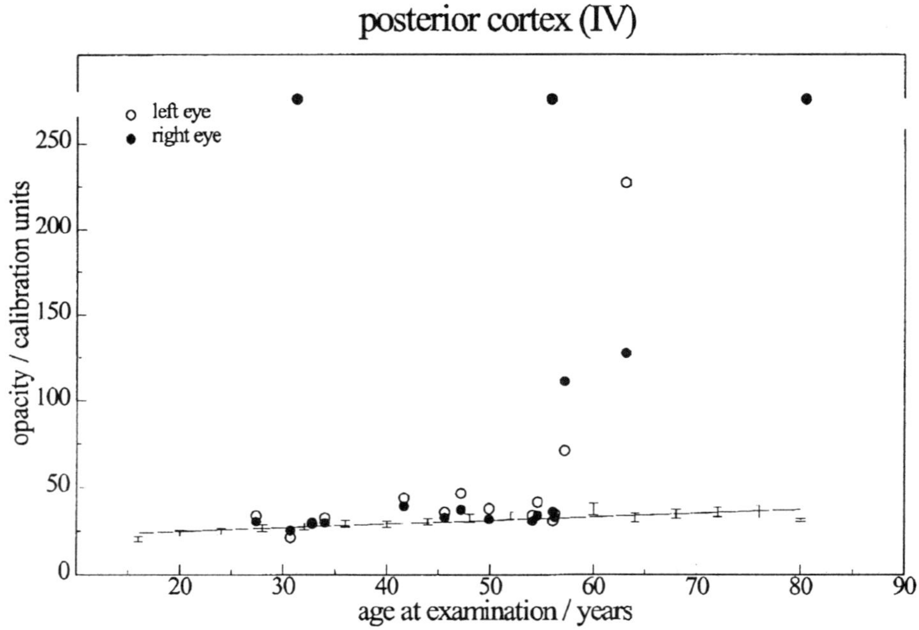

Figure 2 d. posterior cortex (IV)

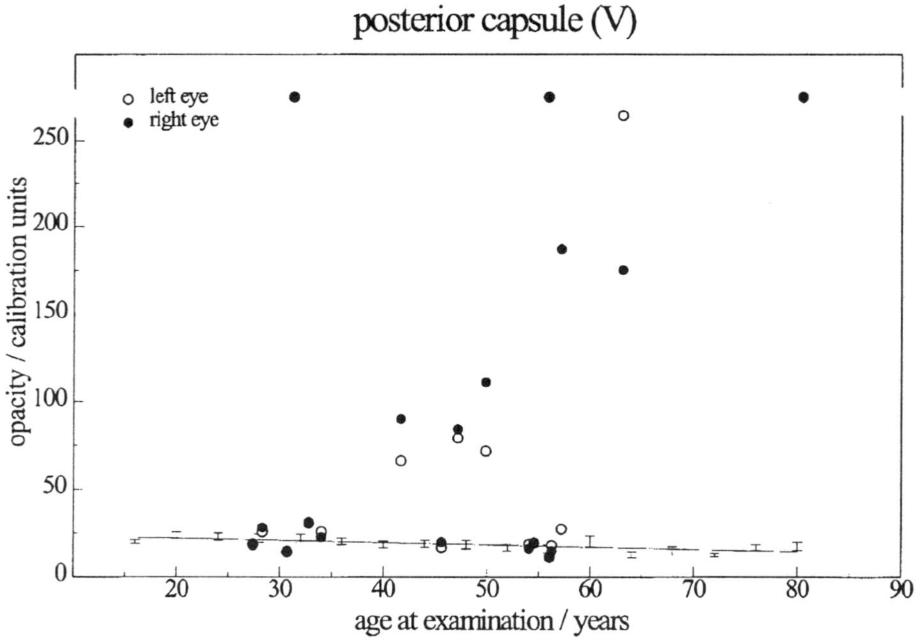

Figure 2 e. posterior capsule (V)

The comparison of the degree of lens opacities with the assigned doses (Figure 3.) shows no distinct relation, although it does indicate a correlation that has not been quantified.

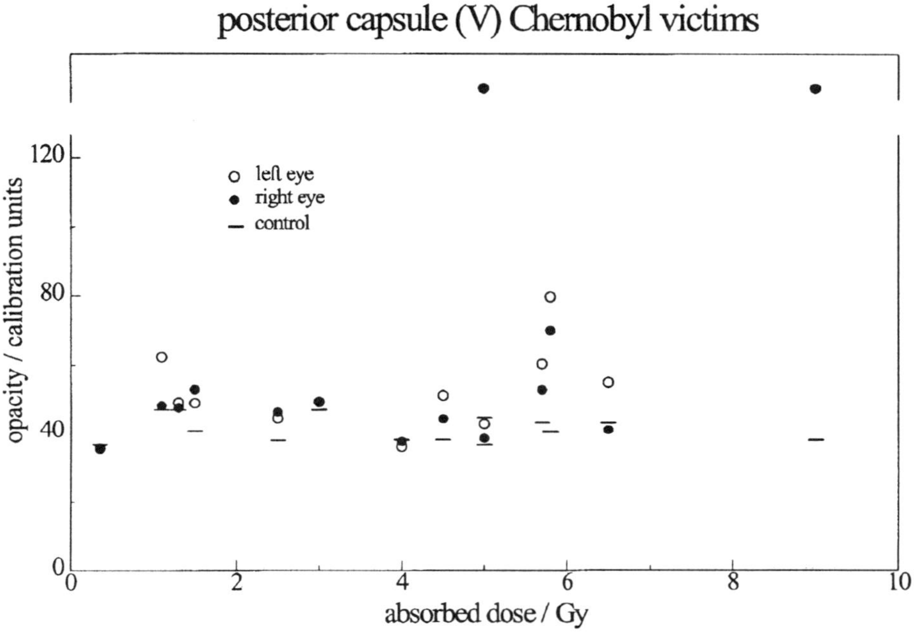

Figure 3. Relation of densitometric data of the posterior capsule (V) to dose

6. Discussion

In contrast to the irradiation damage in the A-bomb victims in Hiroshima and Nagasaki which were predominantly exposed to γ-rays and neutrons, our patients were mainly exposed to a mixture of ambient γ-radiation and β-radiation emitted by a multitude of fission products. This led to irradiation of the skin, partly with extreme doses, and to lower, concomitant exposures of the bone marrow and the gastrointestinal tract. A correlation between the development of posterior subcapsular opacities and assigned dose, or dose estimated in terms of chromosomal aberrations, is suggested in our results. It has not been quantified in this study, however, because the doses represent estimates of the effective dose. It is the equivalent of a whole body dose and as such has a very weak correlation to the dose in specific tissues - such as the ocular lens - because of the highly non-uniform exposure situation. Due to the inhomogenous irradiation there is little expectation of a distinct relation between the dermatological and the ophthalmological findings, and such a correlation has, in fact, not been found. This is in line with the observation of substantial differences between the degrees of opacity in the two eyes of some of the patients as shown in Figure 1a,b.

Acknowledgment: Diagnosis and treatment of the patients at the Department of Dermatology and the Department of Ophthalmology, University of Munich, was made possible by a generous grant of the Bavarian Broadcasting and Television Services, which was administered by the Bavarian Red Cross.

7. References

1. CEC (Commission of the European Communities) (1991) Treatment and Biological Dosimetry of Exposed Persons, in K. Chadwick and G. Gerber (eds.) *Post-Chernobyl Action*, Radiation Protection Series EUR-12558 EN.

2. Egner P. (1998) Entwicklung eines elektronischen Scheimpflugsystems zur Untersuchung von Linsentrübungen, thesis, Ludwig-Maximilians-University of Munich.

3. Egner, P., Roos, H., Kellerer, A.M. (1994) Development of an Electronic Scheimpflug System for Cataract Studies Among the 224Ra Patients, in G. van Kaick, A. Karaoglou, A.M. Kellerer (eds.), *Health Effects of Internally Deposited Radionucleides: Emphasis on Radium and Thorium,* World Scientific Singapore, EUR 15877 EN, 275-280.

4. Peter, R.U., Braun-Falco, O., Birioukov, A., Hacker, N., Kerscher, M., Peterseim, U., Ruzicka, T., Konz, B., Plewig, G. (1994) Chronic cutaneous damage after accidental exposure to ionizing radiation: The Chernobyl experience. *Journal Am Acad Dermatol*, **30**, 719-723.

5. Salassidis, K., Schmid, E., Peter, R.U., Braselmann, H., Bauchinger, M. (1994) Dicentric and translocation analysis for retrospective dose estimation in humans exposed to ionizing radiation during the Chernobyl nuclear power plant accident. *Mutation Research*, **311**, 39-48.

6. *United Nations Scientific Committee on the Effects of Atomic Radiation: Sources, Effects and Risks of Ionizing Radiation (UNSCEAR)* (1988) United Nations, New York.

THE INCIDENCE OF EYE DISORDERS AMONG CHERNOBYL CLEAN-UP WORKERS

A. A. EGLITE, G. J. OZOLA, E. V. CURBAKOVA
Institute of Occupational and Environmental Health of Medical Academy of Latvia, Centre of Occupational and Radiological Medicine, Dzirciema 16, LV- 1007, Riga, Latvia

1. Background

The accident of the Chernobyl Nuclear Power Plant (NPP) on the 26th of April 1986 is so far the biggest accident of nuclear energy that created a new problem for Nuclear Medicine and gave a new opportunity for science to study the wide effects of small doses of ionising radiation to big human populations.

This accident has also become a problem for Latvia, because nearly 6000 people took part in clean-up works of the Chernobyl accident from 1986 till 1991. The doses documented for the clean- up workers are variable- they are estimated to be between 0.01 - 0.5 Gy although the specialists working on the precision of received doses think that they could be even 2 or 3 times higher.

The difference between Latvian Chernobyl accident clean-up workers and clean-up workers from other countries contaminated with radionuclides that make Latvian Chernobyl clean-up workers to be a unique cohort for studies is the fact that because Latvian Chernobyl clean-up workers have only had a low ionising radiation exposure during an exact period of time and then had been moved to regions free of radionuclides [1, 2].

The eye disorders related to ionising radiation are among the less studied pathologies, although the diseases of nervous system and organs of sense have become the most significant pathology of Latvian Chernobyl clean-up workers during the last four years.

Therefore the aim of work is to evaluate the incidence of eye disorders among Chernobyl clean-up workers in order to provide more information to different specialists helping them to understand this problem deeper.

The following tasks have been stated:

1) to analyse the morbidity of Chernobyl clean-up workers in order select persons with eye pathologies;
2) to analyse and evaluate the structure of eye pathology;
3) to analyse the incidence of eye pathology among Chernobyl clean-up workers in comparison with control group.

A. K. Junk et al. (eds.),
Ocular Radiation Risk Assessment in Populations Exposed to Environmental Radiation Contamination, 43–49.

2. Materials and methods

Diagnoses of all eye diseases were confirmed by specialists of the Centre of Occupational and Radiological Medicine of P. Stradina Clinical Hospital. Data from the "Latvian State Register of Occupational diseases and persons that have received radiation in Chernobyl NPP accident clean-up works" were used. Epidemiological monitoring in forms of epidemiological survey and statistical analyses were used.

On the first stage - data about the diseases of clean-up workers were extracted from the Register and analysed in order to select persons with one ore more eye pathology (table 1) [3].

TABLE 1. The most frequent eye diseases of Chernobyl NPP accident clean-up workers

N	ICD-9	Diagnosis
1.	361.3	Ruptura retinae sine ablatione
2.	362.0	Retinopathia diabetica proliferans
3.	362.1	Angiopathia retinae
4.	362.2	Retinopathia proliferans
5.	362.5	Degeneratio (dystrophia) maculae luteae
6.	362.6	Degeneratio (dystrophia) retinae periferica
7.	362.81	Haemorrhagia retinae
8.	365.0	Glaucoma
9.	366.0	Cataract
10.	367.0	Hypermetropia
11.	367.1	Myopia
12.	367.2	Astigmatism
13.	367.4	Presbyopia
14.	372.0	Conjunctivitis
15.	372.2	Blepharoconjunctivitis
16.	373.0	Blepharitis
17.	376.2	Exophthalmus incretorius
18.	376.21	Exophthalmus thyreotoxicus
19.	376.3	Exophthalmus
20.	377.42	Neuropathia nervi optici ischaemica
21.	379.0	Scleritis
22.	379.01	Episcleritis
23.	379.20	Vitreal degeneration

The group under investigation was formed by following criteria :

1) men and women ;
2) participants of the Chernobyl NPP accident clean-up works from 1986 till 1990 y.;
3) one ore more eyes pathology (table 1).

On the second stage - the incidence of eye pathology among Chernobyl clean-up workers in comparison with control groups was analysed.

The group under investigation was formed by following criteria:
1) men;
2) participants of the Chernobyl NPP accident clean-up works in 1986.;
3) age of 1 subgroup: 30 - 40 years (100 persons);
age of 2 subgroup: 41 - 50 years (100 persons);

Control group (patients with occupational diseases) was formed by following criteria:
1) men;
2) not involved in Chernobyl NPP accident clean-up works;
3) the same occupations as clean-up workers (drivers, tractor drivers etc.);
4) age of 1 subgroup: 30 - 40 years (100 persons);
age of 2 subgroup: 41 - 50 years (100 persons).

3. Results and discussion

On the first stage - Register's data about the diseases of clean-up workers were analysed in order to select persons with one ore more eye pathology (table 1). There were 571 (11.46%) persons with eye pathology from 4841 clean-up workers registered till January, 1, 1996. First stages results are presented in table 2. As we can see in table 2 the structure of eye pathology is as follows:

Angiopathia retinae is most typical eye pathology for Chernobyl clean-up workers; followed by the myopia as a second most common pathology and cataract as third. Conjunctivitis and dystrophia retinae are also very common in this group. Our results are similar with results of Ukrainian and Belorussian authors [4, 5].

On the second stage - the incidence of eye pathology among Chernobyl clean-up workers in comparison with control groups were analysed. Results are presented accordingly in tables 3, 4.

TABLE 2. Structure of Chernobyl NPP accident clean-up workers eye diseases

N	Diagnosis	Year of participating in clean-up works				Summary	%
		1986	1987	1988	1989		
1.	Angiopathia retinae	178	71	23	5	277	41.47
2.	Myopia	84	46	10	3	143	21.40
3.	Cataract	38	10	8	-	56	8.38
4.	Conjunctivitis	25	9	3	1	38	5.69
5.	Dystrophia retinae	21	11	2	-	34	5.09
6.	Hypermetropia	17	10	3	2	32	4.78
7.	Astigmatism	16	7	-	2	25	3.74
8.	Presbyopia	10	6	5	-	21	3.14
9.	Blepharitis	7	2	1	-	10	1.50
10.	Blepharoconjunctivitis	4	4	1	-	9	1.35
11.	Contusio bulbi	4	-	-	-	4	0.60
12.	Glaucoma	-	-	2	-	2	0.30
13.	Occlusio vasorum retinae	-	-	2	-	2	0.30
14.	Keratitis	-	-	2	-	2	0.30
15.	Retinopathia diabetica prol.	-	-	2	-	2	0.30
16.	Endophthalmitis purulenta	-	-	1	-	1	0.15
17.	Other eye diseases	-	-	1	-	1	0.15
18.	Orbital foreign body	-	-	1	-	1	0.15
19.	Corneal scar	-	-	1	-	1	0.15
20.	Retinosclerosis	-	-	1	-	1	0.15
21.	Other diseases of the eye lid	-	-	1	-	1	0.15
22.	Amblyopy	-	-	1	-	1	0.15
23.	Nubecula cornea	-	-	1	-	1	0.15
24.	Macula cornea	-	-	1	-	1	0.15
25.	Leucoma cornea	-	-	1	-	1	0.15
26.	Episcleritis	-	-	1	-	1	0.15
Summary		404	176	75	13	668	100

TABLE 3. Analysis of eye pathology of Chernobyl clean-up workers in comparison with control group (age group - 30 - 40 years)

N	Diagnosis	Clean-up workers n = 100	Control group n = 100
1.	Angiopathia retinae	14	1
2.	Myopia	8	10
3.	Cataract	2	-
4.	Contusio bulbi	2	-
5.	Dystrophia retinae peripheral.	2	-
6.	Hypermetropia	1	-
7.	Amblyopia	1	1
8.	Conjunctivitis	1	-
9.	Astigmatism	-	5
10.	Trichromasy	-	2
11.	Glaucoma	-	1
12.	Pterygium	-	1
13.	Neuritis nervi optici	-	1
14.	Enophthalmus	-	1
15.	Blepharoconjunctivitis	-	1
16.	Blepharitis	-	1
Summary		31	25

As can be seen from table 3 in the age group of 30 - 40 years angiopathia retinae was more common among Chernobyl clean-up workers than in control group, but numbers of myopia were similar in both groups of this age.

TABLE 4. Analysis of eye pathology of Chernobyl clean-up workers in comparison with control group (age group - 41 - 50 years)

N	Diagnosis	Clean-up workers n = 100	Control group n = 100
1.	Angiopathia retinae	14	8
2.	Cataract	7	4
3.	Myopia	5	6
4.	Conjunctivitis	3	2
5.	Keratitis	2	-
6.	Leucoma corneae	1	1
7.	Dystrophia macula lutea	1	-
8.	Chalacion	1	-
9.	Macula corneae	1	-
10.	Contusio bulbi	1	-
11.	Presbyopia	1	5
12.	Astigmatism	-	2
13.	Retinopathia diab. prol.	-	1
14.	Amblyopia	-	1
15.	Neuritis nervi optici	-	1
16.	Corneal scar	-	1
17.	Phacosclerosis	-	1
18.	Hypermetropia	-	1
19.	Cysticercus	-	1
20.	Ablatio retinae totalis	-	1
	Summary	37	25

As shown in table 4 angiopathia retinae was revealed more frequently among Chernobyl clean-up workers than in control group for age group 41 - 50. The number of angiopathia retinae in this age group was similar to that of age 30 - 40 years, but we also revealed an increased number of cataracts in group of age 41 - 50 years (cataract - on the second place), that we can partly explain by influence of age and another factors, perhaps ionising radiation. Number of myopia was also similar in both groups of 41 - 50 years.

In order to evaluate the trends of common eye pathology incidence of eye pathology for clean-up workers in age group from 30 to 50 years (200 persons) were analysed in comparison with control group (table 5).

TABLE 5. Analysis of eye pathology of Chernobyl clean-up workers in comparison to control group (age group 30 - 50 years)

N	Diagnosis	Clean-up workers n = 200	Control group n = 200
1.	Angiopathia retinae	28	9
2.	Myopia	13	16
3.	Cataract	9	4
4.	Conjunctivitis	4	2
5.	Macular degeneration	3	1
6.	Contusio bulbi	3	-
7.	Keratitis dendritica	2	-
8.	Presbyopia	1	5
9.	Amblyopia	1	2
10.	Leucoma corneae	1	1
11.	Hyperopia	1	1
12.	Macula corneae	1	-
13.	Astigmatism	-	7
14.	Proliferative diabetic retinopathy	-	1
15.	Neuritis nervi optici	-	2
16.	Corneal opacity	-	1
17.	Phacosclerosis	-	1
18.	Cysticercus	-	1
19.	Ablatio retinae totalis	-	1
20.	Trichromasy	-	2
21.	Glaucoma	-	1
22.	Pterygium	-	1
23.	Chalacion	-	1
Summary		67	63

Statistical analyses revealed that clean-up workers have a higher risk to develop angiopathia retinae than the control group (table 5), relative risk is estimated to be ~ 3. Clean-up workers more frequently developed pathologies as cataract, conjunctivitis and dystrophia retinae. With respect to myopia our analyses show that morbidity in the group of investigated persons and morbidity in control group is similar. This could be partly explained by higher frequency of myopia as pathology of eyes refraction in population as well as by influence of various hazardous factors at work (bad working conditions, overloads, shift work etc.).

4. Conclusions

For the first time in Latvia analysis of the prevalence and structure of eye pathology of Chernobyl NPP accident clean-up workers were performed. It has been revealed that during last 10 years most common eye pathologies for Chernobyl NPP clean-up workers has been angiopathia retinae (41.5 %), myopia (21.4 %) and cataract (8.4 %). Angiopathia retinae is showing a trend to increase in the group of Chernobyl NPP accident clean-up workers and this allows to make parallels between the development of angiopathia retinae and a common answer reaction of an organism to wide range diapason of small doses of radiation as well as the influence of other harmful accident's factors.

Our investigation does not allow to distinguish ionising radiation effects from another harmful factors as reasons for increased number of eye pathology.

5. References

1. Eglite, M. (1996), *Electromagnetic radiation: ionising and non-ionising radiation* and its influence on the *human organism,* Institute of Occupational and Environmental Health of Medical Academy of Latvia, Riga, pp. 1 - 26.
2. Curbakova, E., Dzerve B., Eglite, M. (1996), Health status and follow-up of the Chernobyl NPP accident clean-up workers in Latvia, *Proceedings of the first international conference on health consequences of the Chernobyl accident,* Minsk, pp. 929 - 934.
3. *Statistic classification of diseases and health problems,* World Health Assembly IDC - 9, Riga, pp. 28 - 33.
4. Semak,G. (1995), The influence of Low doses of radiation on vascular pathology of eyes, Swedish international development cooperation agency, report, pp. 5 - 15.
5. Jabojedov, G., Umovist, N. (1992), The particularities of the organ of vision state in persons, having been exposed to the radiation effect, *Theses of rep. of the Intern. Symp.*, Yaremcha, p. 9.

RADIATION CATARACTS IN HIGH DOSE LIQUIDATORS WHO DEVELOPED ACUTE RADIATION SYNDROME

V.G. BEBESHKO, V.M. GAYDAY, Y.V. GAYDAY,
A.N.KOVALENKO, D.A. BELYI
Scientific Centre for Radiation Medicine
Melnikova Street 53, Kiev, 254050, Ukraine

1. Introduction

All eye tissues are liable differently to a radiation damage but many proceedings have been devoted chiefly to the radiation injury of the lens for several reasons. First, the lens is the most radiosensitive eye structure and is considered as a critical organ. Second, its pathological changes lead to essential reduction of visual acuity. Recent publications have shown that the doses ranging between 0.6-1.5 Gy may cause radiation cataract [1].

The latency for the onset of lens opacities due to exposure to radiation is dependent the absorbed dose and the age and may vary largely from less than 6 months to 12 years [2, 3, 4, 5, 6].

2. Methods

The annual examination of the eye function during post-accident years was done starting from 1986 in 90 male patients who had endured acute radiation syndrome (ARS) of first to third degree of severity and 40 patient with absorbed doses less than 0.5 Gy. All patients were irradiated in the result of the Chernobyl accident. The clinical description of these patients has shown in table 1. More than 90 % of our patients served in the Ministry of Internal Affairs or worked at the Chernobyl NPP and had an annual all organs system examination with well formalised medical documentation. So it was possible to obtain the base level of eye status. No patient had cataract formation before the accident.

All patients were exposed to external beta and gamma irradiation. The contribution of internal irradiation was negligible [7].

The eye examination consisted of visual acuity, biomicroscopy with split lamp, ophthalmoscopy, perimetry, refraction, tonometry. Cataract stages were estimated by Vishnevskyi's classification [2]. All data were collected by one Moscow-trained investigator and estimated in collaboration with other well experienced military ophthalmologist. The background literature and design of the study were the

A. K. Junk et al. (eds.),
Ocular Radiation Risk Assessment in Populations Exposed to Environmental Radiation Contamination, 51–56.

responsibility of other authors.

TABLE 1. The clinical characteristics of the patients under the examination ($M \pm \sigma$)

Groups	Absorbed doses less than 0.5 Gy	ARS 1	ARS 2	ARS 3
Number of patients	40	40	40	10
Age in 1997, years	38.3 ± 11.1	38.8 ± 7.3	38.4 ± 8.7	39.9 ± 11.2
Absorbed dose, Gy	0.29 ± 0.17	1.07 ± 0.54	2.49 ± 0.84	4.6 ± 1.52
Doses range, Gy	0.1 - 0.5	0.1 - 3.3	4.9 - 0.5	3.0 - 7.1
Medical history:				
diabetes mellitus, %	15	7.5	10	20
essential hypertension, %	50	52.5	30	10
coronary heart disease, %	7.5	10	17.5	30
cerebral atherosclerosis, %	15	22.5	25	30
arteriosclerosis obliterans, %	7.5	0	0	0
systemic corticosteroids, %	0	0	0	0
Ophthalmological history:				
complains about vision, %	50	40	42.5	80

3. Results

3.1. CATARACT FORMATION

The generalised data are submitted in table 2, except one patient born in 1961 who survived ARS of forth degree due to estimated 8 Gy of absorbed external γ- and β-dose. He is the only one who survived after so high irradiation in the result of the Chernobyl accident. First signs of his radiation cataract were revealed at the end of 1986, that is exactly 6-8 months after irradiation. As shown in table 1 the number of typical radiation - posterior subcapsular cataracts - correlates with ARS severity. Other cataracts such as nuclear, coronary, stratified and corticonuclear, does not depend on ARS severity.

In general 10-years after the accident all of our patients in the group of third degree ARS of 3 degree developed posterior subcapsular cataract, 30 % after second degree ARS and 5 % after first degree ARS (Figure 1). In the group of patients with absorbed doses less than 0.5 Gy there were no cases of posterior subcapsular cataracts found.

The clinical findings correlate well with prior publications [1, 2, 4] on irradiation doses, terms of the radiation cataract forming and cataract growth, and corresponds to the "dose-effect" relation.

The less dose of ionizing radiation the slower cataract develops, opacifications appear later and may stop to progression before cataract operation is demanded.

It is important to note that many patients after second degree ARS having received total body doses around 2 Gy did not yet develop typical radiation cataracts 10 years after the Chernobyl accident. This may be explained by individual differences in radioresistance or ongoing latent periods for cataract formation. As the given doses are total body doses, calculated as effective doses to the bone marrow by estimating of gamma doses only the do not reflect the exposure of the eye.

TABLE 2. Main eye pathologies in patients examined 10 years after the Chernobyl accident

Ophthalmologic diseases or symptoms	Number of examined patients				Total
	Absorbed doses less than 0.5 Gy	ARS confirmed, degree of severity			
		1	2	3	
Chronic conjunctivitis, blepharitis	5	4	4	2	15
Telangiectases of eyelids skin and conjunctiva and eyeball	0	2	3	4	9
Degeneration of uveal tract anterior part	0	1	3	3	7
Typical radiation (posterior subcapsular) cataracts	0	1	6	10	17
Conglomerations of vacuoles in lens posterior pole or combinations of vacuoles with dotted opacities	0	1	6	0	7
Nuclear, coronary and stratified cataracts	5	5	2	0	12
Multiple diffuse dotted opacities of different lens' localisation	9	10	10	2	31
Corticonuclear cataracts	7	6	7	4	24
Atrophy of optical nerves,	0	1	2	1	4
Angiopathy (dystonic, hypertonic, diabetic and others), retinal angiosclerosis	15	14	20	7	56
Macular degeneration	9	8	12	5	34
Glaucoma	1	3	1	1	6
Vitreous destruction	1	2	3	1	7

The quantitative dynamic of radiation cataracts is reflected in table 3.

TABLE 3. Post-accident dynamics of radiation cataracts number in patients who suffered ARS

Groups of patients	Case number				
	1987-1988	1989-1990	1991-1992	1993-1996	Total
Absorbed doses less than 0.5 Gy	0	0	0	0	0
ARS degrees					
First	0	0	1	2 (1)	2
Second	0	3	7 (4)	12 (5)	12
Third	4	8 (4)*	10 (2)	10 (0)	10

* In brackets - the number of new radiation cataracts cases

Revealed cases of lens small dimensions opacities are demanded a special attention. The quantity of this opacities does not match to frames of age-specified. These multiple diffuse dotted, small flaky and as lump opacities gave an occasion to diagnose powdered cataracts. Such cataracts were found in the patients after ARS of different severity degrees.

Senile (nuclear, cortical and anterior subcapsular polar) cataracts that patients had had before the accident evolved faster than usual. So the radiation exposure may accelerate this growth.

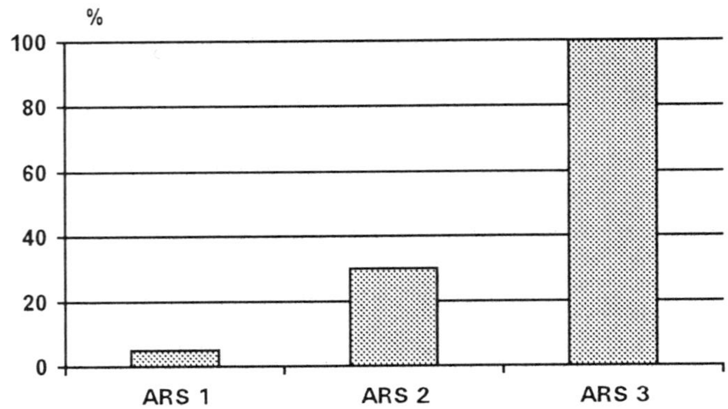

Figure 1. The prevalence of radiation (posterior subcapsular) cataracts in patients who suffered from ARS (10 years after the Chernobyl accident)

3.2. RETINAL PATHOLOGY

Second to any kind of lens changes angiopathies of retina were detected at the end of 1996 (48 %) (Figure 2). These findings are mainly secondary to cardiovascular diseases.

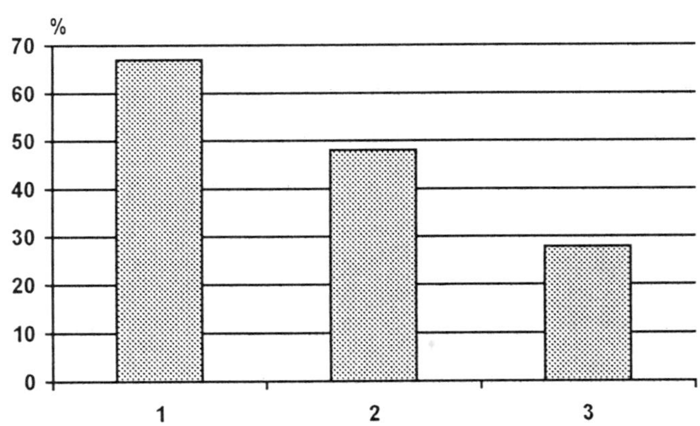

Figure 2. The prevalence of cataracts, all different types and all theirs combinations (1), prevalence of retinopathy (2) and macular degeneration (3) in patients who suffered from ARS of different degrees of severity

A ratio of the retinal arteries to veins in calibre less than 3 to 2 was defined as dystonic retinopathy. This ratio is changed due to retinal vein dilation and atony as in hypotony, or retinal artery hypertonic contraction as in hypertony. Vein dilation of 150 to 200 micrometer and artery contractions of 50 to 70 micrometer were assessed by calibrometry [8].

Signs of arteriosclerosis and hypertonic retinopathy such as "Salus"-phenomenon (the sign of arterial hypertension sclerotic stage: retinal veins decline after its cross retinal arteries), positive Guist phenomenon (the sign of hypertonic retinopathy: serpentine veins in the field of yellow spot) and positive sign of "silver wire" indicated on severe and non-reversible pathology.

In 28 % of our patients macular degeneration was diagnosed. Macular drusen arising from Bruch's membrane are referred to as macular degeneration. Drusen were found in the retina of the posterior pole, but also in peripheral retina and at the optic disc.

3.3. OPTIC NERVE PATHOLOGY

Progressive optic nerve atrophies were found in two patients. The fireman B. born in 1954 received a dose of 3.3 Gy and had to be treated for second grade ARS had initial signs of atrophy of the right optic nerve. A follow-up was negative: 10 years after the accident the right eye function, including visual acuity, visual field and adaptation to darkness ware severe broke down and corresponded to the clinical picture of expressed atrophy of optic nerve.

4. Conclusion

The majority of patients that had suffered from ARS after the Chernobyl accident had pathological changes in eye tissues and different diseases that lead to break of eye functions and to disablement (in the case of non-operated cataract and serious impair of visual acuity). This may be considered as radiation long term consequences.

Medical (cataract operation) and social (professional reorientation, pensions) rehabilitation is a particular part for ophthalmologic patients treatment.
In the treatment of radiation cataracts of 3, 4 and 5 degree of severity a surgical operation applied. If expressed macular degeneration had occurred operations for choroid vascularization were used.

The eye pathologies detected in these patients 10 years after the radiation exposure following the Chernobyl accident dictates to continue the examination of these individuals in the future.

References

1. Ito C. (1996) Atomic bomb damage and health care for a-bomb survivors in Japan, in International symposium in commemoration of the 50th Year of the Atomic Bombing. Proceedings. Hiroshima International Council for Health Care of the Radiation-Exposed (eds). Hiroshima, pp. 73-81.
2. Vishnevskyi, N.A., Abdullaeva, V.M., Ivanova, E.A. (1961) Initial signs and classification of radiation cataracts, *Vestnik ophthalmologii* **5**, 65-68.
3. Volkov, V.V. (1970) *Beta-radiation Damages*, Military Medical Academy, Leningrad, 168 p.
4. Guskova, A.K. and Bayisogolov, G.D. (1971) *Radiation Disease in Man*, Medicine, Moscow, 384 p.
5. Kovalev, I.F. (1960) Initial mechanisms of radiation damage of lens and their role in development of secondary pathological processes and in genesis of radiation cataracts, in *Effect of Ionizing Eradiation on Animals*, Kiev: Zdoroviya, pp. 33-39.
6. Shigematsu, I., Chikako, I., Kamada, N. (1995) *Effects of A-bomb radiation on the human body*, Harwood academic publishers, Bunkodo Co., Ltd., Tokyo, 419 p.
7. Guskova, A.K., Baranov, A.E., Barabanova, A.V. (1989) Diagnosis, clinical picture and therapy of acute radiation disease in persons exposed to radiation during the accident at the Chernobyl nuclear power station. I. Conditions of irradiation, dose levels, bone marrow syndrome and its therapy, *Therapeutic archive*, **61**, 95-103
8. Handbook of ophthalmology (1978) Medicine, Moscow, 376 p.

OPHTHALMO-PATHOLOGY IN VICTIMS OF THE CHERNOBYL CATASTROPHE - RESULTS OF A CLINICAL EPIDEMIOLOGICAL STUDY

V. BUZUNOV, P. FEDIRKO
Research Center for Radiation Medicine, Kiev, Ukraine

1. Introduction

Longitudinal epidemiological monitoring may help objectively assess population health damage arising from the Chernobyl nuclear power plant (NPP) accident. For this reason, a system of long-term clinical and epidemiological monitoring of victim health has been established [1]. It is hoped that analysis of data arising from this project will lead to a more comprehensive evaluation of the medical consequences of the Chernobyl accident, a better understanding of radiation-induced health effects in general and a broader knowledge of the role of radiation and non-radiation environmental factors in long-term human health.

2. Patients and Methods

Representative groups of exposed individuals were created utilizing generally accepted epidemiological and statistical considerations. The total population included 40,000 individuals, 12,500 of which were workers at the Chernobyl NPP. An additional 10,000 were evacuees (among them 6,500 adults and 3,500 children), 10,000 were inhabitants of radiation contaminated territories, 3,000 were children born from individuals in these three groups and 4,500 were control individuals. Selection of individuals for inclusion into the registry was conducted by a group of epidemiologists taking into account age, sex, occupational factors. Dosimetric information was collected and processed by qualified specialists. Additional information relating to residence and non-radiation risk factors was collected and processed by another specialist group.

Standardized protocols for medical examination of adults and children were utilized. All patients, regardless of health, were similarly examined.

The Clinical and Epidemiological Registry (CER) was established for collection, long-time storage and processing of results of standardized medical studies. A computerized data base was developed for record storage and dissemination.

An important component of the CER program is an ophthalmological examination. Initial eye studies focused on the development of lens opacities. Criteria

A. K. Junk et al. (eds.),
Ocular Radiation Risk Assessment in Populations Exposed to Environmental Radiation Contamination, 57–67.

utilized for lens examination included the potential for maximum early diagnoses of lens changes, maximum objectivity, rapidity and minimum cost. The following methods of lens examination were considered: examination in ambient light; slit lamp biomicroscopy; slit lamp photo documentation, slit lamp biomicroscopy with measure of the intensity by the Tyndall effect; slit lamp biomicroscopy with comparison to standardized description of lens changes; Scheimpflug imaging; retroillumination photo documentation and laser light imaging.

While examination by ambient light is rapid and cheap, this method has very low diagnostic capability and is quite subjective. Slit lamp biomicroscopy is rapid, relatively low cost and has the advantage of a higher diagnostic capacity but analysis is also subjective. The addition of photo documentation permits more objectivity but requires a longer examination time and has a relatively high cost for equipment and supplies. In addition, it is difficult to obtain consistent images of standard quality. Slit lamp biomicroscopy with tyndallometry is more objective than biomicroscopy alone and has a high relative diagnostic capability but requires instrument calibration. Furthermore, it is difficult to compare results because the measurement zone is not localized. Slit lamp biomicroscopy with comparison to standardized descriptions of lens changes is relatively rapid, cheap and has high diagnostic capability. The method is sufficiently objective. Difficulties due to the complexities of personnel training and the possibility of errors during data entry are disadvantages. Scheimpflug imaging is objective and has high diagnostic capacity but, at the time of this study, the technology did not permit detection of lens changes out of the plane examined. In addition, considerable expense and examination time is required. Retroillumination photo documentation is rapid and objective but does not permit precise depth localization of opacities and requires relatively expensive equipment. While potentially useful, laser imaging is still in its infancy.

Slit lamp biomicroscopy with comparison to standardized description of lens changes was ultimately utilized because it provides the potential for maximum early detection of radiation-induced lens changes, is sufficiently rapid and offers acceptable objectivity and cost. Although Scheimpflug imaging is attractive, its implementation would extend the examination time to such a degree that sufficiently large numbers of individuals might not be examined. Furthermore, at the time this study was initiated, Scheimpflug methodology did not permit analysis of certain lens opacities out of the image plane.

The following parameters were utilized in standardized lens examinations: morphological description of lens changes, the degree of change, localization by lens layer, precise three-dimensional localization and geometric area of change.

Ophthalmoscopy with comparison to a standard description of the retina were considered as retinal and optic nerve imaging methodologies. As in evaluation of lens images, basic criteria included the potential for early diagnoses of retinal and optic nerve changes, maximum objectivity, rapidity and minimum cost. Ultimately, ophthalmoscopy with comparison to a standardized description of retinal changes was adopted because it permitted quick, low cost exams with sufficient sensitivity and objectiveness.

Slit lamp biomicroscopy was utilized in conjunction with standardized descriptions of changes to assess pathologies of the conjunctiva, cornea, anterior chamber and iris.

Refractive exams were also conducted with standard methods. A number of additional methods were used in a sampling mode. All the patients were interviewed to obtain information about level of radiation exposure, other occupational factors, peculiarities of nutrition. All examiners were required to receive a preliminary specialized individual course of instruction and training followed by additional periodic training.

Patient exams were standardized and included detection of visual acuity, subjective refraction, tonometry and standard list of ophthalmologic methods of examination. Biomicroscopy and ophthalmoscopy were conducted under maximum dilation. Patients and examiners were randomly assigned. Each patient received an independent evaluation by two examiners followed by comparison of results. Additional examinations were conducted by P. Fedirko. All examinations and processing of results were blind.

Between 1992 and 1997 8,682 individuals were examined, 2,951 were examined more than once. 6,087 workers within the Chernobyl zone, who were exposed to the highest ionizing irradiation exposure among examined individuals, were evaluated. Ophthalmological examinations were conducted on 1,071 workers at the Chernobyl NPP in 1992-1993, 1,115 in 1994, 1,344 in 1995, 1,916 in 1996 and 641 in 1997. Of these, 1,887 individuals had dosimetry. Irradiation dose below 0.05 Gy was documented at 93 individuals, 0.05-0.10 Gy in 236 individuals, 0.10-0.25 Gy in 500 individuals and >0.25 Gy in 1,058 individuals. Irradiation doses are different for individuals working around the Chernobyl NPP at different time periods. Individuals who worked there in 1986 were exposed to the highest irradiation doses. 95% of individuals working there in 1988 and later had documented irradiation doses at or below 0.05 Gy. Statistical analysis was provided with calculation of the Relative Risk with all necessary coefficients, correlation analysis was included, variation statistical methods used.

3. Results and Discussion

In 1992-1993, analysis of 1,071 individuals revealed 1,429 pathological eye conditions (average of 1.33 per subject). In 1994, 3,183 pathologies were reported in 1,115 persons (average of 2.85 per subject). During 1995, 3,462 documented eye pathologies were found in 1,344 patients (average of 2.58 per subject) while in 1996, 5,395 were identified in 1,616 patients (average of 4.01 per subject). In 1997, 1841 diagnoses were made in 641 individuals for an average of 2.87 per subject. An overview of eye pathologies documented in this group is given in Table 1.

Retinal pathologies were most common (34.15% of cases in 1992-1993, 34.59% in 1994, 32.39% in 1995 and 34.9% in 1996). Refractive abnormalities were second most common (32.6% in 1992-1993, 26.83% in 1994, 30.16% in 1995 and

28.99% in 1996) Cataract was the third most common ocular abnormality accounting for 22.8% in 1992-1993, 12.63% in 1994, 20.1% in 1995 and 14.16% in 1996.

Among diseases of the retina, angiopathies were most frequent (22.8% in 1992-1993, 26.61% in 1994, 22.04% in 1995 and 25.67% in 1996) followed by macular dystrophies (10.22% in 1992-1993, 7.13% in 1994, 9.71% in 1995 and 8.56% in 1996). Presenile and senile cataracts were more common that classical radiation induced cataracts, accounting for 19.73% of all diagnoses in 1992-1993, 12.63% in 1994, 18.89% in 1995 and 13.36% in 1996. These opacities were noted to develop at a relatively young age.

Among abnormalities of refraction, hyperopia was most common (13.16% of diagnoses in 1992-1993, 9.27% in 1994, 10.05% in 1995 and 9.77% in 1996). Myopia and astigmatism were diagnosed less frequently. 2.24% of abnormalities noted in 1992-1993 and 5.19% in 1996 were vitreal pathologies.

TABLE 1. Ophthalmological disorders in Chernobyl NPP clean-up workers between 1992-1997

Disease, ICD code	Examination period				
	1992-1993 abs (%)	1994 abs(%)	1995 abs (%)	1996 abs(%)	1997 abs(%)
malignant eye tumors (190)	0(0%)	0(0%)	0(0%)	1(0.06%)	0(0%)
Benign tumors of eyelid (216.1)	2 (0.19 %)	23(2.06%)	17(1.26%)	37(2.29%)	10(1.56%)
Benign eye tumors (224)	0(0%)	0(0%)	1(0.07%)	5(0.31%)	4(0.62%)
Retinal angiopathy & angiosclerosis (362.1)	327 (30.53%)	847 (75.96%)	763 (56.77%)	1385 (85.71%)	471 (73.48%)
Macular degeneration (362.5)	146(13.63%)	227(20.36%)	336(25%)	462(28.59%)	153(23.87%)
Infant, juvenile and presenile cataract (366.0)	77(7.19%)	205(18.39%)	424(31.55%)	403(24.94%)	137(21.37%)
Senile cataract (366.1)	205(19.14%)	163(14.62%)	230(17.11%)	318(19.68%)	119(18.56%)
Radiation cataract (366.8)	1(0.09%)	19(1.7%)	34(2.53%)	24(1.49%)	6(0.94%)
Hyperopia (367.0)	188(17.55%)	295(26.46%)	348(25.89%)	527(32.61%)	200(31.2%)
Myopia (367.1)	157(14.66%)	161(14.44%)	187(13.91%)	268(16.58%)	101(15.76%)
Astigmatism(367.2)	53(4.95%)	79(7.09)	150(11.16%)	194(12%)	67(10.45%)
Presbyopia (367.4)	69(6.44%)	317(28.43%)	357(26.56%)	571(35.33%)	195(30.42%)
Chronic conjunctivitis (372.1)	20(1.87%)	344(30.85%)	193(14.36%)	402(24.88%)	127(19.81%)
Blepharitis (373.0)	18(1.68%)	122(10.94%)	77(5.73%)	142(8.79%)	22(3.43%)
Optic nerve atrophy (377.1)	5(0.47%)	4(0.36%)	7(0.52%)	7(0.43%)	6(0.94%)
Vitreous diseases (379.2)	32(2.99%)	175(15.69%)	153(11.38%)	280(17.33%)	97(15.13%)

Analyses of these ocular pathologies suggests that the most common abnormalities are those usually associated with advancing age, namely retinal vessel abnormalities, macular degenerations and cataracts.

The extent of ophthalmic pathology increased with time following exposure. For example, angiopathies were diagnosed in 30.53% of cases in 1992-1993 and 85.71% of cases in 1996 ($X^2=850.49$, $p<0.001$). Similarly, the incidence of macular degeneration increased during comparison of each subsequent year with the previous one (1992-1993 vs. 1994: $X^2=83.16$, $p<0.001$; 1994 vs. 1995: $X^2=17.94$, $p<0.001$; 1995 vs. 1996: $X^2=4.98$, $p<0.05$). Overall incidence increased from 13.63% in 1992-1993 to 28.59% in 1996. Cataract incidence increased as well (26.33% in 1992-1993 vs. 45.62% in 1996: $X^2=92.85$, $p<0.001$). The frequency of vitreal pathologies increased from 2.99% in 1992-1993 to 17.33% in 1996 ($X^2=130.45$, $p<0.001$). An increase in chronic conjunctivitis was observed in 1994 ($X^2=259.32$, $p<0.001$).

Reported ophthalmic pathologies can be divided into two groups. The first includes specific radiation injuries of the eye, especially radiation cataracts and "syndrome kashtanu"(chestnut) and "syndrome dyfrakcijnoj gratky" (diffraction maize) [2,3].

Radiation cataracts were diagnosed in 64 clean-up workers, 59 of which worked at the Chernobyl NPP or in the alienation zone in 1986, mostly during the first days after the accident. Five individuals worked at the plant in 1987 and was examined of the author before the incident of cataract was registered during of the Follow-up study. Confirmed irradiation doses in these individuals ranged from 0.02 to 2.00 Gy. The highest number of radiation cataract cases was found in 1994 and 1995 (absolute risk 0.025 per 1000 and 0.015 per 1000 respectively). New cases continued to be identified in 1996 and 1997 suggesting that the latency period for radiation cataract development can exceed 10 years.

"Dyfrakcijnoj gratky syndrome" was revealed only in irradiated individuals immediately near the active zone of the destroyed reactor. Although of some scientific and clinical interest, there are only small numbers of affected individuals. "Kashtanu syndrome" was identified only in those individuals in the city of Prypjat during the first days after the Chernobyl accident. Only late forms of the syndrome are currently observed. As this pathology is relatively rare, it was included with other macular degenerations.

As previously mentioned, age-related eye pathologies were most common and generally found at an earlier age than commonly detected in the general population. The influence of radiation exposure on their development must be considered [4]. To further analyze this finding, subject age at the time of examination was examined as were the relationship(s) between radiation dose and the year(s) during which these individuals spent time at Chernobyl.

In 1996, cataract was more frequently diagnosed ($X^2=5.64$, $p<0.05$) in individuals with documented irradiation doses of 0.25 Gy and higher in comparison with those receiving documented irradiation doses up to 0.10 Gy (Table 2). Absolute risks in 1995 and 1996 were higher in the group with irradiation dose of at least 0.25 Gy in comparison with the group where irradiation doses were below 0.05 Gy.

TABLE 2. Absolute risk for cataract development in Chernobyl clean-up workers with different documented irradiation doses, per 1,000/year.

Examination period	Irradiation dose, Gy			
	up to 0.05 Gy	0.05 to 0.1 Gy	0.1 to 0.25 Gy	0.25 Gy and more
1992-1993	380	290	260	280
1994	440	340	340	390
1995	470	380	310	580
1996	400	340	480	500

Relative risks are depicted in Table 3. Preliminary data indicates this trend continues in 1997 for individuals with irradiation dose of 0.25 Gy and more in comparison with individuals with irradiation dose of 0.05 Gy (Relative risk = 1.58).

TABLE 3. Relative cataract risk for individuals with irradiation doses of 0.25 Gy and more in comparison with individuals with irradiation doses of 0.05 Gy or less.

Period of examination	1992-1993	1994	1995	1996
Relative risk	0.74	0.89	1.23	1.25

As cataract frequency increases with advancing age, risk was analyzed in individuals below 40 years old at the time of exam. (Table 4).

TABLE 4. Absolute risk of cataract development in Chernobyl NPP clean-up workers, age below 40 at examination, with different documented irradiation doses, per 1,000/year.

Examination period	Irradiation dose, Gy		
	up to 0.05 Gy	0.1 to 0.25 Gy	0.25 Gy or greater
1992-1993	0	0	80
1994	0	170	170
1995	0	240	260
1996	0	210	150
1997	0	330	340

Attributed risks for this age group with documented irradiation dose of at least 0.25 Gy in comparison with individuals who received irradiation dose up to 0.05 Gy was 0.08 in 1992-1993, 0.17 in 1994, 0.26 in 1995, 0.15 in 1996 and 0.34 in 1997.

As expected, the risk of developing cataract is higher in individuals with higher irradiation doses. Because average irradiation doses in individuals who worked in the irradiation zone in 1988 were lower than that of those who worked there in 1986 and 1987, differences in cataract frequency and relative risk among these groups were analyzed.

Individuals who worked in the Chernobyl NPP or the alienation zone in 1986, 1987 or 1988 were analyzed for cataract frequency in 1992-1993. Workers from 1987 had a higher frequency than those who worked there in 1988 ($X^2=8.49$, $p<0.01$). Similarly, individuals examined in 1995 who worked at the Chernobyl NPP in 1986 had a higher frequency of cataract in comparison with those who worked there in 1988 ($X^2=5.72$, $p<0.05$). Combination of data from individuals worked at the Chernobyl NPP in 1986 or 1987 compared to those who worked in 1988 also revealed a higher frequency of cataract in the former group (X^2=5.56, $p<0.05$). After examination in 1996, the frequency of cataract continued to be higher (X^2=4.93, $p<0.05$) in those workers who took part at the clean-up work during 1986 or 1987 years. When workers in 1987 and 1988 were compared, the trend continued (X^2=5.3, $p<0.05$). Even in 1997, cataract frequency was higher (X^2=8.19, $p<0.01$) in the group of individuals who worked in the alienation zone around the Chernobyl NPP in 1986 as compared to 1987.

Absolute risks of cataract in those who worked at the Chernobyl NPP at different times is shown in Table 5. Relative and attributed risks for those who worked at the Chernobyl NPP in 1986 in comparison with 1988, age group below 50 at the time of examination, is shown in Table 6.

TABLE 5. Absolute risks for cataract development in Chernobyl clean-up workers at different times, per 1,000/year.

Examination period:	Year of work		
	1986	1987	1988
1992-1993	250	440	80
1994	340	380	160
1995	480	280	170
1996	440	470	250
1997	460	260	500

TABLE 6. Relative and attributive cataract risk for Chernobyl clean-up workers in 1986 in comparison with 1988, age group below 50 at time of examination

Period of examination	1992-1993	1994	1995	1996
Relative risk	1.55	1.27	2.64	1.57
Attributive risk	0.05	0.04	0.19	0.10

The average level of morbidity for individuals who worked at the NPP in 1986 (age below 50 at the time of examination) is 245.42 per million; average annual growth = 45.41 per million, average rate of excess = 18.5. The average level of morbidity for individuals who worked at the NPP in 1988 (age below 50 at the time of examination) is 171.74 per million; average annual growth = 50.89 per million, average rate of excess = 29.63.

Calculation of trends, taking into account time from the moment of irradiation, e.g., calculated trend for clean-up workers in 1986 or 1988 for 7, 8 and 9 years after working in the zone of the Chernobyl NPP, indicates that average level of morbidity is 358.33 per million for all participants in 1986; average annual excess = 112.75 per million, average rate of excess = 31.45. Similar values for workers in 1988 were 305.57, 166.65 and 54.54 respectively.

In 1996, macular degeneration was more frequent (X^2=14.16, $p<0.001$) in individuals with documented irradiation doses of 0.25 Gy and more in comparison with those who received documented irradiation doses up to 0.1 Gy (Table 7). As seen in Table 7, absolute risks in 1992-1993, 1995 and 1996 were also higher in the group with irradiation dose of 0.25 Gy and more in comparison with the group where irradiation doses were below 0.05 Gy (relative risks depicted in Table 8).

TABLE 7. Absolute risk for development of macular degeneration for Chernobyl clean-up workers with different documented irradiation, per 1,000/year

Examination period	Irradiation dose, Gy			
	up to 0.05 Gy	0.05 to 0.1 Gy	0.1 to 0.25 Gy	0.25 Gy or more
1992-1993	170	130	140	200
1994	250	130	230	220
1995	320	320	290	360
1996	100	240	330	350

TABLE 8. Relative risks of macular degeneration for individuals with irradiation dose of 0.25 Gy and more in comparison with individuals with irradiation dose of 0.05 Gy.

Period of examination	1992-1993	1994	1995	1996
Relative risk	1.18	0.88	1.13	3.5

To exclude the influence of age, the risk of macular degeneration in individuals below 40 years old at the time of examination is shown in Table 9.

TABLE 9. Absolute risk of macular degeneration development for Chernobyl clean-up workers, age below 40 at the time of examination, with different documented irradiation doses, per 1,000/year.

Examination period	Irradiation dose, Gy		
	up to 0.05 Gy	0.1 to 0.25 Gy	0.25 Gy or more
1992-1993	0	90	130
1994	0	60	110
1995	0	120	230
1996	0	210	230
1997	0	170	200

Attributive risks for those below 40 years old with documented irradiation dose of 0.25 Gy or more in comparison with the age group below 40 with irradiation dose up to 0.05 Gy were 0.13 in 1992-1993, 0.11 in 1994, 0.23 in 1995 and 1996 and 0.2 in 1997. Thus, risk of development of macular degeneration at a younger age is higher in individuals with higher irradiation doses. Absolute risks of development of macular degeneration in individuals who worked at the Chernobyl NPP at different times is shown in Table 10.

TABLE 10. Absolute risks for macular degeneration in Chernobyl clean-up workers, per 1,000/year.

Examination period	Year of work		
	1986	1987	1988
1992-1993	140	100	80
1994	220	180	110
1995	320	330	110
1996	310	330	200
1997	260	300	250

Relative and attributive risks for individuals having worked at the Chernobyl NPP in 1986 in comparison with 1988, age group below 50 at the time of examination, is shown in Table 11.

TABLE 11. Relative and attributive risks of macular degeneration for Chernobyl clean-up workers in 1986 in comparison with 1988, age group below 50 at the moment of examination.

	Period of examination			
	1992-1993	1994	1995	1996
Relative risk	1.13	1.51	2.25	1.26
Attributive risk	0.01	0.05	0.15	0.05

Average morbidity level of macular degenerations among workers in 1986 was 22.92%, annual growth = 8.98% as compared to 9.99% and 1.39% respectively, for workers in 1988. Study results for 1996-1997 show that morbidity level for macular degeneration is 252.52 per million; average annual growth = 32.91 per million, average rate of excess = 13.03 for 1986 workers. Average morbidity values for 1988 workers is 149.02 per million, average annual excess = 42.82 per million, average rate of excess = 28.56 per million. However, for individuals, age below 50, average morbidity level was 196.12 and 100.1 per million; average annual growth was 33.41 and 7.73 respectively for those who worked there in 1986 and 1988. Thus, morbidity growth was only observed in the group of individuals who worked at the Chernobyl NPP in 1986.

Calculation of trends for the same cohorts taking into account time from the moment of irradiation, calculated trend for clean-up workers in 1986 and 1988 for 7, 8 and 9 years after their work in the zone of the Chernobyl NPP, indicated that the average level of morbidity was 229.17 per million for 1986 workers, average annual growth = 90.1 per million, average rate of excess = 39.32. For 1988 workers, these indices were 187.03, 69.45 and 37.13, respectively. Thus, the average level of macular degeneration morbidity and the rate of excess morbidity is higher in the group exposed to higher irradiation doses.

The frequency of retinal angiopathy was high in all groups examined. Absolute risks for groups with different external irradiation doses is shown in Table 12. Retinal vessels pathology was already present at initial exam in all groups. At subsequent exams, frequency sharply increased in all groups. Risk of retinal angiopathy for individuals aged 50 or less at the time of examination is shown in Table 13.

TABLE 12. Absolute risk for development of retinal angiopathy for Chernobyl clean-up workers with different documented irradiation doses, per 1,000/year

Examination period	Irradiation dose, Gy			
	up to 0.05 Gy	0.05 to 0.1 Gy	0.1 to 0.25 Gy	0.25 Gy or higher
1992-1993	130	270	320	320
1994	920	750	890	760
1995	630	700	690	770
1996	830	640	850	820

Thus, the risk of retinal angiopathy in younger age groups is great regardless of irradiation dose. Absolute risk for development of retinal angiopathy in individuals having worked at the Chernobyl NPP at different times is shown in Table 14.
As can be seen from this data, angiopathy risk is elevated regardless of time of work. Excess morbidity was observed only in the initial stage of the study. Because of the high frequency of angiopathy, subsequent increases in the frequency of angiopathy related morbidity is not expected.

TABLE 13. Absolute risk for development of retinal angiopathy for Chernobyl clean-up workers, age below 50 at the time of examination, with different documented irradiation doses, per 1,000/year.

Examination period	Irradiation dose, Gy		
	up to 0.05 Gy	0.1 to 0.25 Gy	0.25 Gy or higher
1992-1993	170	170	260
1994	1000	870	700
1995	300	580	660
1996	740	760	700
1997	670	750	800

TABLE 14. Absolute risk for development of retinal angiopathy for Chernobyl clean-up workers at different times, per 1,000/year.

Examination period	Year of work		
	1986	1987	1988
1992-1993	350	310	80
1994	790	720	920
1995	700	630	610
1996	800	800	700
1997	850	840	1000

4. Conclusion

A great variety of ocular pathological changes were found in a representative group of individuals irradiated as a result of the Chernobyl NPP accident. An increased ocular morbidity during the period of this study was noted. Diseases of the retina, refractive abnormalities and cataracts were most common.

Delayed development of eye pathologies continues in the study group. It was shown that the latency period for irradiation cataract can exceed 10 years. Following considerable periods after irradiation, an increase in eye diseases was noted, the composition of which is more typical of an aged human population. Even at initial study periods, pronounced retinal angiopathy morbidity was noticed across all age groups. Soon afterwards, cataract morbidity increased. This morbidity continues, although the rate of morbidity excess has diminished somewhat. At about the same time, frequency of macular degeneration began to increase, although compared to cataracts, the rate of morbidity excess has not decreased. It was found that the frequency of cataracts and macular degeneration is higher in groups of individuals exposed to higher irradiation doses. Risk of cataract and macular degeneration development in individuals below 40 years old is higher for those who were exposed to irradiation in doses of 0.25 Gy or greater. The rate of excess of macular degeneration morbidity 7-9 years after participation in the Chernobyl NPP clean-up was higher in those who worked there in 1986 and were thus exposed to higher irradiation doses.

The results obtained allow to suppose that radioactive action can lead to earlier development of involutional and dystrophic processes in eyes.

5. References

1. Buzunov, V. A., Fedirko, P. (1995) Eye morbidity of persons included into the National register of sufferers due to Chernobyl accident, *Ophthalmol. J* **5-6**, 286 -290.
2. Fedirko, P. (1995) Clinical peculiarities of eye diseases in victims of irradiation as a result of the Chernobyl atomic accident, *Data of Scientific Research,* **3**, . *60.*
3. Fedirko, P. (1997) Clinical peculiarities of retinal diseases in people suffered from the Chernobyl catastrophe, *XI Congress of the European Society of Ophthalmology, Hungary, Budapest, June 1 - 5, 1997 Final Program and abstract book*, Budapest, 1163.
4. Poljchov, A.M., Vojtenko, V. M., Kobzar, I. V., Nyaga, A.I. (1994) Valuation of the route of aging of liquidators, *Chernobyl and Health of Population*, **3**, 54 - 55.

CONDITION OF EYE AND PARAMETERS OF FREE RADICAL PROCESSES IN ORGANISM IN THE LIQUIDATORS AFTER THE CHERNOBYL ACCIDENT

S. V. SOSNOVSKY, V. F. DANILICHEV, N. N. ZYBINA,
L. I. NESTERUK*, A. E. BELOZEROV*
Military Medical Academy, Lebedeva, 6, Saint-Petersburg, Russia
**Helmholtz Institute of Eye Diseases*
Sadovaya-Chernogriazskaya, 14/9, Moscow, Russia

1. Abstract

Eightyfour liquidators from the age of 28 to 58 were examined. The control group consisted of 22 men in the age of 28 to 52 years. A certain increase of infringement of lens transparency without typical attributes of radiation cataract is revealed in the experimental group. Electrophysiological investigation (EPI) shows a certain reduction of amplitude of a-wave of macular electroretinogram (ERG) on green stimulus. Amplitude of flicker-ERG 30 Hz, amplitude of main component and lengthening of interpeak time interval of flicker-ERG 10 Hz are revealed. These changes indicate a tendency of decreasing retinal function in paramacular and in a smaller degree in peripheral zones in liquidators. Contrast sensitivity is definitely reduced in liquidators for achromatic, red, green and blue stimuli on all spatial frequencies. Luminous and color sensitivity to stimuli of different color in liquidators is definitely reduced in all central visual fields, but is highest in the paracentral zone. We investigated 14 parameters for activity of free radical processes and antioxidant system in peripheral blood in both groups. Definite increase of production of the reactive oxygen species and disbalance of a glutathione link of antioxidant protection are revealed. Authentic correlation dependences are revealed: strong direct correlation - between a level of superoxide dismutase and amplitude of the first component of flicker-ERG 10 Hz, moderate direct correlation - between a level of glutathione reductase and amplitude of a main component of flicker-ERG 10 Hz, between a level of reduced glutathione and interpeak time interval of flicker-ERG 10 Hz. In consideration of large spontaneous activity of free radical processes in the normal retina the received results indicate a deterioration.

A. K. Junk et al. (eds.),
Ocular Radiation Risk Assessment in Populations Exposed to Environmental Radiation Contamination, 69–80.

2. Introduction

Among medical problems, stipulated by Chernobyl, the medical rehabilitation of people, who had taken part during the clean-up work after the accident at the Chernobyl nuclear power-plant (so called "liquidators") occupies a very important place today. Disease rates among the liquidators considerably exceed that among the population of Russia [1].

Within the last years the leading specialists in radiobiology, clinical radiology and radiation hygiene formed the new hypothesis on pathogenesis of post-Chernobyl pathology. The liquidators were subjected to the influence of a unique complex of extreme stress-producing factors such as low doses of radiation, chemical agents of deactivation, psychological stress [2, 3, 12]. Combination of these factors leads to infringement of some important regulatory systems in the organism and formed the negative background for the development of somatic pathologies. One of the universal mechanisms to form such pathologies are free radical processes, initiated in the body by reactive oxygen species [6]. Overproduction of free radicals or lack of antioxidants may lead to oxidative cell damage. In case of high radiation exposure, the role of free radicals causing pathology is considered to be a confirmed fact. Even 10 years after the accident, despite of low doses of radiation, the liquidators demonstrate free radical production and high levels of oxidative destruction of macromolecules [13].

Thus, various diseases in liquidators are influenced by complex and unfavorable factors including radiation and chemical components. As a result they develop pre-clinical pre-morbid functional disorders as shown in non-ophthalmologic studies [2, 7, 8]. Concerning the eye, it has to be mentioned that no research in this respect was found in the publications available to us. The analysis of literature shows that the majority of authors used simple clinical methods such as direct and/or indirect ophthalmoscopy, skiascopy, biomicroscopy [9, 10]. For functional examination, visual acuity testing by Sivtsev-tables and perimetry were used, classical, but rather unsophisticated diagnostic methods.

In addition to the methods mentioned above, we were able to apply further objective and state of the art psychophysiological methods known for their high sensitivity.

The risk of free radical damage in the eye is extreme [11]. It is stipulated by 3 factors. First, the eye is continuously subjected to light, capable of provoking free radical processes [14]. Second, retinal membranes are especially receptive to free radicals as they contain high amounts of unsaturated lipids and thiol-esters [15]. Thirdly, retina is a tissue intensively supplied with oxygen and blood, which creates the particular prerequisites for activation and deactivation of free radical processes.

3. Material and methods

71 liquidators without any visual complaint were examined, their age varied from 28 to 53 years. A control group of 22 sound persons, their age ranging between 28 and 50 years, was established. As inclusion criteria for both groups, a visual acuity with correction not below 40/50 and ametropia not over 5 diopters was requested. Individual

effective gamma radiation dose by dose registration cards in the experimental group was within the limits of 5.6 mGy to 1.25 Gy.

In addition to the standard ophthalmologic examination, including

- visual acuity test (Syvtsev-tables [16]),
- perimetry (Goldmann perimeter, Carl Zeiss Jena, Germany),
- subjective and objective refraction,
- slit-lamp biomicroscopy (SL-3M, LOMO, Russia),
- direct binocular ophthalmoscopy (fundus-camera RCM-310, Carl Zeiss Jena, Germany),
- color sensitivity (Yustova-tables [17]).

The following EPI were performed (MBN-electroretinograf, MBN, Russia):

- Ganzfeld electroretinogram (ERG),
- macular ERG to red and green stimulus,
- flicker ERG to frequencies of 10 and 30 Hz.

The following parameters were considered for further evaluation of electrophysiological data: a- and b- wave amplitudes as well as implicit times of a- and b-waves for Ganzfeld and macular ERG as shown in figure 1; for the flicker ERG at 10 Hz a- and b-wave amplitudes as well as a-b and b-b interpeak time intervals (figure 3). In the 30 Hz flicker ERG b-wave amplitudes and b-b interpeak intervals were evaluated (figure 2).

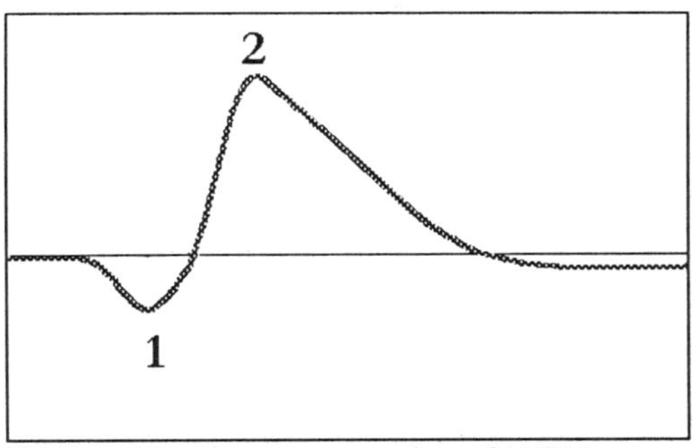

Figure 1. Components of Hanzfeld ERG:
1. a-wave; 2. b-wave

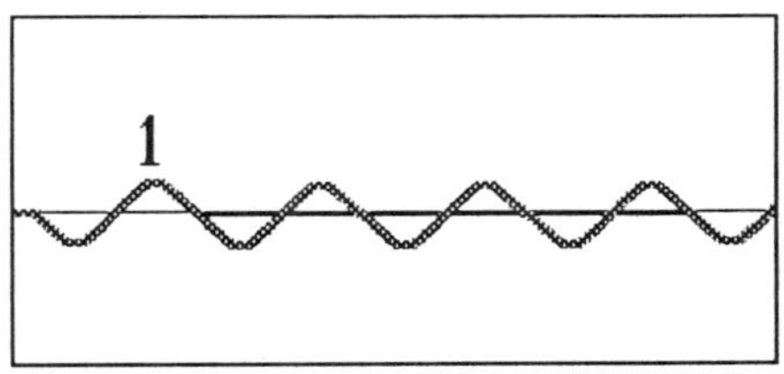

Figure 2. Components of flicker ERG to 30 Hz
1. b-wave

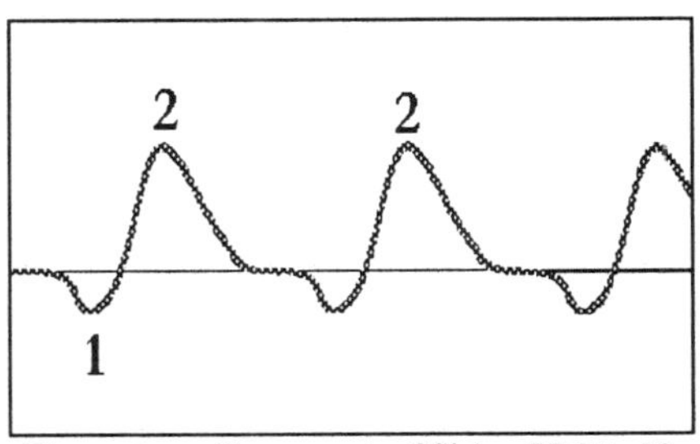

Figure 3. Components of flicker ERG to 10 Hz
1. a-wave; 2. b-wave

Central sensitivity testing was studied by application of IBM-based program "Ocular" (Nesteruk L. I. et al. [18]) This program allows to study the retinal sensitivity in the central area (20 degrees from the fixing point). The exams are conducted monocular. Subjects are placed 30 cm in front of the computer monitor. For detection of sensitivity thresholds, red, green and blue stimuli of 1mm diameter were presented in increasing brightness in a gray background on different points of the screen (figure 4). The gray screen background of 1 cd/m^2 ensures mesopic conditions to suppress answers of the rod system.

We estimated differential thresholds of physical brightness of stimulus in different areas of central eyeshot:
* area 2 degrees from the fixing point;
* summary threshold of area 0 to 5 degrees;
* summary threshold of area 5 to 20 degrees;
* area 20 degrees from the fixing point.

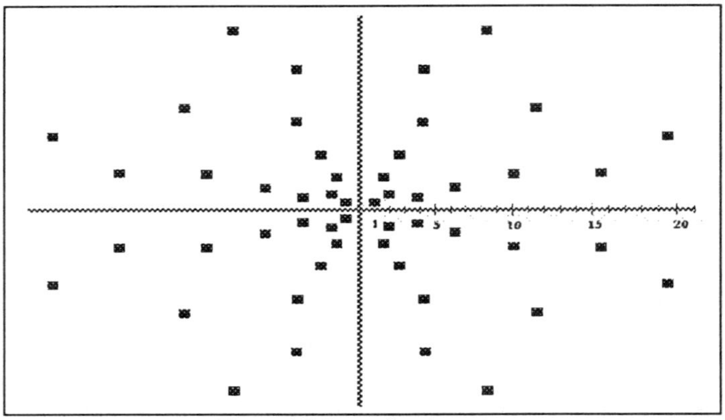

Figure 4. Scheme of testing points

While determining thresholds of luminous sensitivity a patient fixes a moment to find a stimulus. While determining thresholds of color sensitivity a patient fixes a moment to discern the stimulus color. The program fixes a threshold of brightness of stimulus (in cd/m^2) on a moment of his detection.

Achromatic and color contrast sensitivity for red, green and blue stimuli were studied by application of IBM-based program "Zebra"(Belozerov A. E. and Shamshinova A. M. [19]). Sinusoidal grids (with black intervals) with the frequencies of 0.5 to 22 cycles/degree were presented on the monitor screen. In total 12 spatial frequencies were examined. The program allows to close pattern by the screen rising from below. Patient fixes a moment, when he stops making out a structure of the grids. The program fixes a contrast threshold to each grid.

In connection with obvious significance of free radical processes in the development of diseases in the liquidators and particularities of molecular structure of retina we defined a number of parameters of oxidative stress among patients.

We defined the following parameters of free radical processes:
1. Level of superoxide (basal and stimulate) [20];
2. Level of hydrogen peroxide (basal and stimulate) [20];
3. Level of reduced and oxidized glutathione [21];
4. Level of glutathione reductase [22];
5. Level of superoxide dismutase [23].

4. Results

Neither in the experimental nor in the control group, changes of eyeshot, retinal pathologies, or decrease of color vision were detected by application of standard methods of ophthalmologic examination. Infringement of vitreous transparency in shape of initial or moderate destruction was revealed equally often in both groups. Infringement of lens transparency was revealed among 32 liquidators in 36 eyes (4 men had the changes in both lenses). We revealed the following lens transparency changes:

* individual dots in cortex - in 6 lenses (4.5%), including 2 persons with changes in both lenses;
* aggregate of dots in cortex - in 6 lenses (4.5%), including 1 person with changes in both lenses;
* combination of individual dots in cortex and individual dots under posterior capsule - in 5 lenses (3.76 %);
* individual spoke opacity in cortex - in 9 lenses (6.77 %);
* individual spot in cortex - in 5 lenses (3.76 %);
* individual dots under posterior capsule - in 5 lenses (3.76 %), including 1 person with changes in both lenses.

Frequency of changes in lens among liquidators was definitely higher, than in the control group ($p<0.001$). But infringement of lens transparency in liquidators could not influence visual functions. Factor analysis did not reveal dependence of lens opacities from individual effective gamma radiation dose.

Three parameters of EPI have statistically reliable differences between experimental and control groups (figure 5):

1. prolonged interpeak interval between a- and b-waves of flicker ERG 10 Hz, ($p<0.01$);
2. reduced b-wave amplitude of flicker ERG 10 Hz, ($p<0.05$);
3. reduced a-wave amplitude of macular ERG to green stimulus, ($p<0.01$).

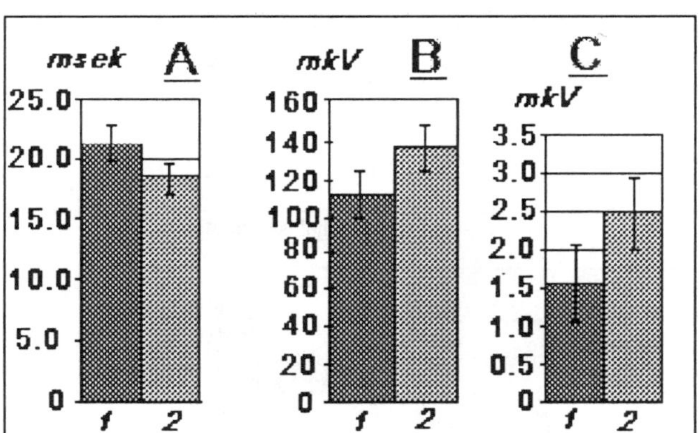

Figure 5. Difference of electrophysiological parameters: A - interpeak time a-b of flicker ERG 10 Hz; B - b-wave amplitude of flicker ERG 10 Hz; C - a-wave amplitude of macular ERG to green stimulus.
1 - Liquidators; 2 - Control

Figure 6 shows the character of luminous sensitivity change in central visual field, while presenting red stimulus. Thresholds in the group of liquidators are definitely higher in all areas ($p<0.001$), but in the paracentral zone in greater degree. Of similar character are luminous sensitivity changes, while presenting blue and green stimuli (Figures 7, 8). While presenting green stimulus the difference in zone 2 degrees was smaller ($p<0.01$), that in other testing zones ($p<0.001$); for blue stimulus probability was identical in all zones ($p<0.001$).

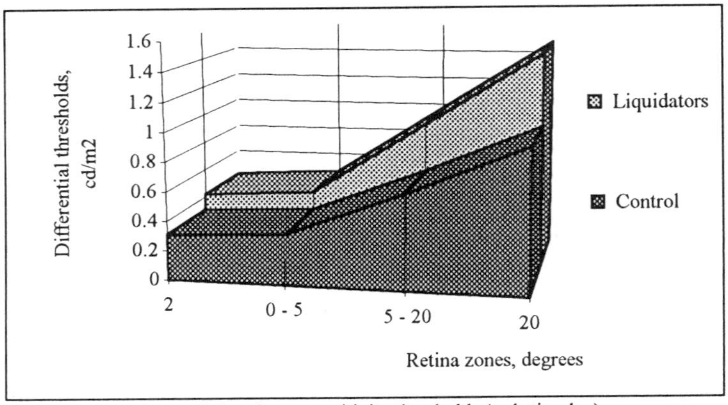

Figure 6. Luminous sensitivity thresholds (red stimulus)

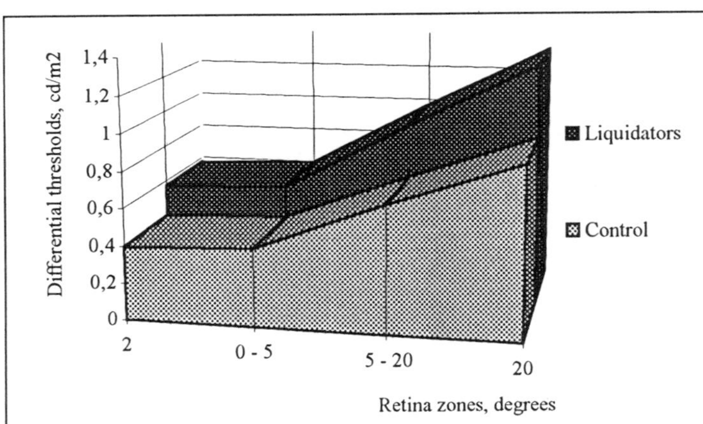

Figure 7. Luminous sensitivity thresholds (blue stimulus)

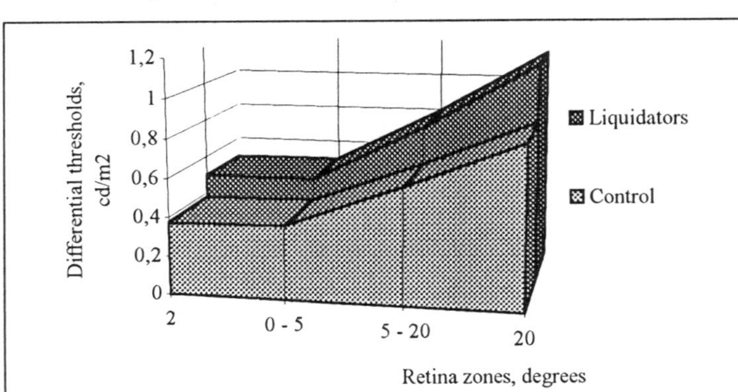

Figure 8. Luminous sensitivity thresholds (green stimulus)

Thresholds of color sensitivity are definitely higher among the liquidators to red and blue stimuli ($p<0.001$ in all zones) (Figures 9, 10).

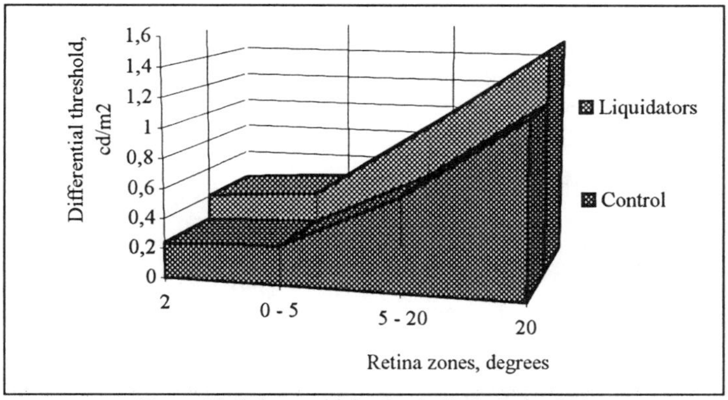

Figure 10. Color sensitivity thresholds (red stimulus)

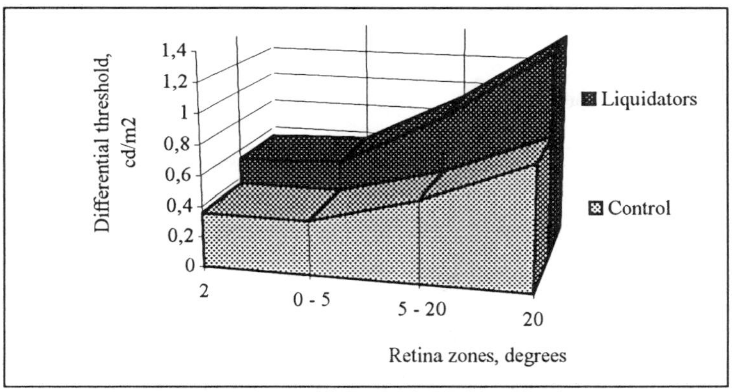

Figure 9. Color sensitivity thresholds (blue stimulus)

Difference between experimental and control groups while presenting a green stimulus is unauthentic (figure 11).

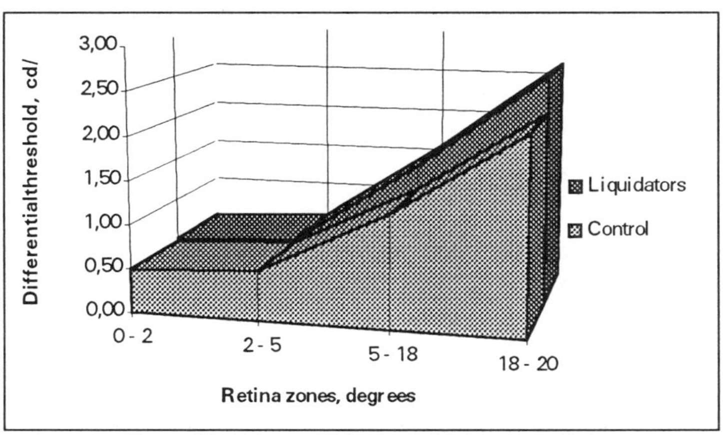

Figure 11.. Color sensitivity thresholds (green stimulus)

Contrast sensitivity among liquidators is definitely reduced on all spatial frequencies while presenting red and blue patterns (Figure 12, 13). Maximum reduction is observed in the field of medium and low spatial frequencies ($p<0.001$). In the field of high spatial frequencies (22 cycles/degree) reduction is smaller, but authentic ($p<0.05$ for red stimulus, $p<0.01$ for blue stimulus).

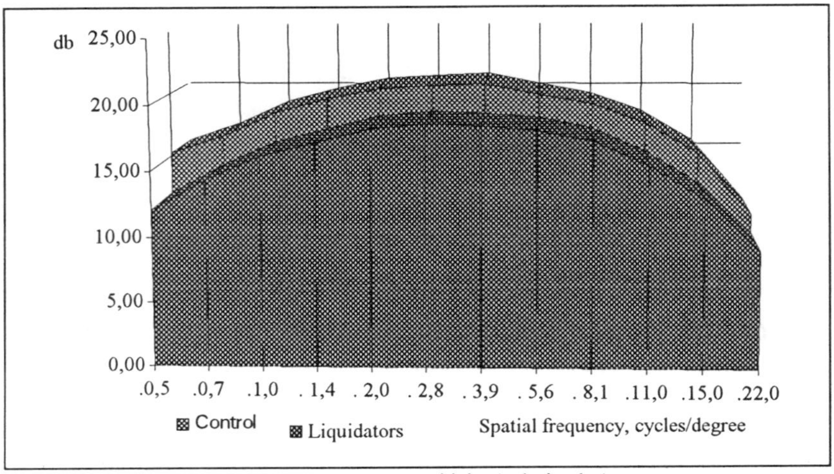

Figure 12. Contrast sensitivity (red stimulus)

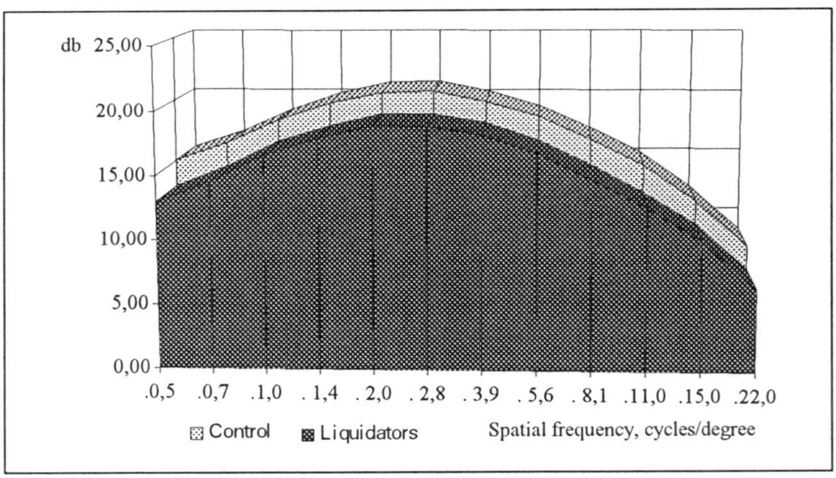

Figure 13. Contrast sensitivity (blue stimulus)

While presenting achromatic and green patterns the reduction of contrast sensitivity had the same character (Figures 14, 15), but in the field of high spatial frequencies (22 cycles/degree) a difference was unauthentic ($p>0.05$).

Correlation analysis did not reveal dependence of investigated parameters of eye from individual dose load. For excepting the influence of lens transparency infringement to subjective functional parameters of eye, we divide liquidators in two groups: with and without lens opacities. Statistical analysis has shown any reliable differences of functional parameters between two group of liquidators. As to electrophysiological investigations, it is known, that lens opacities cannot influence to results of EPI [24] (excepting pattern-ERG and pattern visual evoked potential).

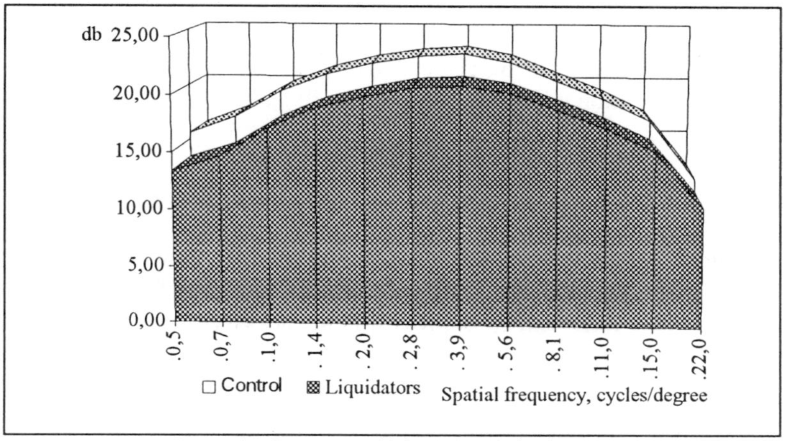

Figure 14. Contrast sensitivity (achromatic stimulus)

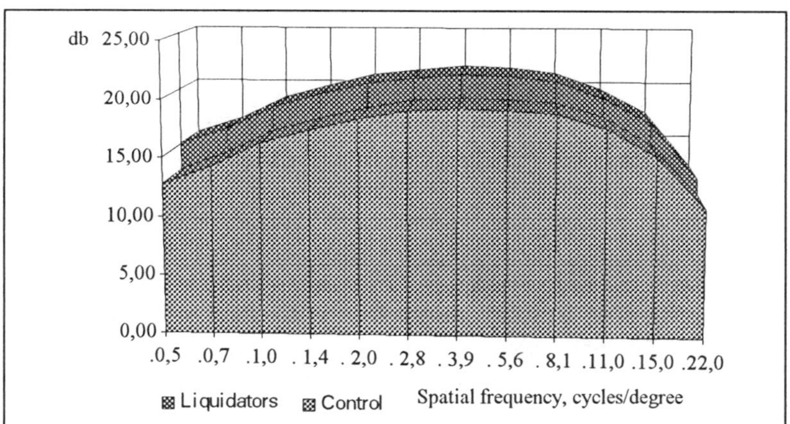

Figure 15. Contrast sensitivity (green stimulus)

Analysis of parameters of free radical processes shows, that the liquidators have a considerably increased production of reactive oxygen species (high level of basal superoxide ($p<0.001$), high level of basal hydrogen peroxide ($p<0.01$)), exhausted reserves of their generations (low level of stimulate superoxide ($p<0.001$), low level of stimulate hydrogen peroxide ($p<0.01$)) and disbalance of antioxidant system in the first place on the level of thiol-disulfide metabolism (high level of oxidized glutathione ($p<0.05$), low level of reduced glutathione ($p<0.001$) and glutathion-reductase ($p<0.05$)).

Correlation analysis of objective functional infringement of vision with changes of free radical processes has shown the following definite moderate correlation ties:
* direct ties - between the level of glutathione reductase and b-wave amplitude of flicker ERG 10 Hz (correlation coefficient 0.57, $p<0.01$);
* inverse ties - between the level of oxidized glutathione and b-wave amplitude of flicker ERG 10 Hz (correlation coefficient -0.58, $p<0.01$);
* direct ties - between the level of oxidized glutathione and interpeak interval a-b of flicker ERG 10 Hz (correlation coefficient 0.63, $p<0.01$).

5. Discussion

Analysis of results of electrophysiological studies allows to draw a conclusion of authentic reduction of electrobiological activity of retina among liquidators first of all in paramacular zone. To a lesser extent oppressed is the activity of retina on peripheral zone. The changes of electrogenesis are revealed on the level of photoreceptors in paramacular zone (reduction of a-wave amplitude of macular ERG to the green stimulus), on the level of bipolars in paramacular and peripheral zones of retina (reduction of b-wave amplitude of flicker ERG 10 Hz), as well as on the stage of interneuronal interactions between photoreceptors and bipolars (a prolonging of interpeak time of flicker ERG 10 Hz). Infringement of retina activity in macular zone by means of EPI is not revealed.
Methods of threshold sensitivity estimation by means of program "Ocular" reveal an oppression of retina functions both in macular, and in paramacular zones. But in paramacula, degree of oppression is considerably higher. The functions of red and blue cone systems are oppressed in greater degree, than of the green.
Contrast sensitivity is an integral parameter of visual analyzer. However, considering functional changes of retina, revealed by electrophysiological investigations and program "Ocular", one can suppose that reduction of contrast sensitivity also has the retina origin. Oppression of contrast sensitivity in the field of medium and low frequencies is typical for disfunction of retina in paramacula and peripheral zones accordingly. Contrast sensitivity to the red and blue patterns is oppressed in a greater degree, than to the green and achromatic patterns.
These data correlate with results of preceding methods.
Increase in contents of oxidized glutathione and shortage of glutathionereductase tell of exhaust in the glutathione metabolism mechanisms on the level of reducing of glutathione. Reduced glutathione is a donor of thiol (-SH) groups for reparations of protein structure, damaged by the free radicals influence. Rhodopsin in retina is one of the proteins, containing SH-groups. The shortage of reduced glutathione may cause deceleration or incomplete reduction of rhodopsin structure in case of its damage by free radicals. Changes in glutathione metabolism and correlation ties, found by us, can be among the possible reasons of infringement of the functions of eye, which we revealed in liquidators. Finding out other reasons requires further deep studies of this problem and is a perspective goal of our research.

6. Conclusion

Reduction of functional parameters of eye is revealed among the liquidators. It is stipulated by oppression of activity in paramacular and to a lesser degree in peripheral retina zones. Reduction of functions of retina among liquidators has no dose dependence. Morphological changes of eye, revealed by means of classical diagnostic methods do not allow to explain discovered functional changes. Reduction of some functional parameters of eye among liquidators correlate with parameters of free radical processes of organism. Disbalance of glutathione link of antioxidant system in blood, revealed among liquidators, can be one of the reasons of changes in the visual function. Combination of biochemical changes and reduction of visual functional parameters allows to speak about sub-clinical level of infringement of eye. It is possible to suppose that revealed shifts of functional parameters of eye among the liquidators appear as a result of influence of some unfavorable factors of Chernobyl accident, which have both radiation, and non-radiation nature.

7. References

1. Tsyb, A. F., Ilyin, L. A., Ivanov, V. K. (1995) Chernobyl radiation risks: estimation of mortality, morbidity and disablement according to National radiation epidemiological register data, in L. A. Ilyin (ed.), *Radio-ecological, medical and social-economical consequences of Chernobyl atomic power-station accident. Rehabilitation of territories and population*, Scientific-medical Center <Holicino> Publishers, Moscow, 37-52.
2. Nikiforov, A. M., Shantyr, I. I., Alexanin, C. C., Romanovich, I. K. (1996) Basic direction of dispensary system of servicemen exposed to radiation after radiation accidents, *Voenno-Medicinsky Zhurnal* **317**, 37-41.
3. Romanenko, A. E. (1992) Radiological consequences and medical and biological problems 4 years after Chernobyl atomic power-station accident, *Vestnik Academii Medicinskih Nayk* **2**, 7-14.
4. Rumiantseva, G. M. (1995) Chernobyl APS accident and psychological distress, in L. A. Ilyin (ed.), *Radio-ecological, medical and social-economical consequences of Chernobyl atomic power-station accident. Rehabilitation of territories and population*, Scientific-medical Center <Holicino> Publishers, Moscow, 59.
5. Zykova, I. A. (1997) Pathogenic particularities of somatic diseases development under combination of radiation influence and stress, in I. M. Markelov (ed.), *Scientific and practice conference <Medical and social aspects of problems of nuclear subjected veterans and ways of solving them>*, Saint-Petersburg, 56-57.
6. Martinez-Cayuela, M. (1995) Oxygen free radicals and humandisease, *Biochimie* **3**, 77, 147-161.
7. Nikiforov, A. M., Chichmarev, J. N., Katachkova, G. D., Fedortseva, R. F. (1995) On factors of somatic pathology forming among the liquidators of consequences of Chernobyl APS accident, in J. L. Chevchenko (ed.), *Actual issues of military and ecological psychiatry*, Military medical academy, Saint-Petersburg, 147-148.
8. Katachkova, G. D., Ovchinnikov, J. V., Zybina, N. N., Agafonova, T. A., Nikiforov, A. M. (1997) Particularities of cardiovascular system changes and free radicals processes in Chernobyl atomic power-station accident liquidators with different cardiac pathology, in I. M. Markelov (ed.), *Scientific and practice conference <Medical and social aspects of problems of nuclear subjected veteransand ways of solving them>*, Saint-Petersburg, 61-62.
9. Petrunya, A. M. (1996) Changes in the organ of vision and in the immunologic status among the liquidators of consequences of accident of Chernobyl atomic power-station and their correction, *Oftalmologichesky Zhunal* 4, 226-230.
10. Day, R., Gorin, M. B., Eller, A. W. (1995) Prevalence of lens changes in Ukrainian children residing around Chernobyl, *Health Phys.* **5**, 632-642.

11. Chvedova , A. A. (1986) *Lipids peroxidation processes in injury of retina membrane structures*, «Medicine» Publishers, Tomsk.
12. Komartsev, V. N., Sosyukin, A. E. (1996) Influence of factors of radiation and non-radiation nature to the health of population of garrisons, stationed on radioactive polluted territory, *Voenno-Medicinsky Zhurnal* **317**, 22-25
13. Emerit, I., Alaoui-Youssefi, A., Cernjavski, L. (1997) Oxidative stress and low dose irradiation in IAEA (ed.), *Low Doses of Ionizing Radiation: Biological Effects and Regulatory Control: Contributed Papers*, IAEA Publishers, Vienna,-4.
14. Kutty, R. K., Kutty, G., Wiggert, B., Chader, G. J., Darrow, R. M., Organisciak, D. T., (1995) Induction of heme oxygenase 1 in the retina by intense visible light: suppression by the antioxidant dimethylthiourea, *Proc. Natl. Acad. Sci. USA* **92**, 1177-1181.
15. Rego, A. C., Oliveira, C. R. (1995) Dual effect of lipid peroxidation on the membrane order of retinal cells in culture, *Arch. Biochem. Biophys.* **321**, 127-136.
16. Volkov, V. V., Gorban, A. I., Galiachvili, O. A. (1976) *Clinical viso- and refractometry*, «Medicine» Publishers, Leningrad.
17. Volkov, V. V., Yustova, E. N. (1995) On diagnostics and classification of variants of color vision in light of new methodical approaches, *Vestnik Oftalmologii* **108**, 19-24.
18. Shamshinova, A. M., Nesteruk, L. I., Endrikhovsky, S. N. (1995) Color campimetry in diagnostics of retina and optic nerve diseases, *Vestnik Oftalmologii* **111**, 24-28.
19. Shamshinova, A. M., Belozerov, A. E., Shapiro, V. M. (1997) New method of contrast sensitivity investigation in ophthalmological practice, *Vestnik Oftalmologii* **113**, 22-25.
20. Pick, A., Keisari, G. (1981) Superoxide anion and hydrogene peroxide production by chemically elicited peritoneal macrophages, *Cell. Immunol.* **59**, 301-308.
21. Kum-Tatt L., It-Koon T. (1974) A new colorimetric method for the determination of glutathione in erythrocytes, *Clin. Chim. Acta* **53**, 153-161.
22. Carlberg, J., Mannervik, B. (1975) Purification and characterization of the flavoenzyme glutathion-reductase from rat liver *J. Biol. Chem.* **250**, 5475-5480.
23. Winterbourn, C. C., Hawkins, R. E. (1975) The estimation of red cell superoxide dismutase activity *J. Lab. Clin. Med.* **85**, 337-342.
24. Galloway, N. R. (1988) Electrophysiological testing of eyes with opaque media, *Eye* **2**, 615-624.

PHYSICAL AND CHEMICAL CHANGES IN MURINE LENS AT EARLY STAGE OF CATARACT DEVELOPMENT INDUCED BY TOTAL GAMMA-IRRADIATION

A. I. DEYEV, A. V. ASEYCHEV, I. A. SITARTCHUK, *B. S. FEDORENKO, Y. A. VLADIMIROV

*Department of Biophysics, Russian State Medical University, Ostrovityanova St. 1, Moscow, 117869 Russia; *Institute for Medico-Biological Problems, Moscow.*

Introduction

Clinicians reveal the cataract when changes in the lens develop an irreversible form and show visible morphological evidence visible. The early stages of cataractogenesis are not readily detectable and represent one of the main impediments to the study of cataractogenesis and the application of an appropriate therapy. The usual indirect approach to this problem is the study in an animal model for cataracts. Quite a good approximation of age related cataract is a cataract induced by single whole body X- or γ-irradiation in sublethal doses 4 to 6 Gy. This model is based on mice as experimental animals which have only a short natural lifespan (approximately two years). The frequence of cataract development and the length of latent period are linear to the exposure dose of γ-rays from 1 to 4 Gy [1]. It is interesting to note that the dose response curve for radiation induced life shortening of mice C57BL/6 is also linear [2]. The cataract initiated by sublethal dose of γ-irradiation progresses for several months and has typical manifestations such as the appearance of fluorescent products in the lens [3], a reduction of gluthatione concentration and changes in protein structure [4].

We started from the assumption that this cataract model is convenient for the identification of some specific molecular precataractous changes and the order in which these changes occur. The purpose of the present study is to investigate the sequence of physical and chemical changes. The changes are related to lenticular antioxidant potential, solubility of proteins and membrane structure with cataract development induced by whole body γ-irradiation.

Materials and Methods

Hybrid mice F1(CBAxC57Bl/6) (virginal females) with a mean initial body weight of 18-20 g were treated with 5 Gy γ-irradiation at a dose rate of 0.08 Gy/sec. Lenses were examined with a slitlamp twice a week after the irradiation and cataracts were graded

A. K. Junk et al. (eds.),
Ocular Radiation Risk Assessment in Populations Exposed to Environmental Radiation Contamination, 81–88.

on a scale of 1+ to 4+ as follows way: 0 - no changes; 1+ - early posterior changes such as clusters of vacuoles and opaque dots in the posterior cortex and the subcapsular region; 2+ - moderately dense posterior cortical opacity and early opacification of the anterior cortex; 3+ - posterior cortex very opaque, moderate nuclear sclerosis; 4+ - completely opaque lens [5]. The lenses were removed immediately after decapitation. The treated animals were of the same age as the controls. The content of GSH was determined by using the 5,5'-dithiobis-(2-nitrobenzoic acid) reaction [6]. We assumed that the reduced glutathione (GSH) content in the lens was equal to the amount of reduced non-protein thiols. Determination of malondialdehyde (MDA), an end product of lipid peroxidation, was based on the formation of a colored complex between MDA and thiobarbituric acid (TBA), by using the following procedure [8]: 1.2 ml of lens homogenate were mixed with 0.125 ml of 80% trichloroacetic acid and the sample was centrifuged at 300 g for 15 minutes. 1.0 ml of the supernatant was mixed with 50 ml of 0.01 M BHT and 0.5 ml of 0.5 % TBA + 0.3 % sodium dodecylsulfate solution. The mixture was placed in test tubes and incubated for 15 minutes at 100°C. The absorbence of the samples was measured at 512, 532 and 550 nm against the controls in which the homogenate was substituted for buffer solution. The concentration of MDA (μmol/g protein) in the lens was calculated by the following equation:

$$MDA = 1.71[D_{532} - 0.5(D_{512} + D_{550})] / P \tag{1}$$

1.71 the dilution coefficient,
ε 0.156 μM^{-1} - extinction coefficient (for 1 cm cuvette) at 532 nm,
P protein concentration, g/l,
D_{532}, D_{512}, D_{550} - the optical density at 532 nm, 512 nm and 550 nm, respectively, measured against the control solution.

The valence of lens proteins was estimated in lens homogenates by the Donnan potential measurement using the experimental set up described previously [9]. The murine lenses or cortices or nuclei were homogenized in 1.0 ml of 10 mM NaCl, 1 mM Tris-HCl, 1 mM dithiothreitol, pH 7.4 and then diluted in the same solution. The radius of cellulose dialysis tubing was 8 mm. The solvent in the two compartments was 10 mM NaCl in 1 mM Tris-HCl, pH 7.4. The volume of the inner protein solution was 1 ml and that of surrounding bath 1 l. The potential (E) was measured within the temperature range 18-25°C, and protein concentration ranged from 2 to 5 mg/ml. The net molecular valence of proteins (Z_p) was calculated by the following equation:

$$Z_p = C_o/C_p[\exp(EF/RT) - \exp(-EF/RT)] \tag{2}$$

C_o molar concentration of the mobile cation or anion
T the absolute temperature

F Faraday constant
R gas constant
C_p molar protein concentration.

C_p was calculated for conditional protein of molecular mass of 20,000. Protein concentration was estimated by the biuret reaction [10].

Water insoluble lenticular proteins were obtained by the centrifugation (twice at 6600 g for 40 minutes, at +4°C) of lens homogenate, which had been prepared by homogenization of 50-60 mg of murine lenses in 1.0 ml of 0.14 M NaCl, 1 mM Tris-HCl, 1mM dithiothreitol, pH 7.4. Protein solubility was defined as the ratio of water soluble protein concentration to total protein concentration in lens homogenate.

The hemolytic activity of proteins was estimated by the addition of the proteins to erythrocyte suspension. The cell suspension was prepared by a two-step centrifugation (for 10 minutes at 1500 g) of oxalate rabbit blood diluted in 0.14 M NaCl, 1 mM Tris-HCl, pH 7.4. The erythrocyte suspension contained 0.1 % cells, v/v. Three samples were incubated simultaneously for 90 minutes at a given temperature with occasional gentle stirring: 1 - erythrocyte suspension with the protein; 2 - erythrocyte suspension without protein (the degree of spontaneous hemolysis in this sample was taken as zero); 3 - erythrocyte suspension diluted in distilled water (the degree of hemolysis in this sample was taken as unity). Then the samples were centrifuged for 10 minutes at 1500 g and the absorbence of each supernatant was measured against buffer at 418 nm. The degree of protein-dependent hemolysis (H) was calculated by the equation:

$$H = A_1 / (A_3 - A_2) \qquad (3)$$

where A_1, A_2, A_3 are the absorbences measured for the first, second and third supernatant, respectively.

Results and Discussion

The development of cataract induced by whole body irradiation was accompanied by typical manifestations: a decrease in the water-soluble protein content, a decrease of GSH level at the end of the third month after irradiation, a drastic increase in MDA content beginning at the end of the second month after irradiation and continuing thereafter (Figure 1).

The earliest observed changes in the lens of irradiated animals consist of a modest (about 20 %) increase of GSH concentration. At first glance, it seems that this result is paradoxical as the reduction of GSH concentration is well known in all types of cataracts. On the other hand, we can interpret this temporal variation of GSH content on the basis of the general theory of regulation. According to current concepts of this theory, the transition process from one stable state to another follows a logical pattern: stable state 1 (normal lens) + pertubation (oxidative stress after irradiation) →

hypercompensation (increase of GSH content) → decompensation (disturbance of GSH level regulation) → state 2 (precataractous lens).

The oppositely directed changes in concentrations of GSH and MDA indicate that lens antioxidant system is the deterrent for free radical processes and the damage or the depletion of this system lead to activation of free radical processes including the lipid peroxidation [11].

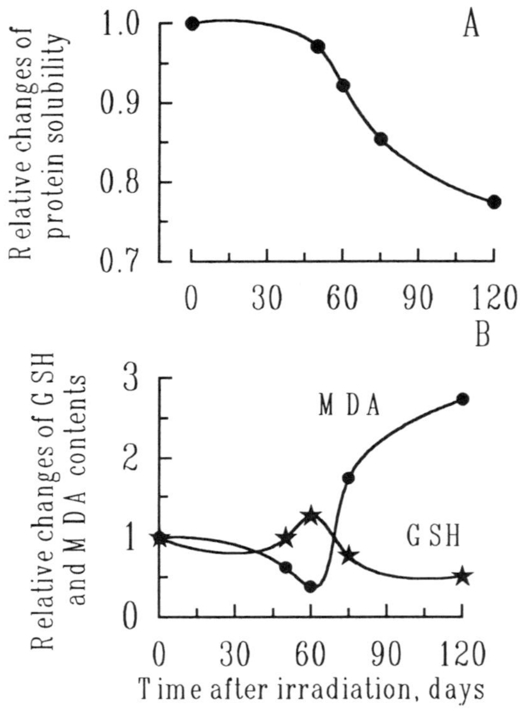

Figure 1. Relative changes of water soluble protein content (A), GSH and MDA content (B) as a function of time after irradiation. The data are plotted as ratio of the sample means (n≥5) in irradiated group to the sample means (n≥5) in control group.

The relation between the GSH level and protein solubility was investigated by using the measurements of both these parameters in the same animals at different times after irradiation. One eye was used for GSH measurement, the contralateral eye was used for protein solubility measuremement. The GSH amounts in both eyes of same animal were considered equivalent since the correlation between the GSH amounts in contralateral murine eyes was equal to 0.997 (n=7, p< 0.001) [7].

The relation between the GSH level and water solubility of lenticular proteins was approximated to a second order polynomial having the correlation coefficient -0.72 (Figure 2). The observed approximation can be explained on the assumption that there is criticial concentration of GSH following which the lenticular proteins start to lose water solubility.

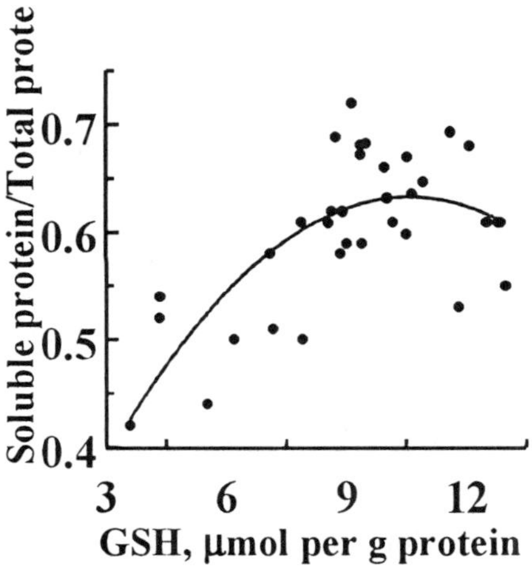

Figure 2. Correlation between the GSH level and water solubility of lenticular proteins (n=35, p<0.01).

The decrease of water solubility of lenticular proteins is attributable to the loss of fixed anion valences on protein surfaces noted in radiation [4] and hereditary [12] cataracts. This rises questions about the nature of charged groups that change as a cataract develops. To address the issue, the net valence of cortical proteins was measured as a function of pH at different stages of cataract development (Figure 3).

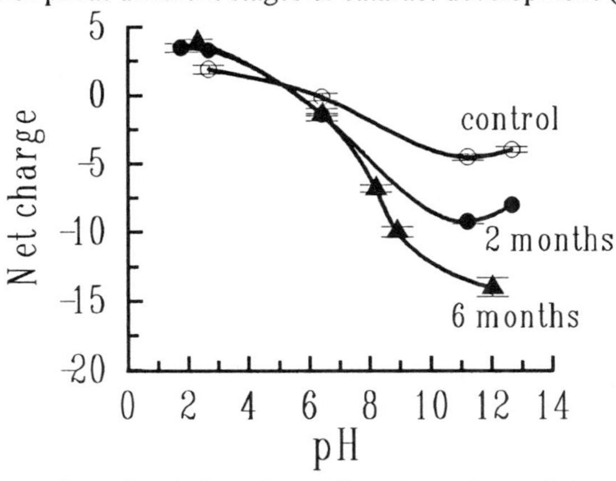

Figure 3. The net valence of cortical proteins at different times after irradiation as a function of pH. The mean molecular mass of protein unit was taken as equal to 20 kD.

It was found that the valences of cortical proteins are determined by the groups having pK about 7 which is rather close to pK of phosphoserine (pK = 7.2). In view of what is known about lens protein phosphorylation [13], we may hypothesize that the reduction of negative valence in cortical proteins after irradiation is a result of deficient phosphorylation of proteins.

These findings completely support the previous assumption that phosphorylation of crystallins plays a key role in lens fiber cell development and maturation [14]. On the other hand it is well known that the activity of proteinkinases depend upon the concentration of cyclic adenosine monophosphate (cAMP) which arises from ATP due to the action of adenylatecyclases localized on the inner surface of the cell membrane . The adenylatecyclases show extreme sensitivity to the action of ionizing radiation [15]. The activity of the adenylate cyclase complex is probably controlled by both its protein structure and the lipid microenvironment in cell membranes, both very sensitive targets of free radical action. Among other factors, the peroxidation of phospholipids leads to an increase in negative valence on lipid surfaces [16]. This is due to the fact that positivly charged amino-groups of phosphatidylethanolamine react with aldehydes released from oxidized fatty acids [17]. The increase of negative valence on the inner surface of membranes or adenylate cyclase complexes can inhibit the transformation of strongly negative charged ATP into cAMP. In turn, the inhibition of adenylate cyclase activity results in cessation of protein phosphorylation.

It has been proposed earlier that proteins binding to the inner surface of cell membranes may lead to membrane rupture and thus impairment of their barrier function [4]. The membrane rupture and disclosure of containing proteins was found in fibers inside local opacifications in clear human post mortal lenses [18]. Fiber disruption induced radiation cataract was assosiated with the appearance of 4 to 10 μm membrane-bound globules [19].

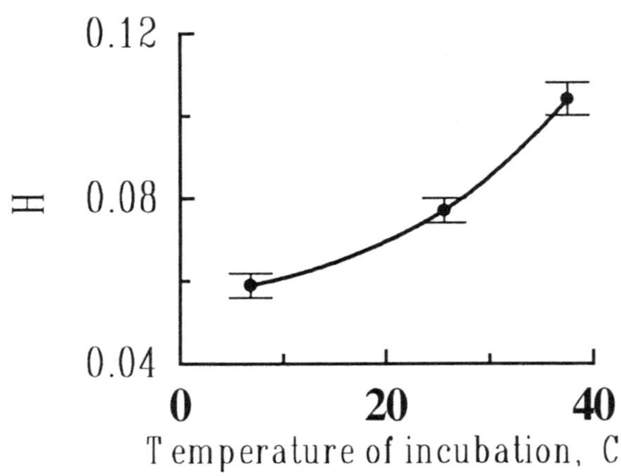

Figure 4. Hemolytic effect of water-insoluble lenticular proteins as a function of temperature.

This rises the question of whether or not the uncharged crystallines have the capacity to be absorbed on membrane surfaces and damage the membranes. In an attempt to answer the question, we used rabbit erythrocytes as a target for the proteins, in order to assess the damaging action on membranes by measuring erythrocyte hemolysis. It was shown that the soluble lenticular proteins in the final concentration of 5 mg/ml did not induce hemolysis during an incubation period of 90 minutes. The insoluble proteins however induced marked hemolysis which increased with increasing temperature (Figure 4). The temperature coefficient Q_{10} of insoluble protein-mediated hemolysis was defined as the ratio H(37°C)/ H(27°C) and was found to be equal to 1.3. The same value of Q_{10} was found for the hemolysis induced by chrysotyl-asbestos particles [20]. A low value of Q_{10} for protein-mediated hemolysis suggests that the adsorption of insoluble proteins on erythrocyte membrane surface induces the hemolytic effect.

In our opinion, damaging effects of insoluble lenticular proteins (Figure 4) on membranes lead to an accumulation of insoluble proteins in lens cortex and the deterioration of membrane function. The result is ionic and osmotic imbalance and cellular disorganization. The clear lens consists of regular and uniform layers of homogeneous transparent cells, while the formation of local irregularities leads to opacification.

Acknowledgements

This study was supported by grant M55300 from the International Science Foundation.

References

1. Fedorenko, B. S. (1991) Experimental studies of biological effectiveness of relativistic energy heavy ions, *Physics of elementary particles and atomic nucleus* **22**, 1199 - 1229 (in Russian).
2. Yuhas, J. M. (1969) The dose response curve for radiation-induced life shortening, *J. Gerontol* **24**, 451-456.
3. Aitmagambetov, M. T., Deyev, A. I., Kabachenko, A. N. and Vladimirov, Y. A. (1989) Study of mice lenses fluorescence at different stages of X-ray cataract by the synchronous scanning method, *Bull. Exp. Biol. Med.* **57**, 347-350.
4. Deyev, A., Vladimirov, Y., Aitmagambetov, M., Kabatchenko, A. and Sitartchuk , I. (1991) Sequence of physical and chemical changes in murine lens with cataract development initiated by total gamma-irradiation, in G. F. J. M. Vrensen and J. Clauwaert (eds.), *Lens Membranes and Aging. Topics in aging research in Europe* **15**, EURAGE, Leiden, 247-259.
5. Merriam, G. R. Jr. and Focht, E. F. (1962) A clinical and experimental study of the effect of single and divided doses on radiation cataract production, *Trans. Amer. Ophthalmol. Soc.* **60**, 35-52.
6. Sedlac, J. and Lindsay, R. H. (1968) Estimation of total, protein-bound, and non-protein sulfhydril groups in tissue with Ellman's reagent, *Analyt. Biochem.* **25**, 192-205.
7. Aseychev, A.V., Tjurin-Kuzmin, A.U., Deyev, A.I., Stebeneva, S.A. and Vladimirov, Ju. A. (1996) The evaluation of hexose monophosphate shunt activity in isolated mouse lens using the registration of the ferrocyanid-ferricyanid system potential, *Chem. Biol. Med..* **3**, 20-27.
8. Asakawa , T. and Matsushida, S. (1980) Coloring conditions of thiobarbituric acid test for detecting lipid peroxides. *Lipids* **15**, 137-140.
9. Ojteg, G., Lundahl, P. and Wolgast, M. (1989) The net electric valence of proteins. A comparison of determination by Donnan potential measurements and by gel electrophoresis, *Biochem Biophys Acta*, **991**, 317-323.

10. Itzhaki, R. F. and Gill, D. M. (1964) A micro-biuret method for estimating protein. *Anal. Biochem.*, **9**, 401-410.
11. Babizhaev, M.A., Deyev, A.I. and Lindberg, L.F. (1988) Lipid peroxidation as a possible cause of cataract. *Mechanisms of Ageing and Development* **44**, 69-89.
12. Aitmagambetov, M. T., Deyev, A. I., Kostenko, E. R.. and Vladimirov, Y. A. (1991) Parameters of lens protein fluorescence quenching in hereditary cataract at the initial stage. *Bull. Exp. Biol. Med.*, **61**, 551-553.
13. Sredy, J. and Spector, A., (1984) The phosphorylation of bovine and human lens polypeptides., *Exp. Eye Res.*, **39**, 653-664.
14. Farnsworth, P., Groth-Vasselli, B., van Inwegen, J., Macdonald, J. C., Mathur, R. and Reddy, M. C. (1991)Tyrosine kinase dependent phosphorylation: its possible role in lens fiber cell development and maturation. in G. F. J. M. Vrensen and J. Clauwaert (eds.), *Lens Membranes and Aging. Topics in aging research in Europe* **15**, EURAGE, Leiden, 303-317.
15. Sobolev, A. S., Orechov, A. N. and Kudryashov, Y. B. (1980) *Radiobiology of cyclic nucleotide system*. Moscow , 14-18 (in Russian).
16. Deyev, A. I., Putvinsky, A. V., Dobretsov, G. E., Roschupkin, D. I., Petrov, V. A. and Vladimirov, Y. A.. (1976) Structural changes in membranes of phosphatidylcholine liposomes by UV - irradiation, recorded by fluorescent probe 1-anilinonaphtalene 8- sulfonate (ANS). *Studia biophysica*, **55**, 199-209 (in Russian).
17. Arnhold, J., Herold, W., Arnold, K., and Deyev, A. I. (1988) Reduction of aminogroups and changes of the surface charge of liposome on methylation and peroxidation., *Studia biophysica*, **128**, 45-50.
18. Vrensen, G., Kappelhof, J. and Willekens, B. (1990) Morphology of the Aging Human Lens. II. Ultrastructure of clear lenses. *Lens and eye toxity research*, **7**, 1-30.
19. Rini, F. J., Worgul, B. V. and Merriam, G. R. (1986) Radiation cataractogenesis in rat lenses. *Bull. N. Y. Acad. Med.*, **62**, 744-752.
20. Sykes, S. E., Morgan, A. and Holmas, A. (1980) The hemolytic activity of chrysotile asbestos, in R. C. Brown (ed.), *The in vitro effects of mineral dusts*, London, 113-119.

OVERVIEW ON EXISTING APPROACHES TO DOSE RECONSTRUCTION

Recommendations for the Ukrainian-American Chernobyl Ocular Study (UACOS)

L.R. ANSPAUGH
Radiobiology Division
University of Utah
40 N. 2030 E. Front Street
Salt Lake City, UT 84112-5860

1. Introduction

Over approximately the last 50 years the reconstruction of radiation doses to hypothetical or actual persons has become a major, ongoing scientific activity. Many dose-reconstruction activities have been undertaken in order to support companion epidemiologic studies of radiation risk or to assist in attempting to achieve social justice [1].

The first major dose-reconstruction study was undertaken for the survivors of the atomic bombings in Japan. Three major steps have occurred in this still-continuing activity: The establishment of tentative 1957 (T57) doses [2, 3], tentative 1965 (T65) doses [4, 5], and the more realistic doses established by the Dosimetry System 1986 [6]. This long-running activity is still not finished, as newer and ever-more sophisticated measurements of residual activities indicate that there are major discrepancies in the neutron doses for the survivors in Hiroshima [7].

In the United States many dose-reconstruction activities have been undertaken in order to assess the dose and possible risks to the general population from the continental testing of nuclear weapons and from the operation of the many sites involved in the production of special nuclear materials. A brief indication of these studies is given in Table 1.

In Europe and Asia the largest activity has been associated with reconstructing and projecting doses as a result of the Chernobyl accident that occurred in 1986, e.g., [18-22].

Finally, with the break-up of the Soviet Union, it has become known that large releases and exposures had occurred from the operation of the Mayak Production Facility in the Urals Region of Russia. The dose-reconstruction study for the Techa River residents had been ongoing since the early 1950s; current results have been published [23-25], and a project to improve the dosimetry data base is ongoing [26].

A. K. Junk et al. (eds.),
Ocular Radiation Risk Assessment in Populations Exposed to Environmental Radiation Contamination, 89–98.

TABLE 1. Major dose-reconstruction studies in the United States concerned with the general population living in the vicinity of sites for the production of special nuclear materials or the testing of nuclear weapons.

Site	Object of assessment	Reference
	Completed	
Nevada Test Site	Hypothetical individuals	[8-10]
	Collective	[11, 12]
	Specific individuals	[13, 14]
Hanford Works	Hypothetical individuals	[15, 16]
	In process	
Hanford Works	Specific individuals	
Fernald Feed Materials Production Centre		[17]
Rocky Flats Plant		[17]
Oak Ridge Site		[17]
Idaho National Engineering Laboratory		[17]
Savannah River Site		[17]

2. Methods of Dose Reconstruction

Over the years many methods of dose reconstruction have been devised and implemented. Methods range widely from old to new, from inexpensive to expensive, from calculational to measurement based, from specific to general, and from roughly approximate to highly accurate. In general, highly accurate methods tend to be rather specific and expensive. Dose-reconstruction methods have been discussed and summarised recently elsewhere [1, 27, 28]; a brief description of the major methods follows.

An outline of the major methods of dose reconstruction is indicated in Table 2. This table is modified from [1] in order to include more methods, particularly those that are more appropriate for workers, as opposed to including only those appropriate for members of the general population. The primary difference among the two population groups in this context is that workers generally were in more controlled environments and had more extensive monitoring of both external and internal exposures.

Of course, the most preferred method would be one that is "biologic" and would allow a direct indication from the individual of what exposure had occurred. For radionuclides such as ^{90}Sr and ^{239}Pu, which stay in the body for very long time periods, it is possible to ascertain the systemic burden based upon bioassay results and, for ^{90}Sr, on whole body counting [29] of the bremsstralung from the beta emitted by ^{90}Y. Samples, particularly of bone, collected at autopsy can also be measured for the content of long-lived radionuclides, again more usefully for ^{90}Sr and ^{239}Pu. Even more valuable would be the analysis of some sample extracted from the person that could be analysed to give a more direct measure of the dose actually received. There is not yet a perfect dosimeter of this type, but two relatively recent developments show great promise.

The first method is the analysis of stable, reciprocal translocations in circulating lymphocytes. Such translocations supplement the well-known measurement of chromosome dicentrics in circulating lymphocytes, which are very useful soon after a significant exposure has occurred. However, the analysis of dicentrics is not useful over

TABLE 2. Methods of dose reconstruction. The methods are arranged roughly in an hierarchy going downward from reliable and preferred to approximate.

Methods
Individual "biologic" analysis
Bioassay (measurement of radionuclides in urine and/or faeces)
Whole or partial body counting to determine radionuclide content
Measurement of samples collected at autopsy
Analysis of stable, reciprocal chromosome translocations in circulating lymphocytes
Electron paramagnetic analysis of teeth
Individual film-badge dosimeters
Individual "environmental" analysis
Area film badges
Area air monitors
Thermoluminescent analysis of samples from home environment
Analysis of environmental residues
Radionuclide-deposition densities, past or present
External gamma-exposure rates, past
Activation products (for neutrons), e.g., ^{36}Cl and ^{63}Ni
Known releases plus models
Models of radionuclide transport in air or water
Models of radiation transport in air or water
Inferred releases plus models
Models of radionuclide transport in air or water
Models of radiation transport in air or water
Known or inferred releases, coupled to global dose factors

long time periods following exposure. On the other hand, it has been demonstrated that reciprocal translocations in chromosomes of the same circulating lymphocytes are stable over at least several decades [27]. The most convenient method of assay of that of "chromosome painting" with the use of fluorescence in situ hybridisation (FISH) [30]. The method is time consuming and expensive. The response of the assay to tritium betas and to gamma rays of various energies has been quantified, but its response to many incorporated radionuclides has not been quantified. The sensitivity of the FISH assay is on the order of 100 mGy, but this depends upon the number of cells that are counted and upon the individual's age, which determines the background incidence of translocations.

The second "modern" method of individual-dose determination is the electron paramagnetic resonance (EPR) analysis of dentine [27, 31]. This method has developed rapidly, as a result of intense interest in its use following the accident at Chernobyl. There are known problems with the method, such as interference of the signal by ultraviolet light for the front teeth and individual differences in sensitivity of response, but methods are rapidly being found to solve these problems. The application of the technique requires the extraction of a tooth, and the analysis is expensive and time consuming, if the problems mentioned above are addressed adequately. The sensitivity of the method is around 50 mGy. The method would not work well for individuals who have had extensive exposure to dental x-rays, although such soft x-ray exposure can be quantified by careful work with depth profiles of dose within an individual tooth.

Most workers in the nuclear industry, even from the earliest days, wore individual dosimeters of some type designed to record external gamma and beta dose. Typically, these individual dosimeters were film badges during the early periods of higher exposures; the design of such film badges has been improved over the years in order to allow for the differential energy response of film. In later times, thermoluminescent dosimeters have been used. Such individual badges provide extremely valuable and reliable information, but in general the resulting data cannot be used directly without careful consideration of bias and uncertainty in the resulting estimates of dose, especially when dose for individual organs is needed [32].

If direct analysis of the individual is not possible, the next more reliable method would be analysis of some material taken from within the individual's environment. For a worker this might be the use of area-radiation monitors, such as film badges, or the use of area monitors that record the concentration of radionuclides in air. For individuals in the general population one technique that has been used quite successfully is the thermoluminescent analysis of materials from homes. In order to be useful the thermoluminescent signal must have been "zeroed out" at some recent time prior to exposure; this is usually done by the firing of bricks and porcelain during the manufacturing process. Such analyses have proved useful for dose reconstructions for the survivors of the atomic bombings in Japan [33], the population living nearby the Nevada Test Site [34], and for the population living downstream of the Mayak plutonium-production facility in the Southern Urals [35]. The sensitivity of the method is approximately 50 mGy.

The analysis of environmental residues is an old, well established technique that has been used since the early days of the study of global fallout and the determination of the resulting dose to man [36]. A major component of such studies was to measure the deposition rate of ^{90}Sr through use of a variety of collectors and to measure the cumulative deposition density of ^{90}Sr by the analysis of soil samples. The deposition density of all other radionuclides, even though they might have decayed long ago, could then be inferred based on what was known about the source term of the releases. Modern calculations using gamma-ray transport codes have allowed the conversion from radionuclide-deposition density to external gamma-exposure rate [37] or external dose rate [38]. Thus, provided that the relative source term of any release is known, it is possible to infer the deposition densities of all radionuclides and the resulting external gamma-exposure rate as a function of time, if the deposition density of any radionuclide is known or if the external gamma-exposure rate was measured at some early time. This technique was used extensively in the dose reconstruction for the residents living near the Nevada Test Site [8, 9, 39, 40]. The accelerator-mass-spectrometry analysis of ^{129}I, half life of 16 million years, as a surrogate for ^{131}I, half life of 8 days, has also been demonstrated as a useful tool for the reconstruction of doses to the thyroid as a result of the Chernobyl accident [41].

The analysis of the neutron-activation product, ^{36}Cl, in samples of concrete taken from Hiroshima has recently provided information on the flux of thermal neutrons at Hiroshima [7]. The next step in resolving the current discrepancy (measurements versus calculations) in neutron doses at Hiroshima is to analyse some product that would respond only to high-energy neutrons. At the present time, ^{63}Ni is the leading candidate for this analysis, and an analytical system has been demonstrated [27, 42].

The remaining methods listed in Table 2 are not usually reliable in the case of episodic releases [1]. However, when releases occur over long time periods, the ability of atmospheric transport models to provide approximately accurate time-integrated predictions is much improved. This method was used for the calculations of thyroid dose from ^{131}I from the Hanford Works; such calculations depended entirely upon the laborious definition of the source term on the basis of process records and the use of an atmospheric transport model [15]. Here, there was no other viable choice, as no known environmental residues were capable of being a surrogate for ^{131}I. [In this case ^{129}I is not a viable surrogate for ^{131}I, as the filters installed at later times to trap ^{131}I eventually released the entrained ^{129}I.] A river model was also used to calculate the dose from radionuclides released to the water at the Hanford Works [16], as the measurements available were not adequate to support an assessment. Sometimes it may be adequate to calculate collective dose only based upon an inferred source term and the use of "global dose factors." Such techniques are discussed in [43] and [44]. If the latter techniques are used, it is not possible to calculate individual doses.

3. Lessons Learned from Prior Dose Reconstructions

3.1. GENERAL

Over the years many dose-reconstruction studies have been conducted. These studies have become increasingly sophisticated as newer methods of reconstruction, verification, and validation have been developed. Many of the "tools" in current use are of fairly recent development, and this development process will continue.

In general, there is no "right" method of dose reconstruction. Methods tend to be site- or problem-specific and tailored to the data available to support the reconstruction. In fact, one might say that the first rule of dose reconstruction is to make maximum use of the data available. Real measurements are extremely useful, particularly in supporting the credibility of the reconstruction. If the measurements themselves are inadequate to support the reconstruction, then the measurements must be saved for validation purposes. Validation is approached by comparing predicted values (of air concentration, deposition density, concentration in vegetation, etc.) to measured values, by comparing several independent types of measurements, and by checking for biological plausibility (i.e., are the predicted doses consistent with the medical observations or lack of observations?).

Methods that have been used vary from completely theoretical (or calculational) to those based on measurements only. It is unlikely that a theoretical only study will yield results of sufficient accuracy, as a large number of assumptions are typically required, and there are too many variables with uncertain influence.

The more successful applications use a combination of approaches, devote a major fraction of effort to verification and validation, and *provide estimates of the central value of reconstructed doses and of uncertainty.*

Dose reconstruction is a very difficult task and is not generally accomplished through the application of textbook methods. An important point is that dose reconstruction should be a continuing activity over the life of any associated epidemiologic study. *There is a deplorable tendency to view dose reconstruction as something trivial and easily accomplished within a short fraction of the time afforded to an epidemiologic study.*

3.2. STUDY OF THE SURVIVORS OF THE ATOMIC BOMBINGS IN JAPAN

Examination of the first major dose-reconstruction study, that of the atomic bomb survivors in Japan, provides some useful insight. The radiation doses for this study have been reconstructed three times. The first was in 1957 [2, 3] and the doses were designated as "Temporary 57" or "T57." The second set of doses was also designated as "Temporary" or "T65" [4, 5]. The T65 doses stood for 21 years even though these doses were clearly intended to be "temporary" by the dosimetrists, the doses were incompatible with other data, and, in several cases, the calculated doses were biologically implausible. In fact, it was not until it was overwhelmingly obvious that the T65 doses contained major discrepancies [45] that work finally began to resolve this important dosimetry question. This lack of attention to dosimetry occurred in spite of the fact that the epidemiologic part of the study was well funded at the rate of several tens of millions of dollars per year.

The eventual improvements in the dose-reconstruction system, known as Dosimetry System 86 [6], depended greatly on experimental data acquired with the use of newly developed techniques and validation of old experimental data. It is fortunate that a small amount of work has continued on this important dosimetry problem, but it is unfortunate that this new work [e.g., 7] indicates that there are serious discrepancies in the neutron doses arising from Dosimetry System 86 for Hiroshima.

In the author's opinion the major failings of the dose reconstructions for the survivors provide the following insights:

- The provision of temporary doses is dangerous—Epidemiologists and/or managers tend to decide that dosimetrists are no longer needed or that further dosimetry study can be postponed indefinitely;
- For a long-term cohort study of major importance, dosimetry investigation and validation should be a continuing process; and
- Dosimetrists and managers must remain open to the application of newly developed techniques and processes.

4. The Dose Reconstruction Required for the UACOS Study Is Very Complicated

The problems encountered in trying to reconstruct the gamma-radiation doses received by the Chernobyl liquidators have been discussed by several Russian authors [46, 47]. These difficulties arise from the fact that few dosimeters were available at the time of the accident, and most of those were not useful at the ranges of doses actually encountered. Also, due to the perceived urgency of the early remedial measures, records of location and time of exposure are not always available or adequate. However, work is continuing on this important problem, and the use of FISH and EPR analyses should provide important additional data.

Even from the very early days following the accident, it was clear that some persons had received very high doses with resulting severe skin injury [46-48]. It was presumed that such skin injury was due to distant beta-radiation sources and from skin contamination; further, it was noted that, "Injuries to skin significantly complicated the clinical course and prognosis of the patients and were the only cause of death in some cases" [48].

In fact, while the problems with gamma dosimetry were eventually solved as time passed, there were hardly any measurements of beta doses to the skin or the eye [47]. The exceptions were limited special measurements carried out by personnel of the Institute of Biophysics. Osanov and Krjuchkov [46] reported on the results of some of these measurements for 28 persons from Military Unit No. 73143 on 2 September 1986. These persons were assigned work on cleaning up pieces of graphite and metal debris on the roof, where the external gamma-exposure rate was 150–200 R h^{-1}. The soldiers were allowed to work for 50 s in groups of four. The exposure calculated for the men was 1 R and this value was entered into the "registration diary." Dosimeters were attached to the clothing of these men: The measured gamma exposures varied from 1.0 to 5.4 R; the measured beta doses (at 70 mg cm^{-2}) varied from 3.6 to 14.1 rad; and the beta-to-gamma ratios varied from 1.7 to 10.4. Further, for thin sources, such as contaminated surfaces of floors, walls, etc., the beta-to-gamma ratio reached values of 100 to 200. The ratios were particularly high when the radionuclides $^{90}Sr/^{90}Y$, $^{106}Ru/^{106}Rh$, and $^{144}Ce/^{144}Pr$ were present.

Thus, at the present time, the beta dose to the eye lens of the various liquidators in the UACOS cohort is virtually unknown, and the methods of assessment that are currently available are inadequate for the task. The proper and adequate solution of this task will require highly focused and directed research and development. In other studies external beta dose (except from rare gases, such as ^{85}Kr) to the skin has not received much attention, as the problem is difficult and skin has not been an organ of oncogenic interest. For example, for the study of residents nearby the Nevada Test Site, beta skin doses were calculated on the basis of an assumed deposition on skin [8], but it was recognised that this method was subject to major uncertainty.

In addition to the major work that must be done to reconstruct gamma doses to the liquidator cohort, it seems clear that the beta dose to the eye lens must be calculated as well. The complicating factors include the size, location, and age of the irradiating sources that affect the beta-to-gamma ratio; corrections that must be made for the wearing of goggles; and corrections that must be made if shielding was worn during liquidation work. In addition, if any dosimeter was worn during the work, it is important to know the location of the dosimeter relative to the shielding in order to make corrections.

5. A Recommended Research Strategy for the UACOS

The difficult problem of beta dosimetry will not be solved easily, and the most straightforward ultimate solution is to develop an assay capable of measuring directly the gamma and beta doses in or near the eye lens. Such a method may indeed be feasible, but it has not yet been proven.

In the meantime the following research strategy is recommended:

- Accumulate all existing dosimetry records pertaining to the Chernobyl Atomic Power Plant environment and to the members of the cohort;
- Develop a calculational approach for external gamma exposures and doses;
- Develop a calculational approach for external beta doses;

- Apply these methods, in conjunction with data from interviews and other sources, on an interim basis with the view that gamma dose is more knowable and verifiable, but that an approximate ratio of beta-to-gamma dose is calculable.
- Collect as many tooth samples as feasible (subject to approvals by all relevant Institutional Review Boards) from cohort members for the measurement of external gamma dose by EPR;
- Collect as many samples of circulating lymphocytes for which analysis by FISH is affordable for measurement of external gamma dose;
- Research, develop, and apply new techniques that would permit measurement of external gamma *and beta* doses in or near the eye lens. Possible new techniques are the assay of micronuclei in lens tissue available from surgery patients and/or FISH assay of skin cells taken near the eye; and
- Based on results from measurements, provide appropriate corrections to the more general calculational procedures.

6. Acknowledgements

This work was funded by the Office of International Health Programs of the U.S. Department of Energy. The author thanks V.V. Chumak, I.A. Likhtarev, T. Straume, and E. Haskell for helpful discussions.

7. References

1. Anspaugh, L.R. (1996) Technical basis for dose reconstruction, in J.E. Till (ed.), *Environmental Dose Reconstruction and Risk Implications,* National Council on Radiation Protection and Measurements, Bethesda, pp. 25–48.
2. Arakawa, E.T. (1960) Radiation dosimetry in Hiroshima and Nagasaki atomic-bomb survivors, *New Engl. J. Med.* **263**, 488–493.
3. Auxier, J.A. (1977) *ICHIBAN: Radiation Dosimetry for the Survivors of the Bombings of Hiroshima and Nagasaki,* U.S. Department of Energy, Washington.
4. Milton, R.C. and Shohoji, T. (1969) *Tentative 1965 Radiation Dose Estimation for Atomic Bomb Survivors,* Radiation Effects Research Foundation, Hiroshima, Technical Report 1–68, 1968.
5. Auxier, J.A. (1982) Development of the dosimetric program, T65D values, in V.P. Bond and J.W. Thiessen, (eds.), *Reevaluations of Dosimetric Factors: Hiroshima and Nagasaki,* U.S. Department of Energy, Washington, CONF–810928, pp. 6–24.
6. Roesch, W.C. (ed.) (1987) *US–Japan Joint Reassessment of Atomic Bomb Radiation Dosimetry in Hiroshima and Nagasaki,* Radiation Effects Research Foundation, Hiroshima.
7. Straume, T., Egbert, S.D., Woolson, W.A., Finkel, R.C., Kubik, P.W., Gove, H.E., Sharma, P., and Hoshi, M. (1992) Neutron discrepancies in the DS86 Hiroshima Dosimetry System, *Health Phys.* **63**, 421–426.
8. Henderson, R.W. and Smale, R.F. (1990) External exposure estimates for individuals near the Nevada Test Site, *Health Phys.* **59**, 715–721.
9. Ng, Y.C., Anspaugh, L.R., and Cederwall, R.T. (1990) ORERP internal dose estimates for individuals, *Health Phys.* **59**, 693–713.
10. National Cancer Institute (1997) *Estimated Exposures and Thyroid Doses Received by the American People from Iodine-131 in Fallout Following Nevada Atmospheric Nuclear Bomb Tests,* U.S. Department of Health and Human Services, Washington.
11. Henderson, R.W. and Smale, R.F. (1992) *Summary of Collective Dose from External Exposure,* Los Alamos National Laboratory, Los Alamos, Report submitted to the Co-ordination and Information Centre, Las Vegas.

12. Whicker, F.W., Kirchner, T.B., Anspaugh, L.R., and Ng, Y.C. (1996) Ingestion of Nevada Test Site fallout: Internal dose estimates, *Health Phys.* **71**, 477–486.
13. Simon, S.L., Till, J.E., Lloyd, R.D., Kerber, R.L., Thomas, D.C., Preston-Martin, S., Lyon, J.L., and Stevens, W. (1995) The Utah leukemia case-control study: Dosimetry methodology and results, *Health Phys.* **68**, 460–471.
14. Till, J.E., Simon, S.L., Kerber, R., Lloyd, R.D., Stevens, W., Thomas, D.C., Lyon, J.L., and Preston-Martin, S. (1995) The Utah thyroid-cohort study: Analysis of the dosimetry results, *Health Phys.* **68**, 472–483.
15. Farris, W.T., Napier, B.A., Ikenberry, T.A., Simpson, J.C., and Shipler, D.A. (1994) *Atmospheric Pathway Dosimetry Report, 1944–1992,* Pacific Northwest Laboratories, Richland, WA, PNWD-2228 HEDR.
16. Farris, W.T., Napier, B.A., Simpson, J.C., Snyder, S.F., and Shipler, D.A. (1994) *Columbia River Pathway Dosimetry Report, 1944–1992,* Pacific Northwest Laboratories, Richland, WA, PNWD-2227 HEDR.
17. Miller, C.W., Smith, J.M., and Denham, L.S. (1994) Dose reconstruction studies at selected nuclear weapons facilities in the USA, in *Assessing the Radiological Impact of Past Nuclear Activities and Events,* International Atomic Energy Agency, Vienna, IAEA-TECDOC-755, pp. 79–85.
18. Balonov, M.I. (1996) Chernobyl dose for population of areas radiocontaminated after the Chernobyl accident, in J.E. Till (ed.), *Environmental Dose Reconstruction and Risk Implications,* National Council on Radiation Protection and Measurements, Bethesda, pp. 207–243.
19. Likhtariov, I., Kovgan, L., Novak, D., Vavilov, S., Jacob, P., and Paretzke, H.G. (1996) Effective doses due to external irradiation from the Chernobyl accident for different population groups of Ukraine, *Health Phys.* **70**, 87–98.
20. Likhtarev, I.A., Kovgan, L.N., Vavilov, S.E., Gluvchinsky, R.R., Perevoznikov, O.N., Litvinets, L.N., Anspaugh, L.R., Kercher, J.R., and Bouville, A. (1996) Internal exposure from the ingestion of foods contaminated by ^{137}Cs after the Chernobyl accident, *Health Phys.* **70**, 297–317.
21. Karaoglou, A., Desmet, G., Kelly, G.N., and Menzel, H.G. (1996) *The Radiological Consequences of the Chernobyl Accident,* European Commission, Luxembourg, EUR-16544.
22. European Commission, International Atomic Energy Agency, and World Health Organisation (1996) *One Decade after Chernobyl: Summing Up the Consequences of the Accident,* International Atomic Energy Agency, Vienna.
23. Burkhart, W. and Kellerer, A.M. (1994) Radiation exposure in the Southern Urals, *Sci. Total Environ.* **142**, Nos. 1-2.
24. Degteva, M.O. (1996) Environmental dose reconstruction for the Urals population, in J.E. Till (ed.), *Environmental Dose Reconstruction and Risk Implications,* National Council on Radiation Protection and Measurements, Bethesda, pp. 155–169.
25. Degteva, M.O., Kozheurov, V.P., Burmistrov, D.S., Vorobyova, M.I., Valchuk, V.V., Bougrov, N.G., and Shishkina, H.A. (1996) An approach to dose reconstruction for the Urals population, Health Phys. 71, 71–76.
26. Degteva, M.O., Kozheurov, V.P., Vorobiova, M.I., Burmistrov, D.S., Khokhryakov, V.V., Suslova, K.G., Anspaugh, L.R., Napier, B.A., and Bouville, A. (1997) Population exposure dose reconstruction for the Urals Region, in S.L. Kellogg and E.J. Kirk (eds.), *Assessing Health and Environmental Risks from Long-Term Radiation Contamination in Chelyabinsk, Russia,* American Association for the Advancement of Science, Washington, pp. 21–33.
27. Straume, T., Anspaugh, L.R., Haskell, E.H., Lucas, J.N., Marchetti, A.A., Likhtarev, I.A., Chumak, V.V., Romanyukha, A.A., Khrouch, V.T., Gavrilin, Yu.I., and Minenko, V.F. (1997) Emerging technological bases for retrospective dosimetry, *Stem Cells* **15**(Suppl. 2), 183–193.
28. National Research Council (1995) *Radiation Dose Reconstruction for Epidemiologic Uses,* National Academy Press, Washington.
29. Kozheurov, V.P. (1994) SICH-9.1—a unique whole-body counting system for measuring Sr-90 via bremsstrahlung. The main results from a long-term investigation of the Techa River population, *Sci. Total Environ.* **142**, 37–48.
30. Lucas, J.N., Hill, F., Burk, C., Fester, T., and Straume, T. (1995) Dose-response curve for chromosome translocations measured in human lymphocytes exposed to ^{60}Co gamma rays, *Health Phys.* **68**, 761–765.
31. Haskell, E.H., Kenner, G.H., and Hayes, R.B. (1995) Electron paramagnetic resonance dosimetry of dentine following removal of organic material, *Health Phys.* **68**, 579–584.
32. Gilbert, E.S., Fix, J.J., and Baumgartner, W.V. (1996) An approach to evaluating bias and uncertainty in estimates of external dose obtained from personal dosimeters, *Health Phys.* **70**, 336–345.

33. Maruyama, T., Kumamoto, Y., Ichikawa, Y., Nagatomo, T., Hoshi, M., Haskell, E., and Kaipa, P. (1987) Thermoluminescence measurements of gamma rays, in [6], Vol. 1, pp. 143–184.
34. Haskell, E.H., Bailiff, I.K., Kenner, G.H., Kaipa, P.L., and Wrenn, M.E. (1994) Thermoluminescence measurements of gamma-ray doses attributable to fallout from the Nevada Test Site using building bricks as natural dosimeters, *Health Phys.* **66**, 380–391.
35. Bougrov, N.G., Vlasov, V.K., Kiryukhin, O.V., and Fatkulbayanova, N.L. (1995) Thermoluminescence measurements of ceramic samples from accidentally polluted territory of Southern Urals, *Radiat. Meas.* **24**, 493–498.
36. U.N. Scientific Committee on the Effects of Atomic Radiation. (1962) *Report of the United Nations Scientific Committee on the Effects of Atomic Radiation,* United Nations, New York, General Assembly, Official Records: Seventeenth Session, Supplement No. 16 (A/5216).
37. Beck, H.L. (1980) *Exposure Rate Conversion Factors for Radionuclides Deposited on the Ground,* U.S. Department of Energy Environmental Measurements Laboratory, New York, EML–378.
38. Eckerman, K.F. and Ryman, J.C. (1993) *External Exposure to Radionuclides in Air, Water, and Soil. Federal Guidance Report No. 12.* Environmental Protection Agency, Washington, EPA 402-R-93-081.
39. Hicks, H.G. (1990) Additional calculations of radionuclide production following nuclear explosions and Pu isotopic ratios for Nevada Test Site events, *Health Phys.* **59**, 515–523.
40. Beck, H.L., and Anspaugh, L.R. (1991) *Development of the County Database: Estimates of Exposure Rates and Times of Arrival of Fallout in the ORERP Phase-II Area. Comparison with Cumulative Deposition-Density Estimates Bases on Analyses of Retrospective and Historical Soil Samples,* U.S. Department of Energy Nevada Operations Office, Las Vegas, DOE/NV–320.
41. Straume, T., Marchetti, A.A., Anspaugh, L.R., Khrouch, V.T., Gavrilin, Y.I., Shinkarev, S.M., Drozdovitch, V.V., Ulanovsky, A.V., Korneev, S.V., Brekeshev, M.K., Leonov, E.S., Voigt, G., Panchenko, S.V., and Minenko, V.F. (1996) The feasibility of using ^{129}I to reconstruct ^{131}I deposition from the Chernobyl reactor accident, *Health Phys.* **71**, 733–740.
42. Straume, T., Marchetti, A.A., and McAninch, J.E. (1996) New analytical capability may provide solution to the neutron dosimetry problem in Hiroshima, Radiat. Prot. Dosim. 67, 568–582.
43. WHO (1983) *Environmental Health Criteria 25. Selected Radionuclides: Tritium, Carbon-14, Krypton-85, Strontium-90, Iodine, Caesium-137, Radon, Plutonium,* World Health Organization, Geneva.
44. IAEA (1985) *The Radiological Impact of Radionuclides Dispersed on a Regional and Global Scale: Methods for Assessment and their Application,* International Atomic Energy Agency, Vienna, Technical Reports Series No. 250.
45. Loewe, W.E. and Mendelsohn, E. (1981) Revised dose estimates at Hiroshima and Nagasaki, *Health Phys.* **42**, 663–666.
46. Osanov, D.P. and Krjuchkov, V.P. (1995) The external doses from gamma-radiation, received by personnel involved in the mitigation of the Chernobyl accident, paper presented at the World Health Organisation's International Conference on Health Consequences of the Chernobyl and Other Radiological Accidents, November 20–23, 1995, Geneva.
47. Kryuchkov, V.P. and Nosovskii, A., (eds.) (1996) Retrospective Dosimetry of Accident Remediation Personnel at the Chernobyl Nuclear Power Plant, SEDA-STIL, Kiev.
48. Barabanova, A. and Nadejina, N.M. (1996) Diagnosis and prognosis of radiation injury to skin, in [21], p. 599.

PHYSICAL AND RADIOBIOLOGICAL CONSIDERATIONS IN EYE DOSIMETRY

M. W. CHARLES
School of Physics & Astronomy, University of Birmingham, Edgbaston,Birmingham, B15 2TT, United Kingdom

Abstract

The most important parameters in radiological protection related to irradiation of superficial tissues are the nature and depth of the cls at risk 11and the depth dose distribution to which they are subjected. This general problem is discussed in the context of exposure of the skin, testes and eye. In the case of the eye a survey of the radiobiological literature concerning animals and humans shows that the epithelial cells of the equatorial region of the lens are those which are involved in cataract induction. The depth of equatorial cells of the lens has been evaluated in the human eye by means of geometrical construction. The relevant dimensions have been determined from a survey of anatomical data supplemented by slit image photography and ultrasonic measurements. In a normal adult working population the minimum depth of equatorial epithelial cells in the lens range from 1.8 to 2.9 mm. The upper and lower values are associated with young and old subjects respectively. Calculations for Sr/Y-90 and Ru/Rh-106 isotropic beta sources give an indication of the range of doses to the target cells which are incurred in a working population - taking account of age dependence and variations in individual eye morphology. Calculations indicate that a planar dosemeter which integrates the tissue dose between depths of 2.5-3.5 mm should give a reasonable measure of the mean equatorial dose. The peak dose may be up to 50% higher. In situations where exposure arises from mixed fission products the dose to the lens is likely to be several times less than the surface/skin dose and several times more than the dose at a depth of 1 cm which is relevant to the evaluation of whole body exposure. The relationship between skin, eye and whole body dose will however be very dependent upon several factors including the particular mixture of radionuclides, the geometry of the source and environment, and the extent of fission product aging. To provide a prognosis in the case of an over exposure each of these factors need to be assessed on an individual basis. Because of the non-uniform exposure of the equatorial cells of the eye lens in beta radiation fields the cataract induction experience of cohorts such as the Japanese bomb survivors may not necessarily be directly applicable to nuclear industry workers exposed to fission and neutron activation products. In the case of acute high dose eye exposures, particularly from weakly penetrating radiations (including hot particle exposures) the possibility of

A. K. Junk et al. (eds.),
***Ocular Radiation Risk Assessment in Populations Exposed to Environmental Radiation Contamination*, 99–113.**

corneal ulceration is likely to be of greatest concern. In the absence of more definitive information it would appear to be defensible to treat this situation, in terms of dose evaluation, in the same way as for skin exposure.

1. Introduction - doses to superficial tissues

For radiological protection purposes the superficial tissues need special consideration because they are subject to external irradiation from weakly penetrating radiations in addition to penetrating radiations which lead to exposure of the majority of deeper lying body organs. In environments contaminated by fission products and neutron activation products the weakly penetrating radiation is primarily composed of electrons arising from beta emitting radionuclides and electrons arising from photon absorption and scattering. The dose to superficial tissues may be very much greater than to deeper lying tissues. Charles [3] for example has measured depth dose distributions in irradiated fuel storage areas (cooling ponds) of British Magnox nuclear reactors using stacks of LiF-in-teflon thermoluminescence (TL) dosemeters. The work areas were contaminated primarily with mixed fission products (Ru/Rh-106, Ce/Pr-144, Sr/Y-90, Cs-134/137, Eu-154/5, Zr/Nb-95, etc) and at lower levels with some neutron activation products such as Co-60, Ta-182, Mn-54, etc The absorbed dose at the surface was typically 4 times higher than the dose at 3 mm. Depth doses could be explained quantitatively in most cases in terms of levels of radionuclides measured using gamma (GeLi) spectroscopy. In some cases discrepancies between measured and calculated depth doses was explained in terms of the presence of the pure beta emitter Sr/Y-90, which was confirmed by radiochemical analysis of surface contamination swabs. Fuel elements were present in the storage ponds, prior to reprocessing, for periods up to 2-3 years and as a result the shorter lived, high energy beta emitters, were depleted compared to short cooled fuel. Figure 1 gives typical results of depth doses measured on a phantom in several locations. The results are expressed relative to the measurements obtained with a commonly used dosemeter (LiF in a PVC sachet) which was used for the nominal measurement of the skin and the eye dose of workers in these areas. The dosemeter produced an average dose evaluation over depths of 150 - 450 microns, somewhat deeper than the 70 microns recommended by the ICRP for the skin and shallower than the depth relevant to the eye lens. One of the conclusions of this study was that in this situation the PVC dosemeter was probably adequate for general skin dosimetry but significantly over estimated eye dose. The use of a thicker window on the PVC dosemeter or a correction factor for the evaluation of eye dose was recommended in order to avoid excessive over estimation. The film badge, which has been widely used as a personal dosemeter in the UK for many years, has a 3 mm plastic filter which makes it a useful indicator of eye dose, although it is designed to be worn on the chest.

Osanov et al [26] carried out similar measurements around the Chernobyl reactor complex in the summer of 1986. Measurements were carried out on phantoms in a number of locations using stacks of LiF TL dosemeters. Direct measurements were made on workers using special 3 - element personal TL dosemeters. Depth dose data showed a wide variation which was related to the geometry of the irradiation and the location. At a distance of 300 m from the destroyed reactor the surface dose on a phantom was about 4 and 30 times more than the dose at 3 mm and 10 mm respectively. In the engine room of units 3 and 4 the surface dose was about 2 and 4 times higher than the dose at 3 mm and 10 mm respectively. Depth doses on personnel (reconnaissance crew and workers who repaired reconnaissance vehicles) showed surface doses which were about 2 - 3 times more than doses at a depth of 2 mm. Figure 2 which shows depth dose data from the roof of unit 3 is typical of the extensive measurements made by Osanov. In this case the doses at depths of less than 5 mm (500 mg cm^{-2}) were interpreted as being due to beta radiation with maximum energies ranging from 1 to 3 MeV and photons with an effective energy of 25 keV. At the time of the measurement the fission products had penetrated into the roof bitumen which had been softened by solar heating. The resultant reduction in beta dose rate was considered to be the reason for the relatively low ratio of surface dose to dose at 10 mm.

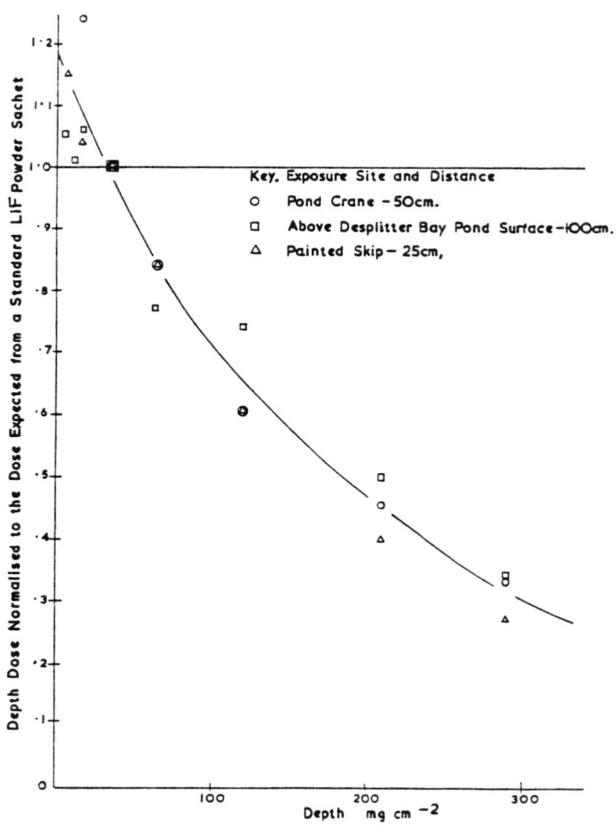

Figure 1. Depth dose data in Magnox reactor cooling pond areas. Measurements have bben normalised to the value obtained with a commonly used 'PVC' sachet' TL dosemeter which evaluates the dose between depths of 150 - 450 microns.

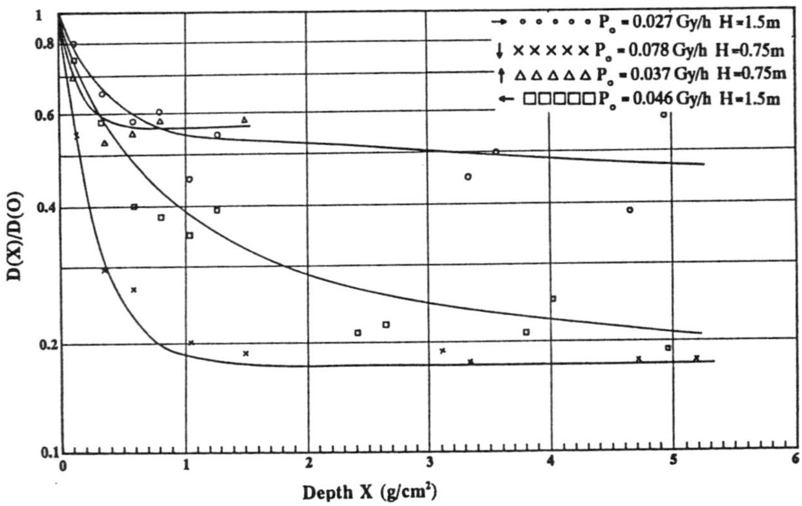

Figure 2. Depth dose data on the roof of unit 3 of the Chernobyl reactor; summer 1986 [26]. The symbols ↑ ↓ → ← correspond to the direction of a normal to the surface of the entrance window of the detector

2. Radiological protection criteria for weakly penetrating radiation

External radiation is termed weakly penetrating if the dose equivalent to the skin or the eye lens are closer to their limits than the effective dose is to its limit [12]. With the current recommended annual dose limits of 500, 150 and 20 mSv for the skin, eye and whole body respectively [17] most beta radiations, other than a few very high energy sources, are weakly penetrating. In situations where the radiation field is dominated by beta radiation the limiting radiological hazard may be due to exposure of the superficial organs which includes the testes as well as the skin and eye (Figure 3). Figure 4 gives some typical depth doses in tissue from plane sources of beta contamination at a tissue - air interface with a superimposed cross section of the eye. Beta radiations with energies below about 0.6 MeV cannot reach the equatorial cells of the lens. As the beta energy is progressively increased the equatorial cells are irradiated and the ratio of eye dose to skin dose increases. The ICRU [13] have recently reviewed the dosimetry of beta radiation for radiation protection in a report which emphasises the importance of skin exposure. The emphasis on the skin is because, on the basis of the latest ICRP dose limits, for isotropic exposure, the dose limit for the skin should adequately protect the lens and the testes for all but a few very high energy beta emitters such as Cl-38, Rb-88 & N-16 with Emax 4.9, 5.3 & 10.4 MeV respectively. These considerations may well be appropriate for radiological protection applications where doses are maintained below the dose limits. In over exposure situations however, such as an acute high dose exposure from fission product contamination, there may be a high probability of overt deterministic damage to all superficial organs. To provide a clinical prognosis a detailed scientific evaluation will be necessary which takes into account more realistic information regarding the depth dose distribution in the exposed tissue and more realistic information on the depth of target cells for the range of early and late effects which may be induced in the skin, eye and testes.

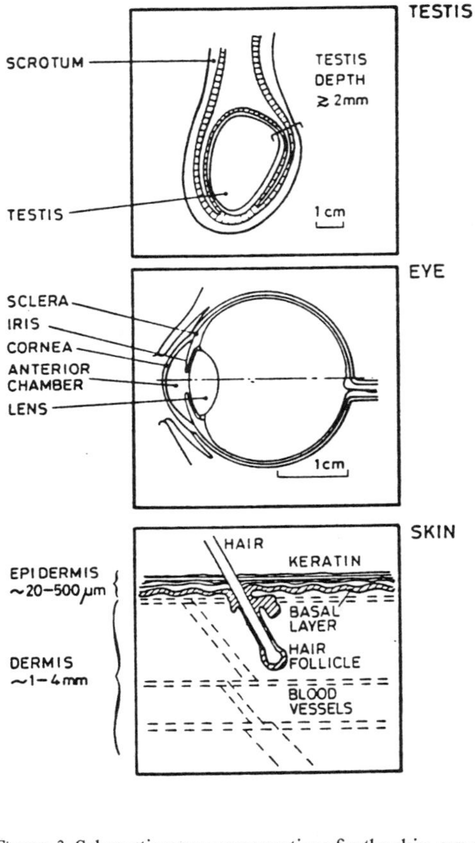

Figure 3. Schematic organ cross sections for the skin, eye and testes.

In the case of an acute exposure of the eye, particularly with weakly penetrating radiation, it is necessary to take account of the very high surface doses which may be received by the cornea even when the lens dose is below the threshold for cataract induction. Merriam et al [24] have reviewed the radiation sensitivity of different parts of the eye and concluded that effects of dose fractionation on corneal ulceration were similar to those for moist desquamation in the skin. The threshold dose for an acute exposure to produce a corneal ulceration is about 20 Gy, which is similar to that for skin ulceration. The cornea is about 500 microns thick and consists primarily of connective tissue. Its anterior and posterior surfaces are lined with single layers of epithelial and endothelial cells respectively. These cells maintain the corneal integrity and play a primary role in repair of corneal damage. If both layers are breached there is the possibility of a severe response, even eye loss. In the absence of more definitive data the use of a skin dosemeter for the control of corneal dose would appear to be appropriate. A specific case of acute corneal exposure is that which might arise from 'hot particles' which are small particles of radioactive material. They represent a skin exposure hazard in all nuclear reactor operations [5]. Recommendations for the limitation of hot particle exposures to the skin have been given by the ICRP [17, 18]. No consideration was given to the hazard posed by hot particles which might be lodged in the anterior part of the eye, possibly because no case seems to have been reported in the scientific literature. The possibility of such exposures obviously exists and needs to be considered. Because of the great fall off in dose with distance around a hot particle the dose to the cornea is likely to be more important than the possible lens dose. In the absence of more authoritative data the ICRP guide lines for hot particle exposure of the skin provide a defensible limitation rationale for hot particle exposures of the eye.

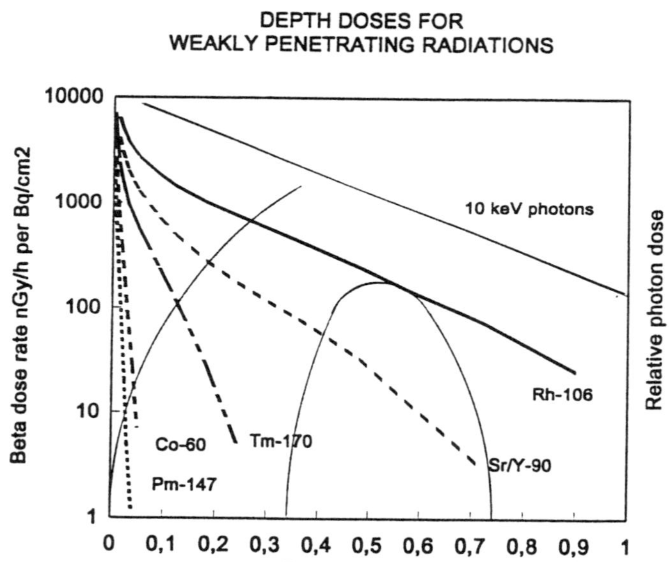

Figure 4. Depth doses in tissue for several thin beta sources at the surface of a semi-infinite tissue-air interface. Superimposed to scale is a cross section of the eye. Beta end point energies (MeV) are: Pm-147, 0.225; Co-60, 0.318; Tm-170, 0.968; Sr/Y-90, 2.281; Rh-106, 3.540. (Data from ICRU 56).

3. Anatomy, radiobiology & dosimetry

It is the skin which most often receives the most significant exposure because important target cells are very near to the skin surface. Epidermal basal cells within 20-100 microns of the skin surface have been implicated in radiation induced skin cancer. Deterministic effects such as early moist desquamation, early dermal necrosis and late damage such as fibrosis have been associated with target cells at depths from

300 - 1000 microns [13, 18]. The ICRP [17] however have recommended that for general applications the dose equivalent should be determined at a nominal depth of 70 microns.

Because of the planar geometry of the skin it is relatively straightforward to interpret skin radiobiology data in terms of the depths of particular target cell populations and to prescribe an anthropomorphic dosemeter design consisting of appropriate thicknesses of planar window and detector. This is not the case for the testes or the eye because of the non-planar morphology of the organs. In these cases it can be useful to define an 'effective depth' as that depth in a planar dosemeter with the same dose as the mean value to the relevant target cell population. For exposure of the testes the limiting biological effect is mutation which can lead to hereditary effects. No separate dose limit is given by the ICRP for the testes but the tissue weighting factor of 0.2 implies an annual organ dose limit of 100 mSv based on the annual effective dose limit of 20 mSv. The ICRP consider that the mean equivalent dose to spermatogonial cells is the relevant dosimetric parameter. These cells are at depths between 2 mm to greater than 15 mm and the effective depth varies from about 3 mm to 8 mm as the maximum beta energy increases from 1 to 3 MeV [9]. For chronic exposure of the eye, cataract induction is considered to be the end point of concern for radiological protection. The most recent statement by the ICRP [15] regarding the effective depth of the lens implies that the equatorial cells of the lens are the target cells for cataract induction and that the depth of the lens can be considered to be 3 mm. In fact, some equatorial cells can be at depths as shallow as 2 mm. So, like the testes, the minimum beta energy which is capable of external irradiation of the target cells is about 0.6 MeV. For beta emitters with a maximum beta energy (Emax) between 2 and 3.5 MeV Charles and Brown [4] calculated an effective lens depth of between 2.5 - 3.5 mm, taking into account shielding by the eyelids and the variations in eye morphology with age in a normal population. The calculation is summarised in appendix A. It was also assumed that the equatorial cells are the target cells for cataract induction and that it is the mean equatorial dose which is the relevant dosimetric parameter. These assumptions are reviewed in appendix B.

4. ICRP statements regarding the eye dose limit

The ICRP annual dose limit for the eye has been changed over the past 50 years probably more than for any other organ, but not necessarily on a logical basis. In ICRP publication 26 [14] the annual dose limit was increased without explanation from 150 mSv to 300 mSv. A critique of this increase [6] led to the setting up of an ICRP task group of which the author was a member. An annual dose limit of 300 mSv over a working lifetime of say 40 years could lead to a lifetime eye dose of 12 Sv. The task group could not find any justification for the increase and indeed, on the basis primarily of the clinical data of Merriam & Focht [22, 23] the task group advised that the annual dose limit should be reduced to 100 mSv. The clinical data appeared to support a dose limit for acute exposure of low LET radiation of about 2 Sv. The clinical data indicated some sparing when the exposure was protracted over a period of up to about 3 years. The task group however considered that this evidence for sparing was not strong and could not be extrapolated to lifetime exposures with any reliability. The ICRP [15] subsequently reinstated the previous annual dose limit of 150 mSv, without explanation and without publishing the task group report. ICRP publication 41 [16] reviewed the dose limits for all deterministic effects and concluded that the then current dose limits (50 mSv whole body, 150 mSv for the eye and 500 mSv for other single organs) provided a substantial margin of safety against deterministic effects for all tissues with the exception of bone marrow, testes and lens of the eye. Since that time the ICRP [17] has recommended a reduction in the whole body (effective dose) annual limit to 20 mSv. This has the effect of restricting allowed doses to the bone marrow and the testes but the reservation made in ICRP publication 41 [16] regarding the acceptability of the 150 mSv annual dose limit for the eye remains.

5. Conclusions

Exposure of the eye lens can be significant in situations where the radiation field is dominated by beta particles from mixed fission products arising from nuclear fuel. There is strong evidence from observations in animals and man to link the exposure of the equatorial cells of the eye with subsequent cataract induction. The depth of these cells decreases with age, being greatest for young myopes and smallest for older hypermetropes. The mean dose to these cells in isotropic beta radiation fields from Sr/Y-90 and Ru/Rh-106 is the same as that which would be measured with a planar dosemeter at a depth of 2.5 - 3.5 mm. Even in an isotropic beta radiation field the equatorial cells of the eye lens will not be uniformly exposed due to the shielding provided by the eye lids and the orbit. The peak dose is about 50 % higher than the mean dose. The mean dose to these equatorial cells, rather than the peak dose, appears to be the relevant dosimetric parameter for use in radiological protection to prevent cataract induction, but evidence is not extensive. Information on threshold doses for cataract induction from studies such as the Japanese bomb survivors, where the exposure of the eye lens would have been relatively uniform, may thus not be directly appropriate for beta radiation exposure.

The non-uniform exposure of the lens which arises due to body shielding (e.g. by the nose and orbit) from beta radiation would be expected to give rise to cataract preferentially in the less well shielded lateral region of the lens equator. An ophthalmological examination of the spatial position of early opacification may thus be a useful indicator of beta radiation exposure. It may even form the basis of a crude biological dosemeter for beta radiation exposure which may provide some much needed validation for the extremely difficult task of eye dose reconstruction in situations such as those encountered by the Chernobyl Liquidators.

Measurements of depth doses in environments contaminated with mixed fission products show that the eye dose may be several times less than the more commonly measured skin dose at 70 microns and several times more than the dose at 10 mm relevant to penetrating radiation. The depth dose data are particularly sensitive to the geometrical orientation of the body/detector with respect to the radiation source and to the physical characteristics of the source which may affect the intensity and the effective energy of the radiation. Any dose reconstruction programme to provide a prognosis in the case of an individual over exposure, or as a basis for epidemiological studies, must take account of these various factors.

In the case of acute, high dose, eye exposures (including localised hot particle exposures) the possibility of corneal ulceration is likely to be of greatest concern, particularly for weakly penetrating radiations. In the absence of more definitive information it would appear to be defensible to treat this situation, in terms of dose evaluation, in the same way as for skin exposure.

References

1. Alter A and Leinfelder P J, 1953. Roentgen ray cataract. Effects of shielding of the lens and ciliary body. *AMA Arch. Ophthalmol.* **49**, 257-260.
2. Britten M J A, Halnan K E and Meredith W J, 1966. Radiation cataract: new evidence on radiation damage to the lens. *Br. J. Radiol.*, **39**, 612-617.
3. Charles M W, 1986. An assessment of the need for improved dosimetry techniques for superficial tissues. *Rad. Prot. Dos.*, **14** (2) 137-140.
4. Charles M W and Brown N, 1975. Dimensions of the human eye relevant to radiation protection. *Phys. Med. Biol.*, **20**, 202-218.
5. Charles M W, 1991. The hot particle problem. *Rad. Prot. Dos.*, **39**, 39-47.
6. Charles M W and Lindop P J, 1979. Skin and eye irradiations - Examples of problems of implementing international recommendations in radiological protection. STI/PUB/521 (Vienna, IAEA) pages 547-561.
7. Chmelevsky D, Mays C W, Spiess H, Stefani F H and Kellerer A M, 1988. An epidemiological assessment of lens opacifications that impaired vision in patients injected with radium-224. *Radiation research* **115** (2) 238-257.
8. Cross W G, 1967. Tables of beta dose distributions. Atomic Energy of Canada Ltd. Report AECL 2793.
9. Facey R A, 1982. Effective depth of spermatogonia in man. II: Calculations for external high energy beta rays. *Phys. Med. Biol.*, **27**, 1357 - 1365.
10. Goldman H and Liechti A, 1938. Experimentelle Untersuchungen ueber die Genese des Roentgenstroms. *Graefes. Arch. Clin. Exp. Ophthalmol.* **138**, 722-736.
11. Grzedzielski J, 1935. Zur Histologie der Roentgenkatarakt. *Klin. Monatsbl. Augenheilk.*, **95**, 360-369.
12. International Commission on Radiation Units and Measurements, 1993. Quantities and units in radiation protection dosimetry. ICRU Report 51. International Commission on Radiation Units and Measurements, Bethesda, Md, USA.
13. International Commission on Radiation Units and Measurements, 1997. Dosimetry of external beta rays for radiation protection. ICRU Report 56. International Commission on Radiation Units and Measurements, Bethesda, Md, USA.
14. International Commission on Radiological Protection, 1977. Recommendations of the ICRP, publication 26. *Annals of the ICRP*, **1** (3).
15. International Commission on Radiological Protection, 1978. Statement from the Stockholm meeting of the ICRP. *Annals of the ICRP*, **2** (1).
16. International Commission on Radiological Protection, 1984. Non-stochastic effects of ionising radiation, publication 41. *Annals of the ICRP*, **14** (3).
17. International Commission on Radiological Protection, 1991a. 1990 Recommendations of the ICRP, publication 60. *Annals of the ICRP*, **21** (1-3).

18. International Commission on Radiological Protection, 1991b. The Biological Basis for Dose Limitation in the Skin. ICRP Publication 59. *Annals of the ICRP* **22** (2)

19. Kimura S and Ikui H, 1951. Atomic bomb radiation cataract: Case report with histological study. *Am. J. Ophthalmol.* **34**, 811-816.

20. Leinfelder P J and Kerr H D, 1936. Roentgen-ray cataract. An experimental, clinical and microscopic study. *Amer. J. Ophthal.*, **19**, 739-756.

21. Leinfelder P J and Riley E F, 1956. Further studies of effects of x-radiation on partially shielded lens of rabbit. *AMA Arch. Ophthalmol.* **55**, 84-86.

22. Merriam G R and Focht E F, 1957. A clinical study of radiation cataracts and the relationship to dose. *Am. J. Roentgenol.***77**, 759-785.

23. Merriam and Focht, 1962. A clinical and experimental study of the effect of single and divided doses of radiation on cataract production. *Tr. Am. Ophth. Soc.*, **60**, 35-52.

24. Merriam G R, Szechter A and Focht E F, 1972. The effects of ionizing radiations on the eye. *Frontiers of Radiation Therapy and Oncology*, **6**, 346-385.

25. Okusawa T, 1933. Die experimentelle Untersuchung ueber durch Roentgenstrahlen verursachten Veraenderungen des Linsenepithels. *Acta. Soc. Ophtha. Japan*, **37**, 79-99.

26. Osanov D P, Krjuchkov V P and Shaks A I, 1993. Determination of beta radiation doses received by personnel involved in the mitigation of the Chernobyl accident, in S E Merwin and M I Balonov (eds.), *The Chernobyl papers, Vol I: Doses to the Soviet population and early health effects studies.* Research Enterprises, Richland Wa USA. pp. 313-346.

27. Pirie A and Flanders P H, 1957. Effect of x-rays on partially shielded lens of the rabbit. *AMA Arch. Ophthalmol.* **54**, 849-854.

28. Roth J, Brown N, Caterall M and Beal A, 1976. The effects of fast neutrons on the eye. *Br. J. Ophthalmol.* **60**, 236-240.

29. Scharff J P, Nekolla E, Egner P, Roos H, Wegener A, Kellerer A M, Spiess H and Stefani F H, 1994. Findings in human lenses 40 years after injection of Ra-224. *Ophthalmic Research*, **26** (S1) 73-78.

30. Supe S J and Korgaonkar, 1969. Biophysical studies of eye lens epithelium. *Science and Culture*, **35**, 524-532

31. Taylor D M and Thorne M C, 1988. The potential for irradiation of the lens and cataract induction by incorporated γ - emitting radionuclides. *Health Physics* **54** (2) 171-179.

32. Von Sallman L, Tobias C A and Anger H O, 1955. Effects of high energy particles, x-rays and aging on lens epithelium. *AMA Arch. Ophthalmol.* **54**, 489-514.

33. Worgul B V, Merriam G R, Szechter A and Dobli Srinivasan B, 1976. Lens epithelium and radiation cataract. *Arch. Ophthalmol.*, **94**, 996-999.

34. Worgul B V and Rothstein H, 1977. On the mechanism of radiocataractogenesis. *Medikon*, **6**, 5-24.

Appendix A: Evaluation of the relevant lens depth

Charles and Brown [4] combined slit image and ultra sonic data to obtain ocular dimensions as a function of age in the range 2-82 years. The 130 subjects included the assortment of myopes, emmetropes and hypermetropes to be found in a normal adult population. The following ocular dimensions were significantly dependent upon age:

Anterior lens radius /mm	16.5 - 0.10 Age ,	r = 0.74	($p<<0.001$)
Posterior lens radius /mm	8.90 - 0.02 Age ,	r = - 0.24	($p\sim 0.02$)
Lens thickness /mm	3.20 + 0.025 Age ,	r = 0.81	($p<0.001$)
Anterior chamber depth /mm	3.40 - 0.015 Age ,	r = - 0.6	($p<<0.001$)
Anterior corneal radius /mm	7.30 + 0.01 Age ,	r = 0.37	($p\sim 0.01$)

There was a highly significant positive correlation between the anterior chamber depth and the anterior lens radius of curvature. There was a highly significant negative correlation between the anterior lens radius of curvature and the lens thickness. There was no correlation between the anterior cornea radius and the anterior lens radius. There was no significant difference in the general results between males and females, and no significant difference between the left and right eye in the same subject.

On this basis it was possible to construct diagrams (figure 5) of the cross section of the eye for a 40 year old emmetrope and the extremes in a 'normal' working population (18-65 years) which can be classified as young myope and old hypermetrope. The minimum distance from equatorial cells of the lens to the anterior surface of the cornea is 2.9, 2.1 and 1.8 mm for myope, emmotrope & hypermetrope respectively. Figure 5 relates to the unaccommodated (relaxed) lens. During accommodation the depth of the equator is reduced by less than about 0.1 mm. The dose to the equator of the eye lens was calculated for isotropic beta radiation fields using the dose distributions of Cross [8]. No account was taken of absorption in air between the source and the eye surface. The shielding provided by the eyelids and the surrounding orbit was approximated by assuming complete absorption of beta radiation passing through the eye lids (figure 6). Table 1 summarises the results for Sr/Y-90 and Rh-106.

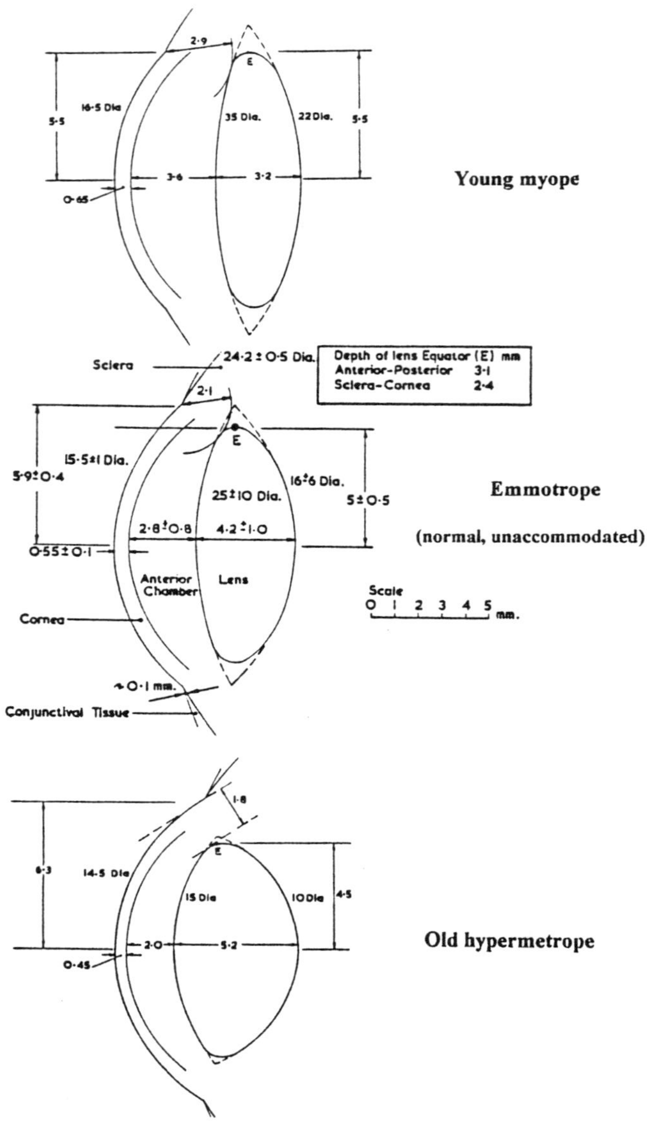

Figure 5. Cross section of the eye based on slit image and ultrasonic measurements

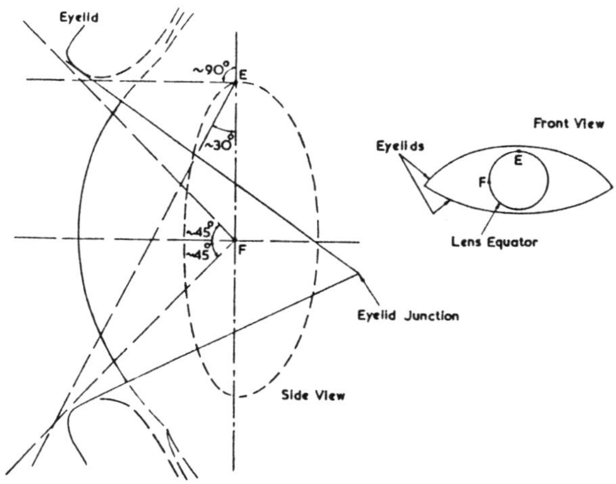

Figure 6. Eye shielding geometry

TABLE 1: DOSES TO THE LENS EQUATORIAL CELLS IN AN ISOTROPIC BETA RADIATION FIELD

			Sr/Y-90	Rh-106
DOSE TO THE EQUATORIAL CELLS OF THE EYE LENS	EMMETROPE	A*	1.0	1.0
		B*	0.2-0.7#	0.3-0.8
	MYOPE	A	0.7	0.9
		B	0.1-0.6	0.2-0.7
	HYPERMETROPE	A	1.4	1.2
		B	0.3-1.0	0.3-0.9
DOSE AT STATED DEPTH IN A PLANAR TISSUE-EQUIVALENT DOSEMETER	4 mm		0.35	0.5
	3 mm		0.65	0.7
	2 mm		1.05	0.95
	1.5 mm		1.35	1.05

A - Excluding eyelid shielding; B - Including eyelid shielding; * - The range corresponds to points E and F (figure 6) which have the minimum and maximum values of equatorial dose

Although the calculations are not precise they are indicative of the non-uniform exposure of the equatorial cells in a beta radiation field and they also indicate that a planar dosemeter which measures dose in the region of 3 mm will give a reasonable measure of the mean equatorial dose.

Appendix B: Radiobiological information regarding the cells at risk and the use of mean equatorial dose for radiological protection

Histological evidence of radiation induced damage to the lens becomes apparent within hours after exposure. These changes occur in the lens epithelium layer on the anterior surface of the lens. This is not unexpected since the epithelial layer is the major site of mitotic activity in the lens. The mitotic activity is greatest in the region called the germinative epithelium which is the outer zone near to the equator and is physically nearest to the anterior corneal surface than any other part of the lens (figure 5). At the equator the epithelial cells differentiate into lens fibres. Studies by von Sallmann et al [32] using the rabbit eye have shown that initial cellular damage is seen in the germinative zone many days before any clinically visible changes can be detected in the animal. Goldman and Liechti [10] appear to have been the first to demonstrate that radiation damage to the equatorial region of the lens is a prerequisite for cataract induction. They utilised a narrow beam of X-rays to irradiate selected portions of the rabbit lens and found that cataract formation occurred only when the equatorial regions of the lens were irradiated. Similar findings from selective exposure of different regions of the rabbit lens have been reported for deuteron [32] and for Sr/Y-90 beta radiations [30]. More recently a range of studies by Worgul et al have strengthened the evidence for the initial involvement of the epithelial cell damage in the induction of radiation cataract in rodents [33, 34].

Evidence for initial radiation induced damage to the equatorial region of the lens has also been reported in histological studies of cataract in man. Early X-ray studies were reported by Okusawa [25], Grzedzielski [11] and Leinfelder and Kerr [20]. Kimura and Ikui [19] found evidence in Japanese bomb survivors following cataract extraction, as did Roth et al [28] in UK neutron radiotherapy patients. The development of cataract in patients receiving injections of Ra-224 for the treatment of tuberculosis or ankylosing spondylitis [7, 29] also strongly implicates the major role played by exposure of the germinative epithelium of the lens. There is preferential uptake of Ra-224 (and other alpha emitters) in the iris and its proximity to the anterior lens surface is such that the germinative epithelium is just within range of the alpha particles emitted from Ra-224 and its daughter products. Taylor and Thorne [31] have shown that the uptake of Ra-224 in the iris is at a level such that epithelial doses can be predicted which are compatible with a causal link between Ra-224 administration and cataract incidence.

Evidence for the primary role of the equatorial region of the lens in radiation induced cataract is therefore compelling. What is not so obvious is the choice of an appropriate dosimetric parameter for limiting lens exposure in radiological protection situations or for the purpose of providing a prognosis in cases of over-exposure. Alter and Lienfelder [1] and Leinfelder and Riley [21] shielded part of the lens of rabbits during X-ray exposure to show that cataract formed only if the equatorial zone was irradiated and not at all if only the central part of the lens was irradiated. The shielding of 1 or 2 quadrants of the lens prevented progression to total cataract even at dose levels up to 4 times that which would produce a total cataract if the entire lens was exposed. Pirie and Flanders [27] found that shielding one quarter of the germinative zone of the rabbit lens produced only minor cortical opacities at dose levels which produced a complete cataract if the whole of the zone was exposed. Evidence from radiotherapy patients also indicates that non-uniform exposure of the lens increases the threshold dose for cataract induction [2]. These findings do not support the use of peak dose (maximum dose) to some limited part of the lens as an indicator of potential cataract induction. Some kind of dose averaging is obviously appropriate. The evaluation of the mean dose to the whole of the peripheral equatorial region of the lens, as carried out in appendix A, is the most straightforward approach and is not incompatible with the available but limited experimental data.

DOSIMETRY, DOSE RECONSTRUCTION AND EPIDEMIOLOGY: LESSONS FROM RADPATH, RADTEST AND RELATED STUDIES

L.J.APPLEBY, E.H.VOICE, F.E.WARNER
SCOPE-RADTEST
Department of Biological and Chemical Sciences, John Tabor Laboratories, University of Essex, Wivenhoe Park, Colchester, CO4 3SQ, UK

1. Abstract

RADPATH and RADTEST are successive SCOPE-ICSU studies of man-made radionuclides in our environment. RADPATH examined the principal sources and biogeochemical pathways of released radioactivity while RADTEST concentrates on the dispersion, deposition and human health effects of fallout from nuclear weapons tests. Together the projects have come up with much valuable data and conclusions on dosimetry, dose reconstruction and the health impact of high and low doses of ionising radiation.

2. Introduction

RADPATH[1] and RADTEST[2] are successive SCOPE-ICSU[3] studies of man-made radionuclides in the world environment. They evolved from the earlier SCOPE project, ENUWAR[4], which researched the environmental consequences of nuclear war. RADPATH (1988-1993), prompted by the Chernobyl reactor accident of 1986, examined the principal sources and environmental pathways of released man-made radionuclides. Chernobyl had provided an unexpected source of data on the large-scale movement of radionuclides in a range of environmental compartments, as well as a unique opportunity to study a major accident's long-term consequences. Both the ENUWAR and RADPATH projects led to the publication of books in the SCOPE series [4, 5, 9].

When assessing Chernobyl's activity release it was clear that while large compared with previous reactor releases it totalled less than one percent of the radioactive fallout from atmospheric nuclear weapons testing in the 1950s and '60s. The subsequent project, RADTEST (1993 -) entered this field, studying the dispersion and deposition of fallout

(1) RADPATH: man-made RADionuclide biogeochemical PATHways
(2) RADTEST: RADiation from nuclear TEST explosions
(3) SCOPE: Scientific Committee on Problems of the Environment
ICSU: International Council of Scientific Unions
(4) ENUWAR: Environmental consequences of NUclear WAR

A. K. Junk et al. (eds.),
Ocular Radiation Risk Assessment in Populations Exposed to Environmental Radiation Contamination, 115–120.

from bomb-testing but moving a step further to focus on the human health consequences. All major testing areas have been considered, including the US Nevada Test Site, the Pacific sites at Enewetak and the Marshall Islands, the South Pacific sites of Mururoa and Fangataufa, the FSU sites at Semipalatinsk and Novaya Zemlya, and the Australian sites at Emu, Maralinga and Montebello.

RADPATH and RADTEST have identified much valuable information relating to dosimetry, dose reconstruction and epidemiology. This paper discusses these developments, looks at the health impact of ionising radiation and considers the implications of risk assessment.

3. Dosimetry

The publication "SCOPE 50" [9] discussed radiation dosimetry, the process of determining the energy absorbed in a specific target from a radiation field. For living organisms this can be complex. For example, in waste disposal operations or in accidents the distribution of radionuclides, and thus the incident field, can be both externally and internally variable in space and time, especially with a mobile animal. Direct or indirect instrumental measurements are seldom possible and computational estimates are usually needed for the dose rate to a given target.

The incident radiation field can be gamma rays, X-rays, beta and alpha particles - and often mixtures of two or more - which have path lengths in tissue ranging from metres down to 0.1mm. The nature and energy of the radiation determines the processes by which energy is absorbed in the target tissue. The theory of energy deposition along the radiation path is complex, and more simple empirical formulae have been developed to describe dose distributions around point sources. Using these to calculate dose rates on a pattern of points within the target, an estimate of the mean dose rate to a given tissue is possible.

For a given absorbed energy dose the different forms of radiation have different effects, related to the ionisation density of the track. This can be defined as the "relative biological effectiveness", RBE of a particular radiation:

$$\mathrm{RBE} = \frac{\text{Absorbed dose of 250 keV X-rays to produce a given biological effect}}{\text{Absorbed dose of specified radiation to produce the same effect}} \qquad (1)$$

But experimentally it is found that the RBE value for a given form of radiation varies with the particular biological effect chosen and also with the dose rate. Hence for a general perception of biological dose an additional Quality Factor (QF) has to be defined, independent of specific biological effect and dose rate.

For all these reasons dosimetric information relating to short-lived fallout nuclides is generally limited, with large uncertainties and errors. If specific quantitative indicators of dose could be found in the human body, confirmation might be possible. Two present techniques based on stable signals are Fluorescent In-Situ Hybridisation (FISH) and Electron Spin Resonance (ESR). In FISH, stable chromosome translocations which are not associated with changed numbers of centromeres per chromosome are visualised, while in ESR radiation-induced persistent changes in tooth enamel and dentin are measured. By their sophistication and complexity these techniques are limited to specialist laboratories.

A biological indicator which could be a stable deterministic endpoint is lens opacification. The special character of optical risk from ionising radiation is that damage may result from changes not part of the progression from DNA damage, which can either be repaired or leads to tumours. With low doses, DNA repair mechanisms may result in lower risks than those estimated by linear extrapolation from high doses. This uncertainty may be illuminated by data from ocular risk.

The difficulties with low doses cannot be resolved by epidemiology when stochastic processes are involved. A discussion on Extrapolation of Dose Response Data for Risk Assessment held at the Royal Society in July 1995 has a number of relevant papers [2, 3].

4. Dose Reconstruction

RADTEST has examined the status of dose reconstruction at the main nuclear test sites. These are Nevada and the Pacific for US explosions, Semipalatinsk and Novaya Zemlya for Russia, Lop Nor for China, Mururoa and Fangataufa for France and the UK's Australian sites. Levels of information vary and the wartime explosions in Japan are not considered.

There are four major dose reconstruction studies:

4.1 ORREP: Off-site Radiation Exposure Review Project.
4.2 The Utah leukaemia case-control study.
4.3 The Utah thyroid cohort study.
4.4 National Cancer Institute fallout study.

ORERP collected and organised documents and offsite fallout data for a dosimetric revaluation of the offsite area [1]. The total collective exposure was estimated at 80,000 person-R, with the largest contribution from the 1953 and 1955 test series.

The Utah leukaemia case-control study was designed to validate earlier indications of excess childhood leukaemia in Southern Utah following weapons tests in Nevada. Median dose for both cases and controls was estimated as 3 mGy.

The Utah thyroid cohort study followed earlier work locating and examining a cohort for thyroid disease including neoplasms. The importance of milk consumption was clear with a mean dose of 12 mGy to non-milk drinkers but up to 100 mGy for milk drinkers. The importance of radioiodine exposure in utero was also clear.

The National Cancer Institute study assessed ^{131}I fallout exposure from the Nevada tests. The estimated collective thyroid dose to the American population was 4 x 10^6 person-Gy.

Of the US tests in the Pacific, radiation doses at Bikini and Enewetak were most important. Results from the very large number of environmental measurements show ^{137}Cs contaminated food to have been the chief source of the radiation dose to humans. Average whole-body doses to Bikini residents between 1971 and 1978 were 2 to 3 mSv per year.

The four most polluting explosions at Semipalatinsk were those in 1949, 1951, 1953 and 1956, accounting for 95% of the radiation exposure of inhabitants near the site. In the Altai region to the North East of the site the collective effective population dose is 42,000 man-Sv.

There is little information on local and regional doses from the nuclear tests on Novaya Zemlya. The local Integrated Research Project covers radiation, seismic, sanitary and ecological conditions but has not yet published its work. Reindeer herders form the critical population in the lichen-reindeer-human foodchain, and their internal dose-rates are estimated to average 1 mSv per year since the 1960s. Doses to urban inhabitants are a hundred times less.

Little is known of dose-reconstruction in China at the Lop Nor site. The average absorbed dose in air outdoors is 0.18 mGy, giving a mean effective dose of 0.044 mSv for populations 400 to 800 km downwind of the test site.

No information is publically available for the French test site in the Sahara. In the South Pacific, French tests at Mururoa and Fangataufa are reported to have given external radiation doses from 1 to 10 microSievert in 1982 and less than 4 microSievert in 1995.

From the whole series of UK tests in Australia at Emu Field, Maralinga and Montebello Island the average individual dose equivalent totalled 0.07 mSv.

Finally, the collective effective dose commitment to the world's population of all atmospheric nuclear weapon testing is estimated to be 3 x 10^7 man-Sv [8].

5. Epidemiology

It appears from RADTEST that doses and dose-rates from local fallout have mostly been restricted to stochastic effects. Nevertheless some cohorts' thyroid and skin doses have reached levels causing deterministic effects, notably in the Pacific and in the first Semipalatinsk test. It seems that in these situations lens opacification could be a stable deterministic endpoint.

Can epidemiology, besides estimating present and future exposure risks, also extend our knowledge of radiation risk factors? To do this, accurate dose estimates for the affected populations are needed, with their health records in a consistent format over a long period.

The population movement should be limited, with little migration, and there needs to be a high level of cooperation. There could be great benefits from such studies.

Two recent University of Utah investigations of cancer and thyroid disease downwind of the Nevada test site have not added greatly to our knowledge of radiation-related risk. RADTEST concluded that it is difficult to quantify the small risk of low radiation doses by studying the exposed populations.

At the US Bravo test in the Pacific most of the dose was from short-lived fission products, with acute effects such as prodromal syndrome, conjunctivitis, skin lesions and epilations. Haematological changes were consistent with the estimated doses.

In the Altai region near Semipalatinsk a register of the irradiated population totalled 40,255 individuals. Much data has accumulated following the test of 29 August 1949, particularly mortality rates and causes of death. For example, men older than 20 years at time of exposure had higher risk of malignant tumour mortality during the next 24 years. Extensive lens opacification has been reported among those receiving doses of 1.5 to 2 Gy. The mortality risk from non-malignant disease was not elevated. The maximum risk coefficients were between 1958 and 1978 - that is, 9 to 29 years after exposure.

Before the tests in Novaya Zemlya the population was evacuated and there were no acute exposures. Fallout deposition, mostly of ^{137}Cs and ^{90}Sr, in territories beyond 60°N led to internal exposures in reindeer breeding communities up to 10 mSv effective dose in areas contaminated to the extent of 3.7×10^9 Bq km^{-3}.

At the three Australian sites collective dose to the local population is estimated at 700 person-Sv, with the plutonium dispersed from non-nuclear explosions causing a long-term problem.

The radiological impact of the French weapons testing totalled around 3% of the world's atmospheric tests. Their local impact was limited by the testing technique and has never given dose rates above 1 mGy per hour.

At Lop Nor unshielded exposures were up to 2 mGy, with internal doses from ^{90}Sr and ^{131}I too low for measurable health effects.

For the world population, the additional dose rates and annual doses have always been only a small fraction of natural exposure, and the overall associated risk remains too small to be observed. For radiation protection in the workplace or in medical treatment, risk assessments must rely on epidemiological data from cohorts in situations untypical for normal circumstances. Differences in effects per unit absorbed dose between acute and chronic exposures are large for most biological endpoints in experimental systems. Thus studies of local exposures from nuclear weapons tests may help to improve the human data base and quantified lens opacification could contribute significantly to dose reconstruction.

6. References

1. Church, B.W., Wheeler, D.L., Campbell, C.M., Nutley, R.V., Anspaugh, L.R. (1990) Overview of the Department of Energy's Off-Site Radiation Exposure Review Project (ORERP), *Health Phys.*, **59**, 503-510.

2. Chadwick, K.H. and Leenhouts H.P. (1995) Multi-step Carcinogenesis and Implications for Low Dose Radiation Risk Philosophy, Extrapolation of Dose Response Data for Risk Assessment, Supplement to Process Safety and Environmental Protection, *Transactions of IChemE*, Part B, **73** (B4), S18-S23.

3. Doll, R. (1995) Assessment of Risk from Low Doses: Contribution of Epidemiology, Extrapolation of Dose Response Data for Risk Assessment, Supplement to Process Safety and Environmental Protection, *Transactions of IChemE*, Part B, **73** (B4), S8-S11.

4. Harwell, M.A. and Hutchinson, T.C. (eds.) (1989) The Environmental Consequences of Nuclear War, SCOPE 28, Vol. II, Ecological and Agricultural Effects, Second Edition, John Wiley and Sons Ltd., Chichester.

5. Pittock, A.B., Ackerman, T.P., Crutzen, P.J., MacCracken, M.C., Shapiro C.S. and Turco, R.P. (eds.) (1989) The Environmental Consequences of Nuclear War, SCOPE 28 Vol. I, Physical and Atmospheric Effects, Second Edition John Wiley & Sons Ltd., Chichester.

6. Shapiro, C.S. (ed.) (1987) Environmental and Human Consequences of Atmospheric Nuclear Tests: A NATO/SCOPE-RADTEST Advanced Research Workshop, held at the International Atomic Energy Agency (IAEA), Vienna, Austria (10-14 January, 1994), Springer, Heidelburg, (submitted).

7. Shapiro, C.S., Kiselev, V.I., Zaitsev E.V. (eds.) (1997) Long-term Consequences of Nuclear Tests for the Environment and Population Health (Semipalatinsk/Altai Case Study): A NATO/SCOPE-RADTEST Advanced Research Workshop, Barnaul, Siberia, Russian (5-9 September, 1994), Springer, Heidelburg, (submitted).

8. UNSCEAR (1993) Sources and Effects of Ionizing Radiation. United Nations Scientific Committee on the Effects of Atomic Radiation, UNSCEAR 1993 Report to the General Assembly, with Scientific Annexes. United Nations, New York.

9. Warner F.E. and Harrison, R.M. (eds.) (1993) Radioecology after Chernobyl (Biogeochemical Pathways of Artificial Radionuclides), SCOPE 50, John Wiley and Sons Ltd., Chichester.

METHODOLOGIES - STRENGTHS AND WEAKNESSES

A View on the Dosimetric Support for the Chernobyl Liquidator Eye Cataract Study

V.V.CHUMAK
Ukrainian Radiation Protection Institute ATS Ukraine
Scientific Center of Radiation Medicine AMS Ukraine
Melnikova 53, 254050, Kiev, Ukraine

1. Introduction

Obviously, any meaningful study of radiation induced health effects depends on knowledge of the doses received by the subjects. Therefore, the design of a dosimetric protocol to support such research is of critical importance. In general, approaches to implement the dosimetry segment of an epidemiological project depend significantly on the particulars of the population under study.

It is commonly accepted that Chernobyl clean-up workers (Liquidators), involved in the early years after the accident, are highly attractive subjects for the study of late radiation effect.. This large population had received, as a rule, moderate doses (although, the highest among the cohorts exposed after Chernobyl) in rather protracted way. The age and gender distribution in this population is more representative (regarding radiation protection issues) than in the A-bomb survivor population.

However, from the dosimetric standpoint, the Liquidator population is very complicated and many problems must be addressed prior to the implementation of the dosimetric protocol for an epidemiological follow up. In contrast to modern nuclear plant worker or radiotherapy patient records, there are very few reliable individual dose data; and, not infrequently, those that are available are incomplete or their quality is doubtful. Moreover, practically all available dosimetric data is related to external whole-body gamma exposure, whereas for some tissues (i.e. eye lens) the beta dose cannot be ignored.

The cohort of Liquidators is very heterogeneous, dictating the application of different approaches to assess . The most rigorous review of the Liquidator population from the point of view of possible sources of dosimetric information is given by Krjuchkov (see this issue) [1]. This review addresses specific issues related to dosimetric support of the eye-cataract study among the Chernobyl Liquidators including the verification of existing dose records, retrospective dosimetric techniques and a possible approach to the beta dosimetry problem.

A. K. Junk et al. (eds.),
Ocular Radiation Risk Assessment in Populations Exposed to Environmental Radiation Contamination, 121–129.

2. Methodologies of dose assessment

Unfortunately, dosimetric support for a cataract follow-up cannot rely directly on the results of dosimetric monitoring at the time of clean-up. To obtain best possible dose estimates, careful verification of the dosimetric registries should be combined with dose reconstruction. . Adequate approaches to retrospective dosimetry should include: an analytical (time-and-motion) estimate of dose, an expert dose evaluation, tooth enamel EPR dosimetry and the application FISH technique using stable chromosome aberrations.

2.1. VERIFICATION OF EXISTING DOSE RECORDS

The information in the State Registry includes many thousands of dose records and therefore cannot be ignored. Since various sources had contributed to the data array, the quality and reliability of those data subsets is variable. However, similarities in exposure conditions and dosimetric practices result in statistical regularities within the data subsets allowing verification of the data by considering partial distributions separately . Insight into the statistical properties of the data will give a sense of the value of the quality and consistency of available dosimetric data. Obviously, statistical analyses of the dose distribution do not allow one to determine the quality of individual records. However, general conclusions regarding the quality of the whole subset of data may be derived from such analyses.

Presently, the verification of extant dose records is proceeding along two primary paths:

i) Descriptive analyze of partial dose distributions and comparison with known characteristics of occupational exposure.
ii) Detection and quantification of the presence of extraneous admixtures in the data set.

In the first instance, dose distributions are analyzed with respect to certain statistical characteristics of occupational exposure. For example, analysis of daily doses (total dose as recorded in the Registry divided by the number of days spent in the 30-km zone) of some military Liquidators had revealed that these values are distributed according to hybrid-log-normal law [2]. The parameters of the distributions as well as their time trends are consistent with the conditions of exposure.

The second verification scheme is based on the effect of altering the entropy of experimental distribution in the presence of unusual admixtures. This method involves simulating the distribution of «pure» data and calculating the entropy curves in the presence of known percentages of admixtures. Such computer experiment allows one to obtain a family of calibration curves corresponding to various percentages of extraneous admixtures. Our investigations demonstrated that this method is quite robust and the results do not depend significantly on the type of admixture (δ-function vs. other types of distributions).

Investigation of the properties of the dose records and evaluation of their quality is underway now. The potential of this effort is the certification of some Liquidator databases (subsets) as having dose records of appropriate quality. The criteria for defining quality are developed jointly by dosimetrists and epidemiologists. Those data arrays, which are certified, could then be used for dosimetric support for the epidemiological study.

The advantages of this methodology are the low cost (comparing to retrospective dosimetry) and high throughput. The shortcoming of this type of verification lies in the fact that the evaluation of the data quality is possible only on sub-cohort level - one cannot estimate the quality and trustworthiness of individual dose values. Another difficulty arises from the need to have clear criteria for categorizing the data. Affiliation and period of work seem to be good keys for categorization. Unfortunately, the State Registry does not contain information about the affiliations of the Liquidators, and, therefore, a special effort employing a questionnaire is needed in order to acquire the necessary information. Obviously, currently the discussed approach is not sufficiently developed to be applied, nonetheless it has great potential to improve the situation with dosimetry of the Liquidators. Within a certain scope, the theoretical and organizational efforts are quite affordable and worth implementation in the nearest future. With respect to its discussed shortcomings, verification of existing dose records may be considered a screening methodology; recognizing that further revision and validation of dosimetric data will be necessary in the course of time.

2.2. ANALYTICAL (TIME-AND-MOTION) ESTIMATION OF DOSES

This methodology is quite traditional and has been widely used for reconstruction of doses following many radiation accidents. However, this approach is endowed with two preconditions: (i) the ability of the person to describe his or her route with desirable accuracy and (ii) knowledge about the dose fields in all the locations visited by the person. The degree of precision when describing the route (time and spatial resolution) is determined mainly by the complexity of dose rate patterns in both time and space). In case of an evacuated population [3], it has been sufficient to reconstruct motions on an hour-by-hour basis with spatial resolution up to several hundreds meters.

The Liquidator situation is quite different. The extreme complexity of the contamination patterns requires a very precise description of the route. This is further complicated by the fact that the information available is sparse and the ability to recall the movements for a majority of Liquidators is very low. Therefore, the scope of application of this methodology is constrained to only those skilled professionals who can describe their movements with great detail or to those who spent time in extremely uniform radiation fields. The methodology developed jointly by Institute of Biophysics (Moscow), Chernobyl NPP (Slavutich) and Scientific Center of Radiation Medicine (Kiev) was designed to estimate doses to NPP workers who were extremely familiar with the topography of the NPP and performed their duties in a highly motivated manner. In addition, the dose reconstruction process is quite elaborate, requiring the involvement of independent experts and eye-witnesses of the Liquidators' activities.

Concluding the discussion, it may be noted that this approach has two obvious advantages: there is no sensitivity threshold (as all other retrospective techniques have) and cost of analyses is relatively low. That said, it has a number of drawbacks and limitations that degrade general attractiveness of this method. First, in many cases it is impossible to recall the route with the desired degree of precision. Second, there remains the possibility of falsification of the migration data, intentionally or not. Such distortion of this information particularly in very heterogeneous radiation fields may be highly misleading .Third, there are significant gaps in the dose-rate data, particularly during the first days after the accident. Recovery of these data by interpolation is often impossible primarily due to the clustered nature of contamination (e.g. in different rooms inside the NPP building). Finally, the major disadvantage of the time-and-motion technique is associated with the limited applicability of this method. According to our assessment, in the best case, doses may be reconstructed in this way for no more than 4,000 persons, while population of Chernobyl Liquidators exceeds 150,000 individuals. All together, this makes analytical dosimetry of the Liquidators a less feasible method than alternative retrospective techniques.

2.3. EXPERT ASSESSMENT OF DOSES

The diversity of the Liquidators as well as the variety of tasks, performed during the clean-up, are causes for distinct differences in the levels of exposure. Normally, experienced experts may predict possible dose by simply knowing the profession, place and time of work of the Liquidator. Clearly, such, rather qualitative, assessment cannot be used as precise dose estimate, however the idea of assessment of dose by evaluation of individual attributes of the Liquidators (without completing a full route list) is sound and appears very attractive.

Currently there are more questions than answers in this area. Although the general guidelines are quite clear, practical implementation is not so trivial. Proper categorization of Liquidator population (see 2.1) would permit assigning a probable range of doses to a given sub-cohort. The inclusion of more detailed dose-modifying factors may allow one to the narrow dose ranges, thereby reducing the «group dose range» to an «individual dose range». These dose-modifying factors may reflect both professional (time and place of work, task, conditions of work etc.) and personal features. The latter includes relevant individual characteristics such as the level of responsibility, so dedicated as to be purposely overexposed for the sake of the mission, patronality (desire to perform work by themselves rather then delegating it to younger and weaker fellows) etc.

The expert dose assessment methodology, as now envisioned, should include two sequential steps: (i) the assessment of the group dose range with respect to profession, location and duration of work, and (ii) the assessment of the individual dose range by including modifying parameters reflecting dose-modifying factors. The task of the expert would be to evaluate individual parameters of the model and assess the consistency of the final results.

The problem in question is how to quantify («calibrate») these dose modifying factors and how to use them for determining the individual dose range. Unfortunately, In The Case Of Chernobyl, the scope of reliable data is very limited and the possibilities of empirically determining the factors are not great. Therefore, certain assumptions should be made based on *a priori* considerations, namely, the experience from other radiation accidents and some empirical Chernobyl data. Since the adequacy of such assumptions is not obvious, the model and results should be validated by independent dosimetric techniques.

Another important issue is development of the questionnaire for interviewing the Liquidators. This form, must be very concise, should match the requirements of the model and address all the important questions. Clearly, the questionnaire should be designed in concert with the development of the expert dose assessment methodology.

Low cost and high throughput should be stressed as important advantages of this approach. The disadvantages of the expert assessment of doses are its inability to assess individual dose as well as the rather high probability of error, which can be anticipated. The main problem of this approach lies in the fact that it is based on an account of the «typical» conditions of work, while often the major contribution to dose is caused by atypical episodes of exposure [4]. Therefore, the expert assessment method, once developed, might be used for rather rough estimations of dose, mainly for screening purposes.

Finally, this approach is currently not sufficiently developed to be applied. Prior to its implementation, the following problems must be addressed: elaboration of a method for the formalized description of occupational history of the Liquidator, design of a cohort-specific questionnaire, and development of a method for deriving an expert assessment of dose.

2.4. EPR DOSIMETRY WITH TOOTH ENAMEL

During the last decade, Electron Paramagnetic Resonance (EPR) dosimetry, considered as one of the most promising methodologies for retrospective dosimetry, has undergone a dramatic evolution. The literature on this topic spans hundreds of articles reflecting an explosion of interest in this problem. A detailed explanation of EPR dosimetry is outside the scope of this paper, but we will focus on most notable problems of this approach.

Presently, the research in field of EPR dosimetry is concentrated on the following: (i) technological improvements; (ii) setting standards, and (iii) addressing confounding factors including the development of approaches to deal with them. Regarding the first aspect, the accuracy, reproducibility and reliability of EPR dosimetry was a subject of rigorous investigations which, resulted in its present status as the most advanced technique appropriate for routine dose reconstruction. Yet, setting standards for EPR dosimetry is not easy. EPR dosimetry is still in the phase of accelerated development and is being used in many laboratories worldwide. The adoption of a single standard protocol should not interrupt research in this area. However, for practical reasons, in some countries EPR dosimetric protocols were officially adopted. For example, the technique developed in SCRM/URPI [5] proved its worth and was adopted by Ukrainian authorities in 1995 for reconstructing individual doses. Since that time the protocol has been used for routine dose reconstruction for several hundred Liquidators.

That said there remain some loose ends in this field. Modifying influences such as the hypersensitivity of dental enamel to soft x-rays or the induction of EPR signals by

UV light may alter results. In addition, an occasional non-linearity of dose-response curves may also lead to either an under- or over-estimation of dose. Lesser, but by no means, negligible effects can be caused by factors such as the decay of transient signals in tooth enamel or a variation of sensitivity as a function of the size of the enamel grains. A proper accounting or mitigation of these effects are required for correct dose determination. In some cases, existing approaches are too complicated to be practical in routine use and further research is needed in order to develop more robust methods for treatment of the mentioned above confounding factors. At its present stage of development, these problems effectively reduce the breadth of application of EPR dosimetry. Clearly solving these problems would expand the limits of EPR utility. An example is that today front teeth (exposed to solar radiation) or molars with reported lifetime x-ray examinations are excluded from the consideration - with time and investigative effort the situation may improve so as to allow inclusion of these samples.

The enhancement of the technological capabilities of EPR dosimetry is another important issue. At the moment, the bottleneck for throughput of the technique is related to the time that it takes to obtain EPR spectra. All other links of this technological chain (sample preparation, laboratory irradiation etc.) can be significantly accelerated by parallel processing of specimens, while acquiring EPR spectra can be done only one sample at a time using very expensive instrument. Therefore, reducing the time needed for recording one spectrum will effectively increase overall throughput of the technique. In this area, gains can be made by employing new, more sensitive hardware, e.g. dielectric resonators. Another, yet not well explored, possibility is recording spectra in different microwave bands. For instance, measurements in Q-band (8-mm wavelength) would require a substantially smaller amount of material. The implementation of adequate software for spectrum decomposition would mark another important step towards complete automation of the process of dose reconstruction.

In more general sense, translating of the dose measured in calcified tissue (essentially that which EPR does) to the doses in critical organs (like red bone marrow or eye lens) is another challenging task. Properly accounting for the energy and geometry of exposure as well as the determination of organ doses may require significant effort, especially with respect to rather complex conditions of the Chernobyl exposure.

The limited availability of samples is the basis of another serious difficulty for EPR dosimetry. Since human teeth cannot be extracted solely for dosimetric purposes, the only way to obtain samples is collecting teeth extracted during routine dental practice. However, the loss of teeth is a random and infrequent event, therefore, the solution is the implementation of a widespread acquisition network which would operate in a passive mode accepting all Liquidators' teeth extracted over many years. Such Nation-wide network is currently being established in Ukraine. This network is centered in Kiev with nodes in each of the seven regions with highest Liquidator population. Once extracted, the teeth, along with ID forms, are accumulated in regional centers and then forwarded to the Central Bioprobe Bank for preprocessing and long term storage. Afterwards, the samples may be retrieved from the repository for EPR analysis and reconstruction of doses. Accumulation of abundant number of samples enable matching the total number of relevant (in terms of epidemiological follow-up) specimens with the presently limited overall throughput of the EPR-dosimetric technique.

Despite of a number of yet unresolved difficulties, the main conclusion to be derived from the above discussion is not a negative. Although some issues require further research and clarification, the general evaluation of EPR dosimetry is very positive. In fact, it is the only retrospective technique, which allows one to reconstruct doses in excess of 100 mGy with an uncertainty of less than 40%. The changes in tooth enamel over a lifetime do not fade nor are there pronounced dose rate effects. In addition, the response of tooth enamel is restricted only to external photon radiation.. With regard to continuing research in the field, the availability of samples remains the major limiting factor in applying EPR dosimetry. Nonetheless, the proposed infrastructure for Liquidator tooth acquisition has the potential to overcome this shortcoming. Ultimately, EPR dosimetry using teeth may be considered the most appropriate methodology for the dosimetric support of follow-up the health outcome studies.

2.5. FISH

Among the many biodosimetric techniques for retrospective dosimetry, fluorescent *in situ* hybridization (FISH) is commonly accepted as the most promising one. Generally, the decline with time of chromosome aberrations is the major constraint in applying cytogenetic biodosimetry long after exposure. However reciprocal translocations which may be detected by FISH are considered to be stable over decades [6]. Compared to EPR FISH is more readily applied because the availability of blood samples makes dose determination possible on virtually all relevant high dose subjects, with perhaps the only exception being patients with a pre-leukemic condition. A shortcoming of FISH is its low sensitivity - only doses in excess of 250 mSv can be determined with 100% error when scoring of 3000 cells (about one man-week of labor) [7]. In addition, variations in individual radiosensitivity, the incidence of spontaneous translocations and a pronounced dose-rate effect make dosimetry even more difficult and uncertain. Another serious drawback is the very high cost of analysis.

An improvement in protocols and inter-laboratory cross-calibrations are necessary to prove the capability of the FISH technique to determine individual doses which are of epidemiological relevance (0.1-1 Gy). In any case, it is not expected that FISH dosimetry will be suitable for routine dose reconstruction. At best, the FISH technique could be used for the selective validation of results derived from other assessment techniques. The FISH technique might also be useful if specimens other than blood lymphocytes are to be scored for translocations. For example, using cells from skin adjacent to the eye would be expected to provide a better organ-specific (eye) dose assessment than any other method of retrospective dosimetry. However, as attractive as this idea may seem it has yet to be employed.

In conclusion, the FISH methodology, despite its being the most useful of the available biodosimetric protocols, still has serious limitations in terms of sensitivity, accuracy and cost. Further developments may improve its capabilities, however it is likely that its application will be restricted to highly selective analyses and verification of dosimetric data from other sources.

3. Conclusions

From the above discussion, one may conclude that there is no single method suitable for the general dosimetric support of the Chernobyl eye-cataract study. While some methods may have good throughput they suffer from insufficient accuracy, while others may be more precise yet have limited application. Therefore, it is necessary to apply a combination of the methods discussed. With a view of the strengths and weaknesses of available techniques, a multistage plan for the dosimetric support of eye-cataract follow-up may be proposed.

As the first step, the existing dose records available in the State Chernobyl Registry and other databases should be verified using the approach described in section 2.1. Those records, which are considered not falsified, may be used as a first approximation of individual doses. The next step should include validating those records by means of retrospective dosimetry. That effort will generate a two-fold output: one, a conclusion about the trustworthiness of the filtered dose records, and, the second, a measure of uncertainty of dosimetric monitoring data. The next step includes a dosimetric screening of the Liquidator cohort using the expert assessment method (discussed in section 2.3). Such analyses, require a survey of the Liquidators. The evaluation of the thousands of responses will provide a rough assessment of possible individual dose ranges. At that point, the results of expert assessment will be checked against existing dose records and the values provided by independent methods. When possible, analytical dose assessment will be conducted. Although having limited application, this methodology is not hampered by a sensitivity threshold and, therefore, may yield a low dose sample to the studied cohort. Towards this end, a major effort should focus on collecting teeth from Chernobyl Liquidators with the goal of wide scale reconstruction of doses using EPR dosimetry. The availability of tooth samples promises very precise dose reconstruction with a high degree of confidence. Therefore, subjects who have donated teeth should be a priority in the dose reconstruction effort. That data in turn can serve as a reference in a variety of applications. Dosimetry using FISH is not considered feasible, unless the technique is modified to assess cells from peri-ocular skin. The first phase of the dosimetric support of the eye-cataract study will end with integration of the results of essentially independent methods. Therefrom the best possible assessment of external gamma-dose will be derived.

In the second phase, another challenge must be addressed, namely the evaluation of the eye lens beta dose using conversion factors from gamma to beta dose. This approach is the only way to solve this difficult problem and deriving appropriate conversion factors is not trivial. Such conversion factors depend on the geometry of the exposure (including the dimensions of the source), the time after release (e.g. nuclide composition of the contamination) and even individual anatomical peculiarities [8]. Clearly, these conversion factors may be calculated under certain assumptions and under idealized conditions however due to the lack of direct measurements, the adequacy of such assumptions is very difficult to assess, if possible at all. In addition, factors such as wearing protective goggles or the contribution of gamma radiation from outdoor deposition areas may have large effects on the beta/gamma dose ratio. According to preliminary assessment, the beta exposure contributed significantly to the eye-lens dose and cannot be neglected. Therefore, the proper evaluation of beta doses should be an important component of eye lens dosimetry.

In general, although dosimetric support of the cataract follow-up is very complex and difficult, it must be addressed in order to obtain any meaningful results from this large-scale and time-consuming study.

4. References

1. Krujchkov, V.P. (in press) Survey and reliability of available database on dosimetry, *in proceedings of NATO Advanced research workshop «Ocular radiation risk assessment in population exposed to environmental radiation contamination», - Kiev , 29 July - 1 August 1997.* **(SEE THIS ISSUE)**
2. Kumazawa, S.; Numakunai, T. (1991) Why do we need dose distribution models? *Radiat. Prot. Dosim* **36**, 2/4, 269-273.
3. Likhtarev,I.; Chumak,V.; Repin, V. (1994) Retrospective reconstruction of individual and collective external gamma doses of population, evacuated after the Chernobyl accident, *Health Phys.* **66,** 643-652.
4. Nossovsky A.,V., ed. (1996) *Retrospective dosimetry of Chernobyl clean-up workers,* Seda-style, Kiev (in Russian)
5. Chumak, V.; Bailiff, I. et al. (1996) The first international intercomparison of ESR-dosimetry with teeth:first results, *Appl.Radiat. Isot.* **47**, 11/12, 1281-1286.
6. Lukas, J.N.; Hill, F.S.; Buck, C.E. et al. (1996) Stability of the translocation frequency following whole-body irradiation measured in rhesus monkeys, *Int. J. Radiat. Biol.* **70**, 309-318.
7. Lloyd, D. (in press) New developments in chromosomal analysis for biological dosimetry, *in proceedings of International Workshop on Retrospective Dosimetry (Physical and Biological Aspects), Tjanjin, 14-17 October 1997.*
8. Charles, M.W. (in press) Physical and radiobiological considerations in eye dosimetry, *in proceedings of NATO Advanced research workshop «Ocular radiation risk assessment in population exposed to environmental radiation contamination», - Kiev , 29 July - 1 August 1997.* **(SEE THIS ISSUE)**

ESTIMATION OF ENVIRONMENTAL BURDENS BY RADIATION.

Radiological Units: From Gray to Sievert

C. BAUMSTARK-KHAN

DLR, Institute of Aerospace Medicine, Radiobiology Section
Linder Höhe, D-51170 Köln, Germany

Abstract

Estimation of environmental burdens by radiation requires profound knowledge on the basics of radiation effects. In order to estimate risks from different kinds of radiation, scientists have to be aware on physical, chemical and biological interactions of electromagnetic waves (X-rays, γ-rays) and particle rays (α-rays, β-rays, neutrons, heavy ions) with biomolecules. These different types of radiation cause different spatial distributions of ionizations and thus can be of different risk potential for humans. Concerning physical quantities and scientific units used for ionizing radiation, an international agreement was made (SI). The special terms including their units (exposure, absorbed dose, equivalent dose, linear energy transfer, relative biological effectiveness and oxygen enhancement ratio) will be explained. Additionally, basic knowledge for comparison (high background areas, exposure to cosmic radiation, medical use of radiation and dato on atomic bomb survivors) is provided.

1. Introduction

As a result of the Chernobyl accident in 1986 the environment was contaminated by radioactive nuclides ($1.85 \cdot 10^{18}$ Bq). Most of the substances released were short half-lived radionuclides (^{131}I, ^{134}Cs and ^{137}Cs). The release of these radiologically important radionuclides to the environment is now estimated at a factor of two to three higher than in 1986. Although the amount of radioactive material has decayed to a great amount, after 10 years considerable radioactivity is still present in the environment (TABLE 1.) and contamination will further remain for a significant time. After 10 years, the major contributors to the low-dose chronic radiation are the remaining caesium radionuclides. The external dose in some isolated spots can still be of the order of 1 mGy per day. In general, the current migration rate is slow and steady and is expected to continue over the coming decades, even as the level of radioactive material in the soil declines. Game and wild foods consumed by people, such as berries and mushrooms, will continue to show elevated ^{137}Cs levels over the next decades. The level of contamination, type of soil, soil moisture, and crop type are important influencing

A. K. Junk et al. (eds.),
Ocular Radiation Risk Assessment in Populations Exposed to Environmental Radiation Contamination, 131–141.

TABLE 1. Release of Significant Nuclides and Remaining Contamination

Nuclide	*Half-life*		*Critical Organ*	*Released in 1986*	*Remaining in 1996*	*Expected for 2056*
	physical	biological		10^{15} Bq	10^{15} Bq	10^{15} Bq
^{90}Sr	28.8 y	very large	Bone	8	6	1.5
^{131}I	8.0 d	120 d	Thyroid	1200 - 1700	0	0
^{134}Cs	2.1 y	110 d	Whole Body	44 48	1.6	0
^{137}Cs	30.1 y	110 d	Whole Body	74 85	68	17
^{238}Pu	87.7 y	very large	Liver, Bone	0.03	0.03	0.02
^{239}Pu	24,110 y	very large	Liver, Bone	0.03	0.03	0.03
^{240}Pu	6,564 y	very large	Liver, Bone	0.044	0.044	0.03
^{241}Pu	14.35 y	very large	Liver, Bone	5.9	3.6	0.2
^{241}Am**	432.2 y	very large	Liver, Bone	0.005	0.08	0.2

Estimate of release decay corrected to 26 April 1986, the day of the accident.
**The activity of ^{241} Am in 1996 has increased as it is a daughter product of ^{241}Pu (half-life 14 years).

factors. These foods may still be contaminated above the strict nationally adopted limits in areas of Belarus, Ukraine, and Russia.

The releases contaminated approximately 17 million people, the exact amount of exposure depended on location, wind and duration of exposure. Immediately after the accident, the highest doses were received within a radius of 30 kilometers from the reactor. The primary groups of interest for studies were the 237 people who suffered from acute radiation syndrome (ARS), the 12,000 children who received large doses to the thyroid gland and the 9,000 children who were irradiated in utero. Of the 28 patients with ARS, who died in 1986, most had skin lesions, which covered more than 50% of the body. 135,000 people which were evacuated during the first few weeks following the accident, were exposed to internal irradiation arising from inhalation of radioiodines, especially ^{131}I and to external irradiation from radioactivity present in the cloud and deposited on the ground [1]. Whole-body doses received from external irradiation prior to evacuation from the Ukrainian part of the 30-km zone showed a large range of variation with an average value of 15 mGy. 800,000 "liquidators" moved in in order to decontaminate the area. Between 17 and 45 percent of these people received doses between 0.1 and 0.25 Gy. The most exposed, with doses of several Gy, were the workers involved immediately after the beginning of the accident and the scientists who have performed special tasks in the sarcophagus [2]. About 270,000 people live in contaminated areas of the former Soviet Union, where more than 555 kBq/m^2 of ^{137}Cs was deposited. During the first few weeks after the accident, due to the consumption of contaminated cow's milk, children in the Gomel region of Belarus appear to have received high thyroid doses up to 40 Sv.

2. Radioactivity and Radiation

2.1. RADIOACTIVITY

Radioactivity is a natural and spontaneous process by which the unstable atoms of an element emit or radiate excess energy in the form of particles or waves. These emissions are collectively called ionizing radiations. Depending on how the nucleus loses this excess energy either a lower energy atom of the same form will result, or a completely different nucleus and atom can be formed.

The fraction of the amount of a radionuclide that undergoes transition per unit time is described by equation 1, where ΔP is the probability of a given nucleus undergoing spontaneous nuclear transition in the time interval Δt.

$$\lambda = \frac{\Delta P}{\Delta t} \tag{1}$$

- The time required to reduce the amount of a radionuclide to one-half the amount originally present is the half-time λ: this physical half-life refers to reduction of activity by radioactive decay;
- biological half-life refers to biological elimination from the body; and
- effective half-life refers to the combined action of radioactive decay and biological elimination.

2.2. RADIATION

Radiation is energy traveling in the form of particles or waves in bundles of energy called photons. The most familiar form of radiation is sunshine, which delivers light and heat. It consists of radiation in a range of wavelengths from longwave infrared to shorter wavelength ultraviolet (UV). Beyond UV are higher energy kinds of radiation which are used in medicine. Collectively these kinds of radiation were refered to as ionizing radiation. Radiation occurs in two forms (rays and particles) at the high frequency end of the energy spectrum.

2.3. INTERACTION OF RADIATION WITH MATERIAL

Ionization is a particular characteristic of the radiation produced when radioactive elements decay. These radiations are of such high energy that when they interact with materials, radiation energy is released into absorbing materials, which causes excitation (which propels an electron to a higher level of orbit in an atom) or ionization (which allows an electron to move away from an atom).

Radiation can cause the loss of any electron from an atom resulting in highly unstable ions called radicals. Most radicals react with neighboring atoms or molecules almost instantaneously (in less than 1/1000 of a second). The human body consists of 70% water. Radiation can break H_2O to produce OH radicals that are known to be the most potent in attacking various biomolecules including DNA, the genetic blueprint. Radiation also can directly hit DNA to produce radicals resulting in DNA strand breaks. This effect is the reason why ionizing radiation is hazardous to human health.

2.4. DIFFERENT KINDS OF IONIZING RADIATION

Different types of radiation (TABLE 2.), such as X-rays and γ-rays, α-particles, β-particles, neutrons and heavy ions, cause different spatial distributions of ionizations. γ-irradiation produces ionizations homogeneously within a cell, whereas neutron irradiation tends to produce clusters of ionization that are believed to cause more serious damage to the cells. Therefore, different kinds of ionizing radiation are evaluated for purposes of radiation protection:

TABLE 2. Different properties of different kinds of radiations

Radiation	Type of Radiation	Mass	Charge	Shielding material	Quality Factor
α	Particle	4	+2	Paper, skin, clothes	20
β	Particle	1/1836	±1	Plastic, glass, light metals	1
γ	Electromagnetic Wave	0	0	Dense metal, concrete, earth	1
X	Electromagnetic Wave	0	0	Dense metal, concrete, earth	1
Neutrons	Particle	1	0	Water, concrete, polyethylene, oil	10

2.4.1. Gamma-Rays

An electromagnetic wave, a γ-ray is similar to ordinary visible light but differs in energy or wavelength. A γ-ray's wavelength is far shorter than UV (ie, it is far higher in energy). γ-rays are produced following spontaneous decay of radioactive materials, such as ^{60}Co and ^{137}Cs as part of their decay process. Like all forms of electromagnetic radiation, the γ-ray has no mass and no charge. γ-rays interact with material by colliding with the electrons in the shells of atoms. They lose their energy slowly in material, being able to travel significant distances before stopping. Depending on their initial energy, γ-rays can travel from 1 to hundreds of meters in air. A ^{60}Co γ-ray can penetrate deeply into the human body, so it has been widely used for cancer radiotherapy.

2.4.2. X-Rays

Over a century ago in 1895, Roentgen discovered the first example of ionizing radiation, X-rays. X-rays and γ-rays, like light, represent energy transmitted in a wave without the movement of material. X-rays and γ-rays have great penetrating power and can pass through the human body. Thick barriers of concrete, lead or water are used as protection from γ- and X-rays. X-rays have the same characteristics as γ-rays, although they are produced differently. When high-speed electrons hit metals, electrons are stopped and release energy in the form of an electromagnetic wave. X rays consist of a mixture of different wavelengths, whereas γ-ray energy has a fixed characteristic according to the emitting radioactive material.

2.4.3. Alpha-Rays

α-particles have a positive electrical charge and are emitted from naturally occurring elements such as uranium and radium, as well as from some man-made elements. Because of their relatively large size, α-particles interact readily with materials they encounter, including air, causing many ionizations in a very short distance. Thus, an α-particle can pass only a short distance in water (less than 1 mm). It has little penetrating power and can be stopped by the first layer of skin or a sheet of paper. Therefore, health effects of α-ray exposures appear only when α-emitting materials are ingested (ie, internal exposure). Inside the body, because they give up their energy over a relatively short distance, α-particles can inflict more biological damage than other radiations.

2.4.4. Beta-Rays

β-decay is a radioactive process in which an electron whose mass is nearly 1/2000 of the mass of a proton or neutron is emitted from the nucleus of a radioactive atom, along with an antineutrino. β-rays are produced following spontaneous decay of certain radioactive materials, such as ^{3}H, ^{14}C, ^{32}P, and ^{90}Sr. Depending on the β-particle's energy (which depends on the radioactive atom), β-particles will travel up to several meters in air. In water a β-ray can traverse different distances (less than 1 mm for ^{3}H to nearly 1 cm for ^{32}P). They can be stopped by a sheet of aluminium or plastic a few millimetres thick. As with α-rays, their major implication for health effects is after their ingestion (internal exposure).

2.4.5. Neutrons

Neutrons are particles which are very penetrating. They come from outer space, from collisions with atoms in the atmosphere, and from the splitting, or fissioning, of certain atoms, mostly of uranium or plutonium, inside a nuclear reactor. In fact, neutrons trigger the nuclear chain reaction to explode an atomic bomb. In the human body neutrons cause various types of cellular damage when they hit the nucleus of hydrogen. At equivalent absorbed doses, neutrons can cause more severe damage to the body than γ-rays. Water and concrete are the most commonly used shields against neutron radiation.

2.4.6. Heavy Ions

Cosmic radiations consist of very energetic particles which bombard the earth from outer space. They are more intense at higher altitudes than at sea level where the earth's atmosphere is most dense and gives the greatest protection.

3. Radiation Definitions and Dose Units

The human senses cannot detect radiation or discern whether a material is radioactive. However, a variety of instruments (ionizing chambers, scintillation counters, γ-counters) can detect and measure radiation reliably and accurately.

3.1. SI: THE INTERNATIONAL SYSTEM OF UNITS OR "LE SYSTEME INTERNATIONAL D'UNITES"

In the late 1970's, an international agreement was made concerning physical quantities and scientific units, including those for ionizing radiation, to be used in future years. Many terms, to which the scientific community had become accustomed were changed, both in name and in size. To ease the transition, since 1979, technical publications adopted the practice of using the old units (which had been in use for many years) followed immediately by the new units in parentheses. Five years later the practice was to use the new units, followed by the old units in parentheses. Eventually, now all publications will be using the new system of quantities and units exclusively [3]. This has already been done by scientists in most parts of the world. In the United States, both the old and new units are still used by government agencies and the non-technical media. The special terms necessary to understand the explanations, including the names, use of the radiation quantities and their units, will briefly be explained (TABLE 3).

TABLE 3. Dose Units

Physical Definition	*SI-Unit*	*Old Unit*	*Conversion Factor (CF) Old Unit/CF=SI*	*Reference*
Activity	Bq (decay/s)	Ci	$2.7*10^{-11}$	[4]
Exposure	C/kg	R	3876	[4]
Absorbed dose	Gy (J/kg)	Rad	100	[5]
Equivalent dose	Sv (J/kg)	rem	100	[6]

Radiation is often measured in these units, depending on what is being measured and why. In international units, these would be Coulombs/kg for roentgen, Grays for rads and Sieverts for rem.

3.1.1. Becquerel (Bq) or Curie (Ci)

When a certain amount of radioactive material is given, it is customary to refer to the quantity based on its activity rather than its mass. The activity is simply the number of nuclear transitions (disintegrations) occurring in a given quantity of radioactive material per unit time. The SI unit of activity is s^{-1}. The special name for the unit of activity is becquerel (Bq), named for Henry Becquerel who is credited with the discovery of radioactivity. The previously used special unit of activity, curie (Ci), named after Pierre and Marie Curie for their discovery of radium, is being replaced by the becquerel. One curie is equal to the disintegrations of 1 g radium (3.7×10^{10} disintegrations per second). One becquerel is equal to one disintegration per second. Thus, the relationship between becquerels and curies is 1 Bq = $2.7 \cdot 10^{-11}$ Ci or 1 Ci = $3.7 \cdot 10^{10}$ Bq.

3.1.2. Exposure or Roentgen (R)

Exposure is quantitatively measured by use of ionizing chambers for X or γ-radiation at a certain place, based on a quantity of ionization (charge) produced by the absorption of X- or γ-radiation energy in a specified mass of air under standard conditions. The SI unit of exposure determines the number of ion pairs, and in the international system (SI), the special unit is coulomb per kilogram. The former unit of exposure was the roentgen (R), named after W.C. Röntgen, who discovered X-rays. The relationship between Coulomb per kg air and roentgen is 1 C/kg = 3875 R or 1 R = 2.58×10^{-4} C/kg.

3.1.3. Gray (Gy) or Radiation Absorbed Dose (Rad)

In a general sense, a dose is a measure of the amount of energy from an ionizing radiation deposited in a mass of some material. Dose is affected by the amount of radiation and the physical properties of the exposed material itself. Specifically, absorbed dose can be related to water, tissue, or material like silicon. The gray (Gy), named after L.H. Gray, who developed the concept of "absorbed dose", is the SI-unit of the absorbed dose. One Gy is the amount of energy deposited in tissues; technically, 1 joule of energy per kilogram of tissue. The Gy replaces the old unit, called rad (radiation absorbed dose, 1 rem is equivalent to 1 R), which was defined as 0.01 Joule absorbed energy per kilogram of any material (also defined as the absorption of 100 ergs per gram of material).

Absorbed dose is often expressed in terms of hundredths of a gray, or centigrays. The relationship between Gy and rad is 1 Gy = 100 rad or 1 rad = 0.01 Gy.

3.1.4. Sievert (Sv) or Roentgen Equivalent Man (Rem)

The unit Gy can be used for any type of radiation, but it does not describe the biological effects of the different radiations. Equal exposure to different types of radiation does not, however, necessarily produce equal biological effects. One Gy of α-radiation, for example, will have a greater effect than one Gy of β-radiation. Other common doses are the effective and equivalent doses, which are adjusted to allow the comparison of different types of radiation. The conventional unit of dose equivalent is the sievert (Sv), named after the physicist R.M. Sievert. One sievert equals one joule per kilogram. The previously used unit, rem, is being replaced by the sievert. Equivalent dose is often expressed in terms of hundredths of a Sv, or cSv. The relationship between Sv and rem is 1 Sv = 100 rem or 1 rem = 0.01 Sv.

The Sv is a unit of radiation dose that is used for radiation protection purposes, in order to account for different radiation quality. The dose equivalent in Sv is numerically equal to the absorbed dose (Gy) multiplied by the quality factor Q, which differs for different kinds of radiation (TABLE 2 and 4).

For most medical applications involving X-ray or γ-emitters, the numerical values of the absorbed dose in Gy and dose equivalent in Sv are numerically roughly equivalent, as the Q-factor is 1. For neutrons and for α-particles or multiple charged particles the Q-factor is 10 Q and 20, respectively (TABLE 4). When an individual is exposed to mixed sources of radiation, the total biologically effective dose is calculated by multiplying the physical dose (Gy) of each kind of radiation by the corresponding Q-factor, after which these amounts are added together. One Sv of radiation produces a constant biological effect regardless of the type of radiation.

TABLE 4. Ionization Density and Q-Factor

LET (keV/μm in water)	*Q-Factor*
3.5	1
7	2
23	5
53	10
175	20

3.2. RADIOLOGIC IMPORTANT RELATIONSHIPS

Q-Factors are important only for radiation protection concepts, where radiation exposure has to be prevented in future. For risk estimations derived from laboratory experiments other relationships are of major importance.

3.2.1. Linear Energy Transfer (LET)

Particles, especially such with uneven spatial distributions, penetrate the irradiated object and simultaneously lose energy (i.e. accelerated heavy ions). For such cases the average amount of energy lost per unit of particle track length, expressed in keV μm^{-1} [5] gives a clue for calculating the amount of specific ionizations. These are the numbers of ion pairs formed per unit of distance along the track of an ion passing through matter. The quality factor Q, used in radiation protection strictly depends on LET for densly ionizing radiation (TABLE 4).

3.2.2. Relative Biological Effecitiveness (RBE)

For comparing different kinds of irradiation (sparsely or densely ionizing radiation), when the activity of the radiation source and the distribution and amounts of contaminations are known, Q-factors are only rough estimations. More accurate for data interpretation is the relative biological effectiveness (RBE; [7]), which can be experimentally determined for certain end-points and certain tissues or organisms, according to equation 2:

$$RBE = \left[\frac{Dose(X - Rays)}{Dose(test - radiation)} \right]_{isoeffect} \tag{2}$$

3.2.3. Oxygen Enhancement Ratio (OER)

For comparing radiation effects on tissues with different metabolic conditions (anoxia, hypoxia, hyperoxia), the oxygen enhancement ratio describes the surplus of effect in presence of oxygen ($+O_2$) over the effect in absence of oxygen ($-O_2$), according to equation 3:

$$OER = \left[\frac{Dose(-O_2)}{Dose(+O_2)} \right]_{isoeffect} \tag{3}$$

4. Radiation and Risk

4.1. COMPARISON OF RADIATION RISK

Ionizing radiation may cause serious health effects in humans. The degree of damage caused by radiation depends in turn on many factors: dose, dose rate, kind of radiation, the part of the body exposed, age and overall health status.

Higher but sublethal radiation doses may produce a delay of many years between a person's exposure and the appearance of the disease. This makes it difficult to correlate the possible agent and a particular cancer. Additionally, humans are very often exposured to doses very close to background levels. In such cases, the radiation-induced effects are too small to be detected with certainty. Thus, risk estimates have their limitations as:

- the doses and dose rates from which risk estimates are derived were much higher than the dose levels in question
- the actual doses received by the atomic bomb survivors (ABS) and some of the medical treatment cases are not known precisely and have had to be estimated
- many other factors like natural levels of cancers, habits, stress and bias effect the estimates.

Most information about radiation and its effects on groups of humans was derived from the following conditions:

4.1.1. High Background Radiation Areas

Around the world there are some areas with populations that have high background radiation levels. Monazite sand deposits are found along certain beaches in Brazil where external radiation levels range up to 50 μGy/hr, which is almost 400 times normal background in the US. On the Southwest coast of India the doses from external radiations by monazite deposits is 5-6 mGy/year, but individual doses up to 32.6 mGy per year have been reported, an area in China has dose rates of about 3-4 mGy/year. In these areas of high natural background radiation no increase in the frequency of cancer is documented for the residing populations, although an increased frequency of chromosome aberrations has been reported.

4.1.2. Cosmic Radiation

Cosmic radiation consist of high energetic particles which bombard the earth from outer space. The atmosphere and the Earth's magnetic fields shield against cosmic radiation, reducing the amount of particles that reaches the Earth's surface. The annual dose from cosmic radiation depends on the altitude people live. Typical cosmic radiation doses for the US are 0.35 mGy/y at sea level, 1.75 mGy/y at 4500 m and up to 25 mGy/y at 15 km altitude [8]. Thus flying can add a few extra μGy to the individual annual dose, depending on the numbers and durations of flights and the altitude, the plane flies. A return-flight New York to London would contribute with about 30 μGy to the annual dose.

4.1.3. Medical uses of radiation

Medical uses of radiation are roughly divided into therapy and diagnosis. Therapy is primarily used for tumor control, but in the past radiation has been used for other treatments as well. Most of the dose is received in a small area of the body. These doses can be several mGy for diagnosis and up to several Gy locally for treatments.

4.1.4. Atomic bomb survivors (ABS) in Japan

Epidemiological data on survivors of the Japanese atomic bomb explosions (ABS) demonstrate a higher incidence of cancer among exposed individuals and a greater probability of cancer as the level of exposure increases. The data are also used to estimate what the effects could be at lower exposures. Based on information obtained from laboratory data obtained by the high dose exposure are extrapolated to low doses, but these extrapolations are acknowledged to be only estimates.

There is some uncertainty in dose estimates for ABS, especially as yields of the bombs and technical issues regarding the characteristics of the radiation can only be estimated. Most radiation exposure was through γ-rays, but there was a small neutron component. In Nagasaki, this neutron component is believed to be virtually negligible, but for Hiroshima, it is somewhat larger, and there is some indication that the neutron exposures in Hiroshima may need revision. Neutrons are believed to have a greater biological effect per unit dose than γ-rays. Many analyses use a weighted total dose, such as the sum of the γ-dose in grays (Gy) and 10 times the neutron dose, in order to approximate an equivalent pure γ-ray dose in Sv.

4.2. PROTECTION FROM RADIATION

The current philosophy of radiation protection is based on the assumption that any radiation may result in human health effects, such as cancer and hereditary genetic damage. Radiation protection standards assume, however, that the effect is directly proportional to the dose, even at low levels. According to this 'linear' theory of radiation effects, if the dose is halved the effect is halved. Most countries have their own systems of radiological protection which are often based on the recommendations of the International Commission on Radiological Protection (ICRP). The authority of the ICRP comes from the scientific standing of its members over more than fifty years and the merit of its recommendations. The three key points of the ICRP's recommendations are

- No practice shall be adopted unless its introduction produces a positive benefit.
- All exposures shall be kept as low as reasonably achievable, economic and social factors being taken into account (ALARA-concept [9]).
- The dose equivalent to individuals shall not exceed the limits recommended for the appropriate circumstances by the Commission.

5. References

1. Likhtarev I.A., Shandala N.K., Gulko G.M., Kairo I.A., Chepurny N.I. (1993) Ukrainian thyroid doses after the Chernobyl accident. Health Physics, 64: 594-599
2. Salomaa S., Sevan'kaev A.V., Zhloba A.A., Kumpusalo E., Makinen S., Lindholm C., Kumpusalo L., Kolmakow S., Nissinen A. (1997). Unstable and stable chromosomal aberrations in lymphocytes of people exposed to Chernobyl fallout in Bryansk, Russia. Int. J. Radiat. Biol. 71: 51-59
3. NCRP Report No 93 (1987): Ionizing Radiation Exposure of the Population of the United States, National Council on Radiation Protection and Measurements, Bethesda, MD, USA
4. NCRP Report No 111 (1991): Developing Radiation Emergency Plans for Academic, Medical or Industrial Facilities, 1991, National Council on Radiation Protection and Measurements, Bethesda, MD, USA
5. NCRP Report No 98 (1989): Guidance on Radiation Received in Space Activities, National Council on Radiation Protection and Measurements, Bethesda, MD, USA
6. NCRP Report No 102 (1989): Medical X-Ray, Electron Beam and Gamma-Ray Protection for Energies Up to 50 MeV (Equipment Design, Performance and Use), National Council on Radiation Protection and Measurements, Bethesda, MD, USA
7. NCRP Report No. 104 (1990): The Relative Biological Effectiveness of Radiations of Different Quality, National Council on Radiation Protection and Measurements, Bethesda, MD, USA
8. NCRP Report No 94 (1988): Exposure of the Population in the United States and Canada from Natural Background Radiation, National Council on Radiation Protection and Measurements, Bethesda, MD, USA
9. NCRP Report No 107 (1990): Implementation of the Principle of As Low As Resonably Achievable (ALARA) for Medical and Dental Personnel, National Council on Radiation Protection and Measurements, Bethesda, MD, USA

IN VITRO BIOCOMPATIBILITY TESTING OF INTRAOCULAR BIOMATERIALS

S.P. DENYER*, S. DROPCOVA*, R.G.A. FARAGHER*, P.R.GARD*, G.W.HANLON*, A.W.LLOYD*, S.V.MIKHALOVSKY*, C.J.OLLIFF*, E. LETKO#, M.FILIPEC#.
**Biomaterials Research Group, University of Brighton, UK.*
#Second Department of Ophthalmology, Prague, Czech Republic.

Abstract

The biocompatible characteristics of intraocular lens materials can be differentiated by *in vitro* testing. Such tests include: bacterial colonisation, protein deposition, cytotoxicity, and cellular adhesion. Using a profile of tests, novel phosphorylcholine (PC)-based biomimetic materials have been evaluated as potential substitutes for poly(methylmethacrylate) (PMMA) in intraocular use. *Staphylococcus epidermidis* attachment (ATP extraction assay), fibrinogen adsorption (ELISA), mouse embryo fibroblast 3T3 adhesion (cellular ATP extraction), primary rabbit lens cell adhesion (cellular ATP), and human peripheral blood macrophage adhesion (antibody detection) tests were employed to compare biomimetic surface behaviour with that of PMMA. In all instances, biocompatibility was improved at least four-fold, and for eukaryotic cell adhesion and proliferation improvements were in excess of ten-fold. In an *in vivo* rabbit eye model, PC-based coatings have been found to reduce giant and diffuse cellular adherence; these characteristics were predicted from the initial *in vitro* cell culture screen. It may be anticipated that any damaging event could alter intraocular behaviour and thereby influence the biocompatibility response. *In vitro* cell culture methods offer a useful tool by which to probe the effects of irradiation on cell-biomaterial interactions; such information may be relevant to the selection and development of intraocular lenses for use following radiation-induced cataract removal.

1. Introduction

Cataract is a major healthcare problem throughout the world [1]. Millions of cases await treatment and this backlog shows no sign of diminishing in the near future. A range of hereditary and environmental factors are responsible for the pathogenesis of cataract including natural ageing, rare hereditary cataract syndromes (Rothmund Thompson syndrome, Werner's syndrome), diabetes, malnutrition and radiological insult [2]. However, regardless of origin, essentially all cataracts are now treated by removal

A. K. Junk et al. (eds.),
Ocular Radiation Risk Assessment in Populations Exposed to Environmental Radiation Contamination, 143–151.

of the natural lens and the insertion of an artificial intraocular lens (IOL) as a replacement. Optimal IOL performance is a major goal of biocompatibilty research within the ocular environment.

A range of complications have been reported following the implantation of IOLs, particularly when the devices are used in uveitic eyes or in the treatment of pediatric cataract [3]. These problems include, unwanted protein deposition [4], a cellular fibrosis resulting from adhesion of viable tissue fragments [5], regrowth of the lens epithelium across the remaining posterior capsule (posterior capsular opacification, PCO) with or without IOL involvement [5,6]; contact damage to the corneal endothelium during implantation [7,8] and a sustained inflammatory response involving humoral and lymphoid components of the immune system [9]. The common denominator of these complications is that they are essentially surface phenomena. This has been recognized for a number of years and a series of simple surface modifications have been attempted. None however has achieved unambigious success[10,11,12].

Recognising the intrinsic biocomatibiltiy of cell surface membranes, Chapman and coworkers proposed that novel polymers based upon the phosphorylcholine (PC) moiety might offer distinct advantages as biomimetic materials [13]. The authors have undertaken a series of studies using one such material, PC1008, to modify the surface of the most commonly implanted IOL material, poly(methyl methacrylate). These studies progressed from simple *in vitro* studies, designed to have application to essentially any surface biocompatibility problem, to more focussed tests intended to reflect the ocular environment. Only after satisfactory performance *in vitro* was PC1008 subjected to a formal *in vivo* trial in a rabbit model. An overview of these studies is reported below.

2 Methods

2.1 PRELIMINARY PHYSICAL CHEMISTRY

2.1.1.Modification of PMMA by physical adsorption of PC1008

PMMA sheets of uniform 1mm thickness, prepared by evaporation from a 10% (w/v) solution of PMMA in Analar grade dichloromethane, were coated with a 0.5 mg ml^{-1} solution of PC1008 (phosphorylcholine-methacrylate copolymer supplied by Biocompatibles Ltd.) in Analar grade ethanol. The PMMA was then air dried under sterile conditions for 10-15 min at room temperature and subsequently stored under sterile conditions.

2.1.2 Dynamic contact angle analysis

Wilhelmy-plate style dynamic contact angle (DCA) analysis was used to verify modification of the standard PMMA surface. Briefly a CAHN DCA-322 dynamic contact angle analyser (Scientific & Medical Products, Manchester UK) was used to determine the contact angle of PMMA and PC1008-modified PMMA. Water (surface tension 72.6 mN m^{-1}) was used as the probe fluid. Immersion and withdrawal speeds were set at 50 μm s^{-1} with an upper dwell time set to zero. Three immersion withdrawal cycles on three separately modified samples were performed in this study. PMMA sample thickness was verified using a precision micrometer and all evaluations were conducted at room temperature.

2.2. PHASE I *IN VITRO* TESTS

2.2.1. Adsorption of fibrinogen

The relative levels of fibrinogen adsorption to PMMA and PC1008-coated PMMA were determined using a three stage ELISA as described below. 0.21 cm^2 discs of both materials were each incubated with 100ng of human fibrinogen in 50 μl of phosphate buffered saline (PBS) pH 7.4 (all from Sigma Chemical Co). The incubation was carried out for 2 h at room temperature. Following adsorption the samples were extensively washed with PBS and excess non-specific binding sites on the surfaces were blocked by incubation with a 4% (w/v) solution of bovine serum albumin (BSA) (Cohen fraction V, Sigma) overnight at 4 °C. Following further washing in PBS the samples were incubated for thirty minutes with a polyclonal goat antiserum directed against human fibrinogen and diluted 1:1000 in PBS. The samples were subsequently washed and the procedure was repeated using sequential 1:500 dilutions of a secondary and tertiary antibody (rabbit anti-goat and goat anti-rabbit) conjugated to horse radish peroxidase (HRP). Antibody binding was visualised using the turnover of the HRP-specific chromogen 2,2'Azino-bis(3-ethylbenzthioline-6-sulphonic acid) (ABTS) in a standard phosphate-citrate assay buffer containing urea and H_2O_2. Non-specific binding was assessed by using the ELISA on both modified and unmodified PMMA in the absence of fibrinogen.

2.2.2 Adhesion of 3T3 mouse embryo fibroblasts

The immortal mouse embryo fibroblast cell line 3T3 was routinely cultured in Dulbecco's modification of Eagles Medium (DMEM, Gibco) supplemented with 10 % (v/v) foetal calf serum (Gibco) at a density of 6000 cells cm^{-2} at 37 °C in 5 % CO_2. Cells were passaged every three days by standard dispersion using Trypsin-EDTA solution (0.25 % Gibco). Viability was routinely checked by trypan blue counting and was always in excess of 90 %. To determine the adhesion of 3T3 fibroblasts to PMMA and PC1008-coated PMMA, 1000 viable cells were seeded onto 0.21 cm^2 discs of both materials in sterile 96 well tissue culture plates. The cells were allowed to attach and divide for 72 h under normal growth conditions. The discs and their adherent cells were then removed and cellular ATP was liberated by incubating each disc with 100 μl of a sterile hypotonic lysis buffer (0.01M Tris-Acetate pH 8, 2 mM EDTA). The ATP solution was then diluted 1:1 with a commercial assay buffer designed for ATP luminometry (0.1 M Tris-Acetate pH 8, 2 mM EDTA) and the amount of ATP in each sample measured using a commercial kit (BioOrbit-Wallac, Turku Finland) and a 96 well plate luminometer (Amerlite, Amersham). The method has been previously described [14].

2.2.3. Bacterial Adhesion

S.epidermidis strain 901, a clinical isolate, was grown in liquid culture in Oxoid No. 2 broth at 37 °C in 5 % CO_2. Bacterial cells were pelleted in a refrigerated centrifuge and washed three times in sterile PBS. The cells were resuspended in PBS and the optical density at 540 nm measured and the bacterial cell concentration adjusted to $3x10^8$ cell ml^{-1}. $1cm^2$ discs of PMMA and PC1008-coated PMMA were incubated with the resultant bacterial suspension for 4 h at 37 °C with constant agitation. The test samples were then removed, washed and the adherent cells quantified using the bioluminescence assay described above, modified to extract ATP with trichloroacetic acid.

2.3. PHASE II *IN VITRO* TESTS

2.3.1. Rabbit lens cell adhesion

AGO4677, a mortal primary rabbit lens epithelial cell strain was purchased from the National Institute of Aging (NIA) repository (Cambden, NJ, USA). The cells were cultured in Minimal Essential Eagles Medium (MEM) with double the normal concentration of non-essential amino acids (Gibco) and 10% (v/v) fetal calf serum (FCS) at a density of 6000 cells cm^{-2} at 37 °C in 5 % CO_2. The cells were never permitted to become confluent under maintenance conditions and were passaged by routine trypsin dispersion. Adhesion of the AGO4677 was assayed by ATP extraction 72 h after 1000 viable rabbit lens cells were plated onto PMMA and PC1008-coated PMMA discs as described for 3T3 fibroblasts above.

2.3.2. Macrophage Adhesion

20ml aliquots of human peripheral blood were withdrawn from a 28 year old healthy male volunteer and the blood defibrinated by agitation with sterile glass beads. Following removal of the fibrin clot the blood was diluted 1:1 with RPMI1640 medium (Gibco) and the mononuclear cells (MNCs) purified by sedimentation on a commercial Ficoll gradient (Lymphoprep, ICN-Flow). After sequential centrifugation at 400 g for 5 min to remove residual Lymphoprep the MNCs were resuspended in sterile Macrophage Serum Free Medium (Gibco) and counted using a haemocytometer. $2x10^5$ MNCs were plated onto each of a series of 1 cm^2 discs of PC1008-treated and untreated PMMA and left to adhere overnight in a sterile 12 well tissue culture dish in a 37 °C incubator under 5 % CO_2. The discs were then each washed three times with PBS and fixed in 4 % (w/v) paraformaldehyde for 10 min at room temperature. The fixed cells were subsequently permeabilised by incubation with a 1 % (v/v) solution of Triton X100 for 2 min. Following quenching of endogenous residual peroxidase activity by a 72 h incubation in 9 % H_2O_2 and extensive washing in PBS a 1:100 dilution of a mouse anti-macrophage monoclonal antibody (Dako Ltd, diluted in PBS +1 % FCS) was added to each disc and allowed to incubate overnight at 4 °C in a humidified chamber. The discs were then washed a further three times in PBS and macrophages visualised using "RapidStain" kit (Sigma). The number of macrophages was determined in 50 randomly selected fields.

2.4. PHASE III *IN VIVO* TESTS

2.4.1. Giant and diffuse cell adhesion

Single-eye surgery was performed on a test series of rabbits (minimum n=6 in each case). PMMA, PC1008-coated PMMA, heparin surface modified PMMA, acrylic and silicone lenses were implanted by standard surgical techniques. All eyes were examined by slit lamp and photographed at one, two, and four weeks after surgery. Giant cell number was evaluated clinically by two independent observers. Diffuse cell adherence was graded by the same observers using an arbitrary scoring system ranging from 0 (none) to 5 (extremely severe). All examinations by the observers were scored blind.

3. Results and Discussion

PC1008 was readily adsorbed to PMMA in a stable physical coating. This was illustrated by the shift in receding contact angle from a baseline of 39° for PMMA to 7° for the PMMA coated with PC1008. Direct visualisation of the PC1008 coat by rhodamine staining showed a coherent bright surface layer consistent with the presence of the copolymer (data not shown).

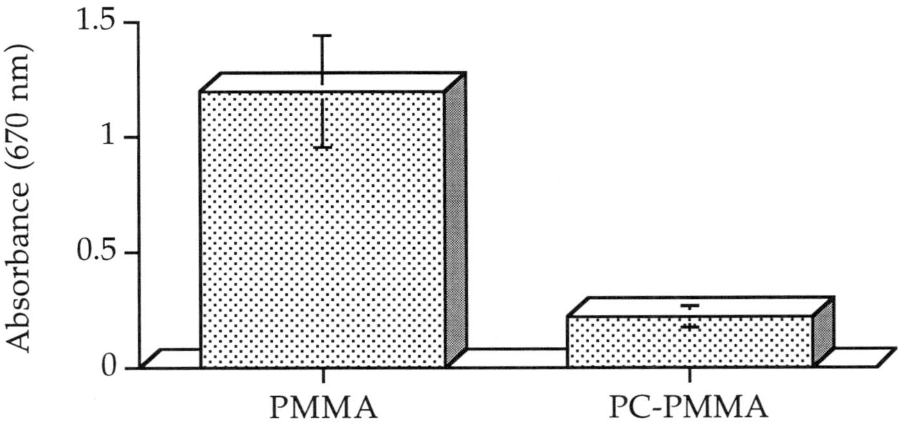

Figure 1. Fibrinogen adsorption to PMMA and PC-coated PMMA. Mean ± sd (n=6)

Initial protein binding determinations using ELISA demonstrated that PC1008 coating reduced the levels of fibrinogen adsorption by 80 % as shown in Figure 1. Similarly quantification of adherent mammalian and bacterial cells by ATP luminometry showed that the modified surface retained significantly less biomass than an unmodified PMMA control (Figures 2, 3). Following its successful performance in these initial tests, the coating was subjected to Phase II screening.

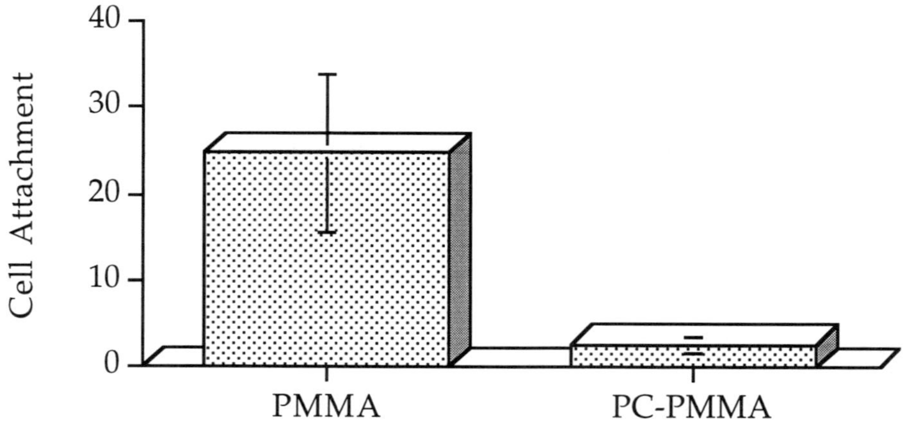

Figure 2. Fibroblast attachment to PMMA and PC-coated PMMA. Mean ± sd (n=6)

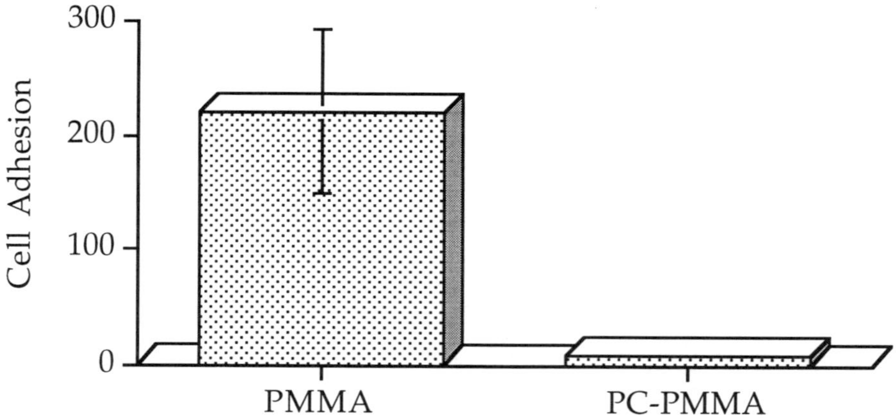

Figure 3. Adhesion of *S. epidermidis* to PMMA and PC-coated PMMA. Mean ± sd (n=6)

The reduction in biomass observed with a permanent cell line (3T3 mouse fibroblasts) was retained when primary rabbit lens epithelial cells were allowed to adhere to the surface (Figure 4). Direct visualisation of adherent human macrophages using an anti-CD68 monoclonal antibody showed a similar trend (Figure 5). The coating was thus subjected to a final Phase III *in vivo* trial.

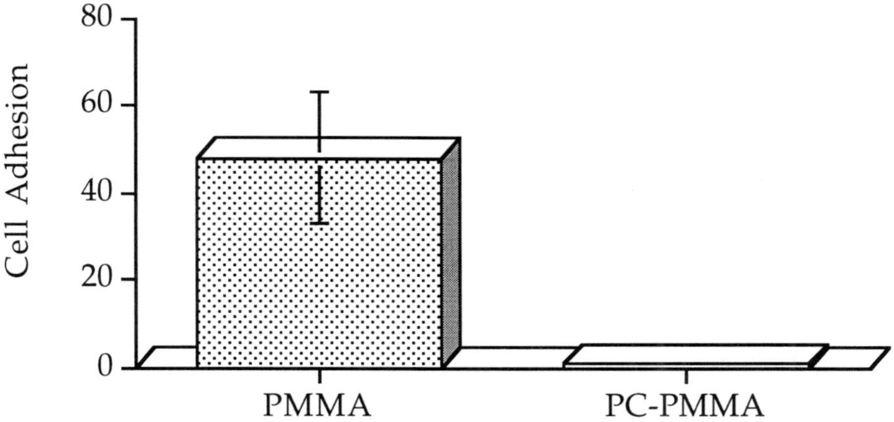

Figure 4. Lens epithelial cell adhesion to PMMA and PC-coated PMMA. Mean ± sd (n=6)

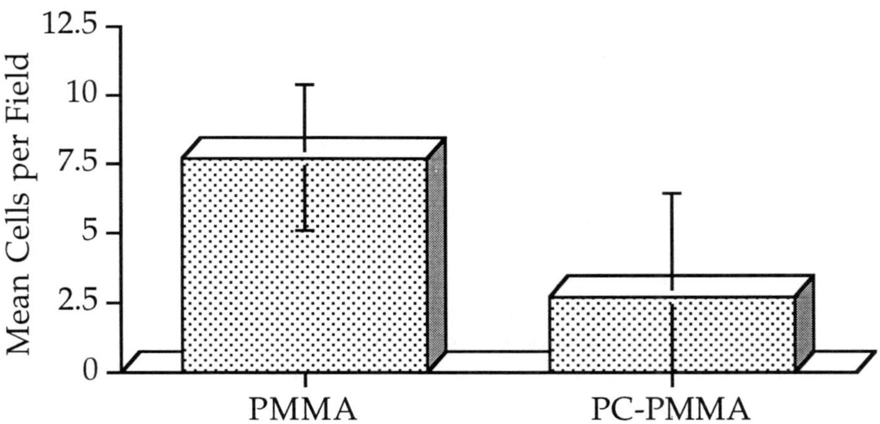

Figure 5. Macrophage adhesion to PMMA and PC-coated PMMA. Mean ± sd (n=25)

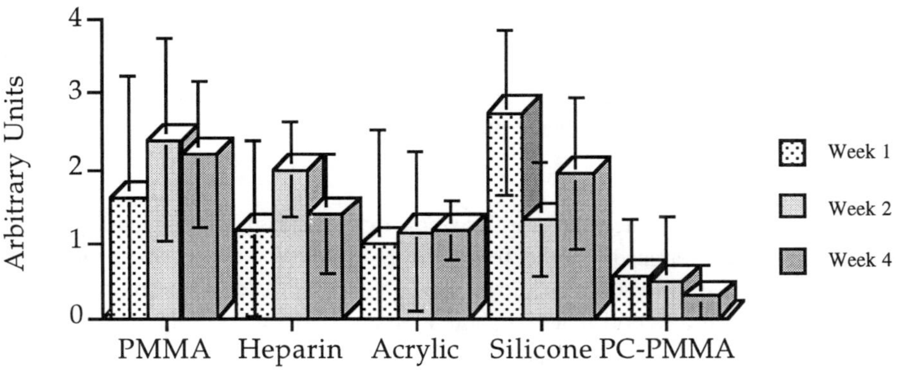

Figure 6. Diffuse cell adhesion to intraocular lenses. Mean ± sd

A series of rabbits were implanted with PMMA and PC1008-modified PMMA IOLs in accordance with existing ARVO guidelines. Specular comparisons of giant and diffuse cell adhesion showed a reduced cellular reaction to the treated surface over the period of the study compared to commercial lens types (Figures 6 & 7). No instances of bacterial endopthalmitis or endothelial barrier failure were noted in either group. Satisfactory surgical technique and a relatively small test pool of animals appear to have contributed to this outcome.

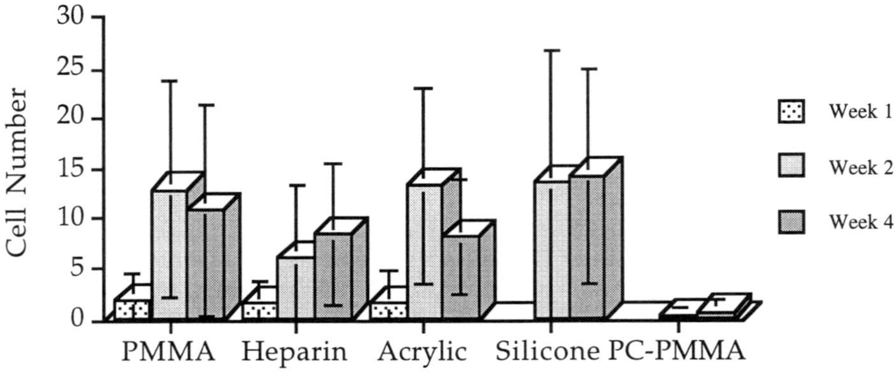

Figure 7. Giant cell adhesion to intraocular lenses. Mean ± sd

The *in vitro* biological screening was deliberately designed to present a series of challenges of increasing sophistication and relevance to the material under test. While this panel of assays has been compiled to be relevent to materials for optical use the general scheme is applicable to the mass screening of materials intended for use in any *in vivo* environment. The key features of the approach are the use of multiple tests in concert and in a step-wise manner. This allows the screens to both inform on one another and, with a suitably stringent design specification, to remove materials which fail to meet project requirements at a relatively early stage. The performance of the coated surface in the final animal trials is very similar to the behaviour seen in the Phase I and Phase II *in vitro* studies. This strongly suggests that the *in vitro* testing regime developed is reflective of the *in vivo* situation. Earlier reports had suggested that single *in vitro* tests could effectively substitute for animal studies [15] but the current investigation, to our knowledge, represents the first systematic attempt to utilise a battery of *in vitro* tests for the same purpose.

This study has demonstrated that modification of a standard PMMA surface with a biomimetic copolymer leads to the formation of a stable coating with considerably enhanced biocompatibiltiy both *in vitro* and *in vivo* for at least one month. Future clinical use of such a hybrid material should reduce the need for IOL explantation and repeated surgery. Should bacterial adhesion follow the same trend *in vivo* observed *in vitro* then the material may be less prone to contribute to endopthalmitis. At a time when the health care policies throughout the developed world are dominated by cost control considerations [16] improved ocular biomaterials offer the welcome opportunity to both improve patient benefit and reduce expenditure.

Acknowledgements

This work was supported under the BIOMIMPOLIOL DTI-MRC LINK Project in association with Biocompatibles International Plc and ChironVision UK. MRC reference number G9231614.

References

[1] Courtney, P.C. (1992) National Cataract Survey. *Eye* **6**, 487-493.

[2] Kritzinger, E.E. (1995) Eye disease in the elderly. *Rev. Clin. Gerontol.* **5**, 383-398.

[3] Rosen, E.S. (1993) Intraocular lenses. *Curr. Opin. Ophthalmol*; **4**, 44-53.

[4] Tang, L., Eaton, J.W. (1993) Fibrinogen mediates acute inflammatory responses to biomaterials. *J. Exp. Med.* **178**, 2147-2156.

[5] Pande M.V., Spalton, D.J., Marshall, J. (1996) In vivo human lens epithelial cell proliferation on the anterior surface of PMMA intraocular lenses. *Brit. J. Ophthalmol.* **80**, 469-474.

[6] Apple, D.J., Solomon, K.D., Tetz, M.R., Assia, E.I., Holland, B.S., Legler, U.F.C., Tsai, J.C., Casteneda, V.E., Hoggatt, J.P., Kostick, A.M.P. (1992) Posterior capsule opacification. *Surv. Ophthalmol* **37**, 73-116.

[7] Intraocular lens implantation. NIH consensus statement. (1979) **2**(7), 37-42.

[8] Bourne, W.M, Nelson, L.R, Hodge, D.O. (1994) Continued endothelial cell loss ten years after lens implantation. *Ophthalmology* **101,** 1014-1023.

[9] Harold, H., Kochounian, B.A., Maxwell, W.A., Gupta A. (1991) Complment activation by surface modified poly(methyl methacrylate) intraocular lenses. *J. Cataract Refract. Surg.* **17**, 139-142.

[10] Umezawa, S., Shimizu, K. (1993) Biocompatibility of surface-modified intraocular lenses. *J. Cataract Refract. Surg.* **17**, 371-374.

[11] Lin, C.L., Wang, A.G., Chou, J.C.K., Shieh, G., Liu J.H. (1994) Heparin surface modified intraocular lens implantation in patients with glaucoma, diabetes, or uveitis. *J. Cataract Refract. Surg.* **20**, 550-553.

[12] Eloy, R., Parrat, C.E., Min Duc, T., Legeay G., Bechteoille, A. (1993) In vitro evaluation of inflammatory cell response after CF_4 plasma surface modification of poly(methyl methacrylate) intraocular lenses. *J. Cataract Refract. Surg.* **19**, 364-370.

[13] Hayward, J.A., Chapman, D. (1984) Biomembrane surfaces as models for polymer design: The Potential for Haemocompatibility. *Biomaterials* **5**, 135 - 142.

[14] Faragher, R.G.A., Nagri, S., Dropcova, S., Mikhalovsky, S.V., Lloyd, A.W., Hanlon, G.W., Olliff, C.J., Denyer, S.P. (1996) Glycocalyx Adsorption Enhances Biocompatibility of Poly(Methyl Methacrylate). in M.D. LeVan (ed.), *Fundamentals of Adsorption* , Kluwer Academic Publishers, Boston MA; pp.285-292.

[15] Rougier, A., Cottin, M., de Silva, O., Rouget, R., Catroux, P., Toufic, A., Dossou K. (1992) In vitro methods: their relevance and complementarity in ocular saftey assessment. *Lens & Eye Toxicity* **9**, 229-245.

[16] Technology foresight panel on health and life sciences. *Progress through partnership* Technology Foresight 4 pp20-22. HMSO 1995.

X-RAY SENSITIVITY AND DNA DAMAGE IN BOVINE LENS EPITHELIAL CELLS IN VITRO

C. BAUMSTARK-KHAN [1], E. HALBE [2] AND H. RINK [2]

[1] *DLR, Institute of Aerospace Medicine, Radiobiology Section Linder Höhe, D-51170 Köln, Germany*
[2] *Radiologic Clinic, Experimental Radiology and Radiation Biology Sigmund-Freud-Str. 25, D-53105 Bonn, Germany*

Abstract

The radiosensitivity of bovine lens epithelial cells cultured in vitro was determined after X-irradiation. On a cellular level survival curves were obtained for immediate plating (IP) and delayed plating (LP) after a recovery period of 24 h and for plating of cells irradiated in the exponential stage of growth (EXP). On a molecular level X-ray induced DNA lesions have been determined. Induction of overall DNA strand breaks in lens epithelial cells and their rejoining was measured by fluorescent analysis of DNA unwinding (FADU), DNA double strand breaks were determined using the non-denaturing elution technique (NE). DNA damage induction is described in terms of dose effect curves, rejoining data are given in terms of rejoining enhancement curves and in terms of damage decay curves, which are best described by the sum of different exponential components.

1. Introduction

The mammalian lens is one of the radiosensitive organs and radiation-induced cataracts are prominent late effects after low-dose exposure. At the anterior lens pole lens epithelial cells are in a mitotically resting state (G_0 phase), whereas cells at the equatorial zone show a relative high proliferative activity. This equatorial zone of the epithelium is the main radiosensitive target of the lens. Irradiation of the proliferating cells leads to aberrant differentiation caused by unrepaired DNA damage. In consequence cataracts develop in the posterior lens part [1, 2]. Young individuals are more sensitive due to their high mitotic rate.

It is well accepted that radiation induced DNA damage leads to cellular inactivation. Double-strand breaks are considered to be the lesions, which are primarily responsible for chromosome aberrations and cell death. Therefore, investigations on a molecular level, determining DNA lesions induced by X-rays have been performed. On

A. K. Junk et al. (eds.),
Ocular Radiation Risk Assessment in Populations Exposed to Environmental Radiation Contamination, 153–162.

the other hand, cellular recovery is based on the complete elimination of such damages. Under these aspects Jose [3] underlined the role of DNA, and Geard and Worgul [4] assessed the effects of γ-rays on sister chromatid exchanges (SCE), chromosomal aberrations, and cellular kinetics in cells from the epithelial monolayer of organ-cultured individual rat lenses. Rink et al. [5] demonstrated the repair capacity in X-irradiated lens epithelial cells and its decrease with aging. Our experiments show the initial amount of DNA strand breaks as well as the rejoining capacity of the cells and correlate these molecular endpoints to cellular survival and recovery.

2. Materials and Methods

2.1. LENS EPITHELIAL CELLS

Diploid bovine lens epithelial cells (cell line: B 24) were cultured under standard conditions (Dulbeccos modified essential medium, 20% foetal calf serum, pH 7.0-6.8, 5% CO_2, 37°C). Cells between subcultures 8 and 20, corresponding to 16-40 cumulative population doublings (CPD) were used.

2.2. CELL LABELLING AND IRRADIATION

Exponentially growing cells were labelled with tritiated thymidine $[^3H]$TdR for three days. After removal of the radioactive medium cells were incubated for an additional period of 24 hours in non-radioactive medium.

2.3. IRRADIATION CONDITIONS

For survival experiments and measurement of overall DNA strand break induction irradiation was performed with an X-ray unit (200 kV, 10 mA) yielding a dose rate of 2 Gy/min. For determination of DNA double-strand breaks labelled cells were exposed to 300 kV X-rays (10 mA, dose rate: 5 Gy/min). Irradiation was performed on ice in order to avoid any DNA repair.

2.4. MEASUREMENT OF COLONY FORMATION FOR CELLULAR SURVIVAL

Cellular radiosensitivity of cultured bovine lens epithelial cells was tested using the colony forming ability test. Growth in the equatorial zone in situ was mimicked by exponentially growing cells. Mimicking the in situ conditions for the lens anterior pole confluent cell layers were irradiated and growth was stimulated afterwards. For immediate plating (IP) cells from confluent layers were plated immediately after X-irradiation. For late plating (LP) experiment, cells from confluent layers were allowed to repair DNA and to recover before they were inoculated (24 h after irradiation). Cells from exponential growing cultures (EXP) were inoculated immediately after X-irradiation. Results are given as survival curves, according to equation (1)

$$S = 1 - (1 - e^{-D/D_0})^n \tag{1}$$

where S is the surviving fraction, D is the dose, and D_0 (=-1/slope) and n (extrapolation number) are constants reflecting radiation sensitivity and repair capability, respectively.

2.5. DETECTION OF DNA STRAND BREAKS

Overall DNA strand breaks were measured using the fluorescent analysis of DNA unwinding (FADU) [6]. DNA double-strand breaks were measured selectively using the non-denaturing filter elution technique developed by Bradley and Kohn [7]. DNA strand break induction was measured immediately after irradiation. The rejoining capacity was determined after incubation of irradiated cells for different time periods.

2.6. DATA EVALUATION AND STATISTICAL ANALYSIS

All experimental data were standardised to $S_D/S_{D=0}$ or $F_D/F_{D=0}$, where F_D and $F_{D=0}$ were the DNA fractions of treated and untreated cells, respectively.

For strand break induction the experimental data (fraction of intact DNA: *FiDNA*) were fitted by a weighted least square regression according to

$$\ln FiDNA = -D/D_0 + \ln n \tag{2}$$

For strand break elimination rejoining enhancement (RE) was calculated for *FiDNA* at a given time minus *FiDNA* at time zero. All data from the samples for time intervals >0 were fitted by regression analysis to $1/RE_{(t)}$ versus 1/time. Extrapolation to time t_∞ (1/t=0) reveals the reciprocal of maximum rejoining enhancement (RE_{max}) and extrapolation to RE_∞ (1/RE=0) gives the half-time of rejoining by $-1/R_t$ [8, 9].

Calculation of the fraction of remaining damage was done according to Weibezahn and Coquerelle [10]. Remaining DNA damage data were fitted to the sum of three exponential functions where half-times τ of different components can be calculated from 1/slope·$\ln 2$. $a_{(I)}$, $a_{(II)}$ and $a_{(III)}$ correspond to the relevant ordinate intercepts [11]:

$$\ln damage = \left(slope_{(I)} \cdot t + \ln a_{(I)}\right) + \left(slope_{(II)} \cdot t + \ln a_{(II)}\right) + \left(slope_{(III)} \cdot t + \ln a_{(III)}\right) \tag{3}$$

3. Results

3.1. CELLULAR SURVIVAL AFTER X-IRRADIATION

Survival curves obtained immediately after X-irradiation are exponential with D_0 values of 1.4 Gy (EXP) and 2.3 Gy for confluent cultures (IP). Survival for delayed plating (LP) resulted in a survival curve with D_0 values of 3.7 Gy (Figure 1.).

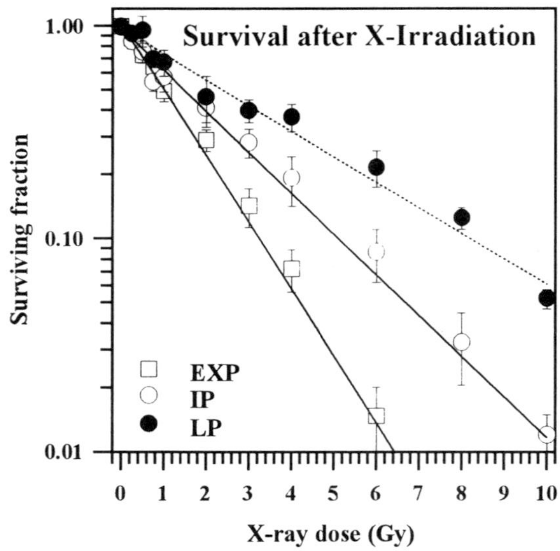

Figure. 1. Survival curves for in vitro cultivated B 24 lens epithelial cells for indicated conditions.

TABLE. 1. Radiosensitivity of in vitro cultivated B10 lens epithelial cells compared to other mammalian cell lines for the indicated conditions.

Cell line	Condition	D_0	n	Ref.
B 24	EXP	1.42	1.03	
	IP	2.28	0.94	
	LP	3.66	0.94	
NHF-23	IP	0.88	1.33	[12]
	LP	1.45	2.02	
GM 730	IP	1.54	1.43	[13]
	LP	2.34	1.46	
AG 1522	IP	1.33	3.04	[13]
	LP	3.20	0.90	
AG 1522	IP	1.27	1.52	[14]
	LP	2.08	1.36	
AT	IP	0.30		[11]
BS	IP	0.5		[11]

bovine lens epithelial cells: B 24
normal human fibroblast: NHF-23, GM 730, AG 1522
repair deficient human fibroblasts: AT, BS

3.2. DNA STRAND BREAK INDUCTION

Induction of overall DNA strand breaks in lens epithelial cells and their rejoining was measured by fluorescent analysis of DNA unwinding (FADU). DNA induction is described in terms of purely exponential dose effect curves with D_0 values of 6.9 Gy (FADU) and 62.4±6.9 Gy (NE), respectively (Figure 2.).

3.3. REJOINING OF DNA STRAND BREAKS

Rejoining data are given in terms of rejoining enhancement curves (Figure 3.). Overall DNA strand break repair shows R_t values of 15-20 minutes (5 Gy: 15 min; 10 Gy: 19 min), the fraction of intact DNA after complete repair ($R_{t=\infty}$) is calculated to be 0.86 (5 Gy) and 0.91 (10 Gy). In consequence, B 24 lens epithelial cells exhibit about 10 % residual damage after repair. For double-strand break repair after 40 Gy X-rays R_t values are in the range of 5-10 minutes, the amount of non-rejoined double-strand breaks is about 8 % (residual damage for $R_{t=\infty}$: 0.92).

Rejoining kinetics are also presented in terms of decay curves, which are best described by the sum of three exponential components. The half-times of these components have been determined as $\tau_{(I)} \approx 4$ min, $\tau_{(II)} \approx 30$ min and $\tau_{(III)} \approx 450$ min (Figure 4., Table 2.). For dsb repair R_t values are in the range of 6-10 min, decay curves can be described by biphasic repair kinetics with half-times $\tau_{(I)} \approx 10$ min and $\tau_{(II)}$ 225 min. These components of damage decay curves are correlated to cell killing.

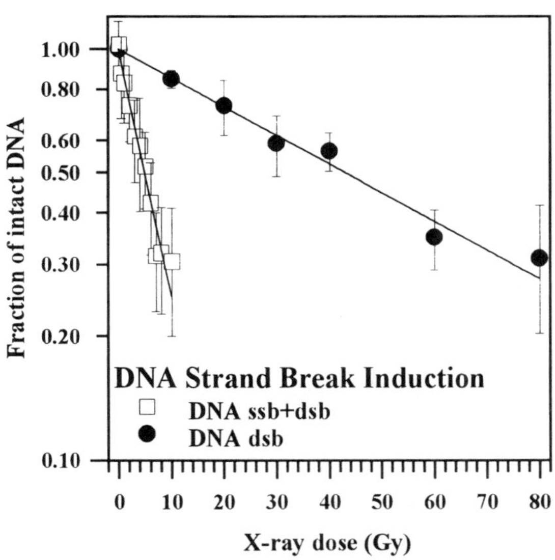

Figure 2. Relative fractions of intact DNA in B 24 lens epithelial cells irradiation. Cells were X-irradiated with varying doses and analyzed using the FADU or non-denaturing filter elution.

4. Discussion

In general radiosensitivity of mammalian cells is the result of initially induced DNA damage and of the cells ability to recover from this damage. The amount of initial damage is a function of dose, the repair processes, however, are influenced by cellular parameters such as the stage of growth and the time period between radiation and plating (IP, LP). These facts are reflected by the survival curves for B 24 lens epithelial cells (Figure 1., Table 1.). Survival curves for lens epithelial cells are purely exponential, the shoulder most oftenly found in other mammalian cell systems is absent. This may be one reason for the high radiosensitivity of lens epithelial cells in vivo.

Induction and repair of DNA strand breaks are molecular events preceeding cellular and recovery. Detection and measurement of DNA damage belongs without any doubt to the most important subjects in radiobiology, especially when induction and repair of damage has to be correlated with biological endpoints, such as cell inactivation and cellular recovery [19-22]. Therefore DNA strand breaks (induction and rejoining) were measured after exposing B 24 lens epithelial cells to X-rays. With the FADU technique it is possible to detect DNA strand breaks after irradiation with X-ray doses in a convenient dose range. With the non-denaturing filter elution DNA double-strand breaks can be measured selectively.

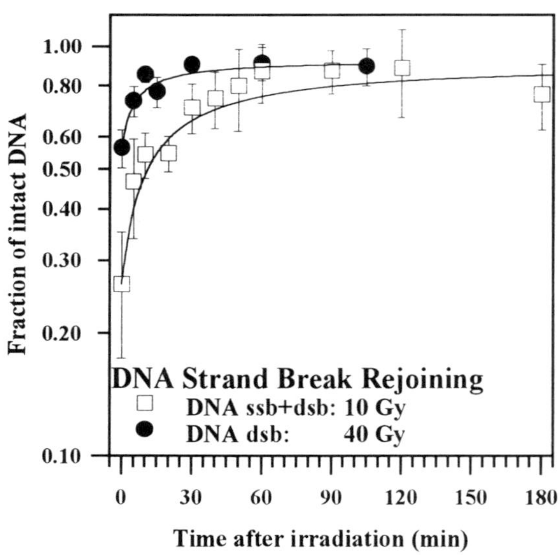

Figure 3. Relative fractions of intact DNA in B 24 lens epithelial cells irradiation with 10 or 40 Gy. Cells were analyzed using the FADU technique or non-denaturing filter elution at various time intervals after irradiation.

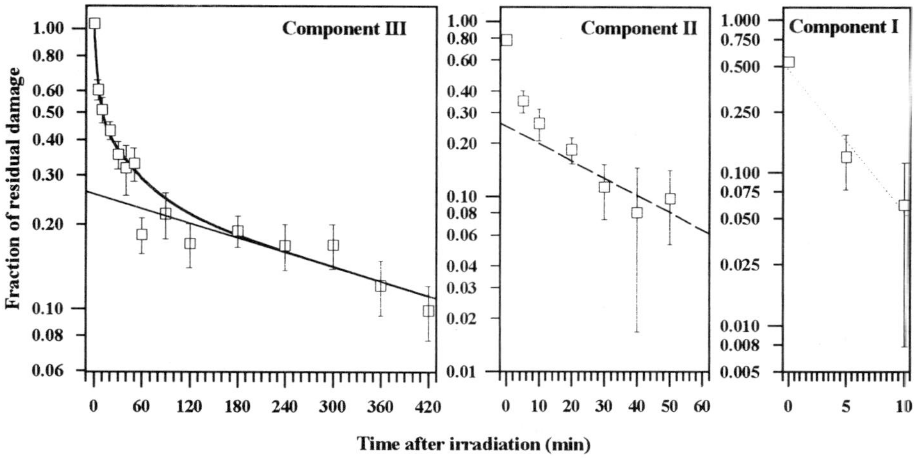

Figure 4. Rejoining kinetics (fraction of remaining damage) of X-ray induced DNA strand breaks. Data from figure 2 were recalculated and standardized according to Weibezahn and Coquerelle [10]. For t≥60 min the curve was fitted by linear regression (component III). After subtraction of component III from the experimental data residual repair kinetics of component II was calculated for incubation times between 10 to 50 min. After subtraction of component II residual repair kinetics of component I was determined for incubation times ≤10 min.

TABLE 2. Analysis of overall DNA strand break rejoining kinetics after X-Irradiation by successive regression yielding half-times (τ) and initial fractions (a) of the exponential components I, II and III

rejoining component						Reference	
I		II		III			
$\tau_{(I)}$ (min)	$a_{(I)}$	$\tau_{(II)}$ (min)	$a_{(II)}$	$\tau_{(III)}$ (min)	$a_{(III)}$	No.	Experiment design
3.20	0.475	30.6	0.251	348	0.256	this study	
1.44	0.658	14.8	0.355	496	0.053	[15]	(A)
2.40	0.710	17.0	0.250	200	0.040	[16]	(B)
2.10	0.700	15.0	0.240	210	0.060		(C)
1.50	0.410	18.0	0.390	170	0.200	[17]	(D)
1.73	0.690	17.0	0.250	218	0.060	[18]	(E)
1.66	0.650	14.2	0.290	194	0.060		(F)

(A)	X-rays	non-growing B 10 lens epithelial cells
(B)	3 Gy of X-rays,	CHO cells
(C)	9 Gy of X-rays,	CHO cells
(D)	internal ß-rays	CHO cells
(E)	9 Gy of X-rays	proliferating CHO cells
(F)	9 Gy of X-rays	non-growing CHO cells

DNA strand break induction as measured in this study follows purely exponential dose-relationships with D_0 values of 6.9 for the determination of overall strand breaks and of 62 for the determination of double-strand breaks. Although single-strand breaks are induced by X-rays about 10-times more than double-strand breaks, the biological consequence of double-strand breaks is more deleterious. They are supposed to be basic events for cell killing and induction of chromosome aberrations, their misrepair is considered to give rise to mutations (deletions, translocations) and thus to transformational events.

It is known, that cells which differ in radiosensitivity also differ in their DNA repair capacity. We, therefore, performed rejoining experiments with respect to incubation time. These experiments show, independent of the X-ray dose a fast DNA repair with half-times R_t from 15 to 20 min (overall strand breaks) and 6 to 10 min (double-strand breaks). Calculations of RE_{max} values point to incomplete rejoining (remaining damage ≈10%) for single- and double-strand breaks.

The lesion decay kinetics recorded for B 24 lens epithelial cells are best described by the sum of three exponential components, as has been shown for CHO cells [11, 16, 17]. Comparison of half-times $\tau_{(I)}$, $\tau_{(II)}$ and $\tau_{(III)}$ with published values for different mammalian cell lines (table II) are in good agreement with the results for B 24 cells.

Based on the fact that the initial fraction (a_{III}: about 0.05) and the half-time of component III were found to be conform with measurements of double-strand break repair using the neutral sedimentation technique [14] it was assumed [16] that the repair component III represents the repair of double-strand breaks whereas components I and II represent either the repair of two different classes of single-strand breaks or the repair of primary single-strand breaks induced by X-irradiation (I) and the occurrence of secondary single-strand breaks caused by incision enzymes during excision repair (II).

Analysis of double-strand break rejoining by use of the non-denaturing filter elution technique revealed a decay curve which can be described by biphasic repair kinetics with half-times $\tau_{(I)}$ ≈10 min and $\tau_{(II)}$ 225 min. This points to different repair mechanisms for double-strand break rejoining as well. Candidates may be either such double-strand breaks which can be subjected to simple rejoining or breaks which are repaired via recombinational repair pathways.

For cell killing, the amount of single-strand breaks in DNA is, however, not as important as the amount of double-strand breaks. The amount of induced damage is not as important as the of non-repaired or mis-repaired breaks. Small amounts of remaining damage have already deleterious effects on cellular survival. On the other hand, rejoining is not synonymous with repair which requires restoration of the original nucleotide sequence.

Obviously, in B 24 lens epithelial cells, double-strand breaks are induced with a high efficiency. They show more double-strand breaks when compared to other cell systems (Table 2): B 24 cells have the capacity to rejoin DNA breaks, although the amount of residual damage after repair ($R_{t=\infty}$) with about 10 % is very high. Another lens epithelial cell line, B 10 was described to express normal amounts of DNA double-strand breaks, the half-life time $\tau_{(III)}$ for repair component III, however, shows more than twice the value obtained by CHO cells [15]. The slower repair of double-strand breaks in B 10 lens epithelial cells additionally implies a relatively high amount of unrepaired double-strand breaks (4-5% at 270 min repair, Table 2.). The data implicate that the remaining damage (double-strand breaks) is responsible for cell death, misdifferentiation and consequently also for radiation induced opacities.

Acknowledgement. This work was performed within the frame work of the EEC Concerted Action on Cellular Ageing and Diseases (EURAGE).

5. References

1. Bergeder, H.-D., Rink, H., Hockwin, O. (1982), Die Röntgenkatarakt. Ein Modell zur Untersuchung der Katakaktogenese. *Klinische Monatsblätter der Augenheilkunde* **180,** 13-16 (1982)
2. Koch, H.-R., Hockwin, O. (1980), Radiation cataractogenesis, in: S. Lerman (ed.): *Radiant energy and the eye.* MacMillan, New York, USA, pp 286-302 (1980)
3. Jose, J.G. (1978), The role of DNA damage, its repair and its misrepair in the ethiology of senile cataract. *Ophthalmic Res.* **10**, 52-62 (1978)
4. Geard C.R., Worgul B.V. (1987), The lens and cataract: clastogenic responses in epithelial cells of the organ-cultured rat lens. *Environ. Mutagen.* **9,** 111-122
5. Rink H., Zblewski R., Baumstark-Khan C. (1986), Repair capacity and aging of lens epithelial cells in vitro, in: Y. Courtois, B. Faucheux, B. Forette, D.L. Knook, J.A. Tréton (eds.): *Modern Trends in Aging Research.* Paris, INSERM **147,** 303-309
6. Baumstark-Khan, C. (1994), Alkaline elution versus fluorescence analysis of DNA unwinding. *Meth. Enzymol.* **234**, 88-102
7. Bradley, M.O., Kohn, K.W. (1979), X-ray induced DNA double-strand break production and repair in mammalian cells measured by neutral filter elution. *Nucl. Acid Res.* **7,** 793-804 (1979).
8. Baumstark-Khan, C. (1990) A calculation method of PLD-recovery based on saturation kinetics, in: E. Riklis (ed.), *Frontiers in Radiation Biology.* VCH, Weinheim, Germany, pp. 513-520
9. Baumstark-Khan, C. (1992) Effect of aphidicolin on DNA synthesis, PLD-recovery and DNA repair of human diploid fibroblasts. *Int. J. Radiat. Biol.* **61,** 191-197
10. Weibezahn, K. F., Coquerelle, T. (1981), Radiation induced DNA double strand breaks are rejoined by ligation and recombination processes. *Nucl. Acids Res.* **9**, 3139-3150
11. Dikomey, E., Franzke, J. (1988), DNA denaturation kinetics in CHO cells exposed to different X-ray doses and after different repair intervals using the alkaline unwinding technique. *Radiat. Environm. Biophys.* **27**, 29-37
12. Baumstark-Khan C, Schneider J, Rink H. (1991), Radiation sensitivity of cultured bovine lens epithelial cells. *Ophthalmic Res.* **23,**:235-239
13. Weichselbaum, R.R., Tomkinson, U., Little, J.B. (1985), Repair of potentially lethal X-ray damage in fibroblasts derived from patients with hereditary and D-deletion retinoblastoma. *Int. J. Radiat. Biol.* **47**, 445-456
14. Bryant, P. E., Blöcher, D. (1980), Measurement of the kinetics of DNA double-strand break repair in Ehrlich ascites tumour cells using the unwinding method, *Int. J. Radiat. Biol.* **38,** 335-347 (1980)
15. Baumstark-Khan, C., Aufderheide, E., Rink, H. (1992). X-ray induced DNA strand break

induction and rejoining in cultured bovine lens epithelial cells, *Ophthalmic Res.* **24,** 220-227 (1992)

16. Dikomey, E., Franzke, J. (1986), Three classes of DNA strand breaks induced by X-irradiation and internal ß-ray. *Int. J. Radiat. Biol.* **50**, 893-908
17. Dikomey, E. (1990), Induction and repair of DNA strand breaks in X-irradiated proliferating and quiescent CHO cells, *Int. J. Radiat. Biol.* **57,** 1169-1182
18. Cox, R., Masson, W.K., Weichselbaum, R.R., Nove, J., Little, J.B. (1981), The repair of potential damage in X-irradiated cultures of normal and ataxia teleangiectasia human fibroblasts. *Int. J. Radiat. Biol.* **39**, 357-365 (1981)
19. Lett, J.T. (1981), Measurement of single-strand breaks by sedimentation in alkaline sucrose gradients. In: E.C.Friedberg, P.C.Hanawalt (eds.), *DNA Repair: A Laboratory Manual in Research Procedures,* Marcel Deker, New York, pp 5151-5154.
20. Ahnstrøm, G. (1988). Techniques to measure DNA single-strand breaks in cells: A review. *Int. J. Radiat. Biol.* **54,** 695-707
21. Radford, J.R. (1988), The dose response for low LET radiation induced DNA double-strand breakage: Methods and measurements and implications for radiation action models. *Int. J. Radiat. Biol.* **54,** 1-11 (1988)
22. Olive, P.L. (1992), DNA organization affects cellular radiosensitivity and detection of initial DNA strand breaks, *Int. J. Radiat. Biol.* **62,** 389-396 (1992)

INDUCTION AND REPAIR OF DNA STRAND BREAKS IN BOVINE LENS EPITHELIAL CELLS AFTER HIGH LET IRRADIATION

C. BAUMSTARK-KHAN [1], J. HEILMANN [2], E. AUFDERHEIDE [3]
AND H. RINK [3]

[1] *DLR, Institute of Aerospace Medicine, Radiobiology Section*
Linder Höhe, D-51170 Köln, Germany
[2] *GSI, Biophysical Unit*
Planckstr. 1, D-64291 Darmstadt, Germany
[3] *Radiologic Clinic, Experimental Radiology and Radiation Biology*
Sigmund-Freud-Str. 25, D-53105 Bonn, Germany

Abstract

RBEs for the induction of DNA strand breaks and the efficiency of repair of these breaks were measured in cultured diploid bovine lens epithelial cells exposed to different LET irradiations. Irradiations were performed either with 300 kV X-rays or at the UNILAC accelerator at GSI. Different accelerated ions were used from Z=8 (O) to Z=92 (U) with kinetic energies from 1.5 to 19.3 MeV/u, LETs ranged from 285 to 16,300 keV/µm and the fluences from $3 \cdot 10^6$ to $80 \cdot 10^6$ particles per cm^2. For strand break measurements the hydroxyapatite chromatography of alkaline unwound DNA (overall strand breaks) was applied. DNA damage occurs as a function of dose, of kinetic energy and of LET. Repair kinetics depend on the fluence (irradiation dose). At any LET value, repair is much slower after heavy ion exposure than after X-irradiation. For ions with an LET greater than 10,000 keV/µm a higher proportion of non-rejoined breaks is found, even after prolonged periods of incubation. At the highest LET value (16,300 keV/µm) no significant repair is observed.

1. Introduction

The lens epithelium is the initiation site not only for the development of senile cataracts but also for radiation induced cataracts. While in the cortex and nucleus radiation interacts with proteins, experimental results from cultured lenses and lens epithelial cells demonstrate that mutagenic and cytotoxic effects might occur in the epithelium. It is suggested that incorrectly repaired DNA damage may be lethal in terms of cellular reproductivity or may initiate mutations or transformations in surviving cells. The occurence of such genetically modified cells, which can not differentiate correctly, may

A. K. Junk et al. (eds.),
Ocular Radiation Risk Assessment in Populations Exposed to Environmental Radiation Contamination, 163–172.

lead to lens opacification. For a quantitative risk estimation of populations to environmental exposure with different types of radiation it is necessary to know their relative biological effectiveness (RBE), because radiations from reactor accidents and fall-out from nuclear testing differ significantly from X-rays. The study of DNA lesions is an important topic in the evaluation of primary damage. Especially the induction and repair of DNA double-strand breaks are essential for the understanding of cellular killing and mutations [1]. This study focuses on the RBEs for the induction of DNA strand breaks in cultured diploid bovine lens epithelial cells exposed to different LET irradiations (for definitions and doses, see [2]). Furthermore, rejoining of strand breaks was monitored as a first step towards more detailed information on repair mechanisms.

2. Materials and Methods

2.1. LENS EPITHELIAL CELLS

Diploid bovine lens epithelial cells (cell line: B 26) were cultured under standard conditions (Dulbeccos modified essential medium, 20% foetal calf serum, pH 7.0-6.8, 5% CO_2, 37°C). Cells between subcultures 8 and 20, corresponding to 16-40 cumulative population doublings (CPD) were used.

2.2. CELL LABELLING AND IRRADIATION

Growing cells were labelled with tritiated thymidine ([^{3}H]TdR) for three days. After removal of the radioactive medium cells were incubated for an additional period of 24 hours in non-radioactive medium.

2.3. IRRADIATION CONDITIONS

Studies on DNA breaks were performed after X-irradiation (300 kV X-rays, 10 mA, dose rate: 5 Gy/min) or after irradiations with heavy ions (UNILAC accelerator at GSI, Darmstadt). Different accelerated ions were used from Z=8 (O) to Z=92 (U) with kinetic energies from 1.5 to 19,3 MeV/u, LETs from 285 to 16,300 keV/μm and fluences from $3 \cdot 10^6$ to $80 \cdot 10^6$ particles per cm^2 (P/cm^2). Irradiation was performed on ice in order to avoid any DNA repair during irradiation.

2.4. DETECTION OF DNA STRAND BREAKS

For strand break measurements a slightly modified version of the hydroxyapatite chromatography of alkaline unwound DNA (overall strand breaks) was used [3]. The procedure was as follows: after removal of the the medium the cells were lysed and the DNA was denaturated by addition of an alkaline solution (NaOH 0.03 mol/l, Na_2HPO_4 0.01 mol/l, NaCl 0.9 mol/l, pH 11.8, ionic strength 0.98) for 30 min at 22°C. After neutralization with HCl solution (0.034 mol/l) this suspension was sonicated (100 W, 15 sec) at ice temperature and SDS solution (0.035 mol/l) was added. For separation of single- and double-stranded DNA, samples were loaded on previously equilibrated hydroxyapatite columns (potassium phosphate buffer, pH 6.8, 0.01 mol/l) and heated to 60°C. Single-stranded DNA (ssDNA) was then eluted with 3 ml of phosphate buffer (pH 6.8, 0.15 mol/l) before double stranded DNA (dsDNA) was eluted with 3 ml of phosphate buffer (pH 6.8, 0.33 mol/l). The eluates were mixed with scintillation cocktail and ^3H activity was measured in a liquid scintillation counter.

DNA strand break induction was measured immediately after irradiation. The rejoining capacity was determined after incubation of irradiated cells for different time periods.

2.5. DATA EVALUATION AND STATISTICAL ANALYSIS

Experiments were repeated at least twice, using up to three parallel samples per experimental point. The fraction of double-stranded DNA (FdsDNA) was obtained from:

$$FdsDNA = \frac{cpm_{(0.33)} - cpm_{(background)}}{cpm_{(0.33)} + cpm_{(0.15)} - 2 \cdot cpm_{(background)}} \tag{1}$$

where $cpm_{(0.33)}$ and $cpm_{(0.15)}$ are the counts in the samples containing single- or double-stranded DNA, respectively, and $cpm_{(background)}$. are the counts in the background sample.

LET values were calculated according to Wulf et al [4]. All experimental data were standardized and fitted to the equations, described by Baumstark-Khan et al. [5]. The effective dose for heavy ion experiments was calculated as:

$$Dose(Gy) = 1.6 \cdot 10^{-9} \cdot LET \cdot P/cm^2 \tag{2}$$

F_0 values from the dose effect curves were used to calculate the relative biological effectiveness (RBE) of heavy ions, compared to 300 kV X-rays. In addition, the effectiveness per particle (P) has been calculated as $\sigma = 1/F_0$.

3. Results

3.1. DNA STRAND BREAK INDUCTION

The measurements of the induction of DNA strand breaks always yielded purely exponential dose-effect curves independent on the detection system. Cross sections were derived from the slopes of least-squares regression analysis. Standardization was achieved by calculating a relative cross section as the ratio of the cross section for the test radiation (heavy ion exposure) and the cross section obtained from corresponding X-ray experiments.

Experiments showed that DNA damage occurs as a function of dose, of kinetic energy and of LET. For particles having the same LET the severity of the DNA damage increases with dose. For a given particle dose, as the LET rises, the numbers of DNA strand breaks increase (Figure 1., TABLE 1.).

3.2. REJOINING OF DNA STRAND BREAKS

The rejoining of DNA strand breaks is considered to be indicative for DNA repair in living cells after exposure to ionizing radiation [6], but it is not proven wheather this repair is genetically correct. After X-irradiation, fast rejoining was found with a half time of about 10 min; only about 5% residual damage was detected after a 1 h of incubation. Extrapolation to t=∞ revealed complete rejoining capacity for the investigated

TABLE 1. Strand break induction in lens epithelial cells by X-irradiation and heavy ions

Radiation		Energy kV		D_0 Gy	-slope	Dose Gy	RBE
X-Rays		300		28.6	0.0350	28.6	1
Particle	Z	Energy MeV/u	LET keV/μm	F_0 10^6 P/cm^2	σ μm^2	Dose Gy-equivalents	RBE
16-O	8	3.4	524	766.8	0.0013	642.9	0.044
		8.7	285	505.5	0.0019	230.5	0.124
40-Ar	18	2.7	2,200	191.7	0.0052	674.8	0.042
		6.1	1,620	189.3	0.0052	490.7	0.058
		10.5	1,150	117.0	0.0085	215.3	0.132
		19.3	790	102.4	0.0098	129.4	0.221
48-Ti	22	4.8	2,500	149.1	0.0067	596.4	0.048
		5.6	2,360	123.5	0.0081	466.3	0.061
		14.3	1,440	89.5	0.0112	206.2	0.139
74-Ge	32	10.1	3,400	47.5	0.0211	258.4	0.111
84-Kr	36	18.0	3,050	50.2	0.0199	245.0	0.117
132-Xe	54	5.4	8,800	78.6	0.0127	1,106.7	0.026
		10.1	7,200	45.6	0.0219	525.3	0.054
		16.5	6,200	30.7	0.0326	304.5	0.094
139-La	57	10.1	8,400	29.9	0.0334	401.9	0.071
208-Pb	82	3.0	14,500	47.0	0.0213	1,090.4	0.026
		6.8	14,300	21.4	0.0467	489.6	0.058
		15.4	14,100	11.7	0.0855	264.0	0.108
238-U	92	1.5	14,200	119.5	0.0084	2,715.0	0.011
		1.9	15,000	142.2	0.0070	3,412.8	0.008
		2.6	15,700	97.4	0.0103	2,446.7	0.012
		4.0	16,300	56.0	0.0179	1,460.5	0.020

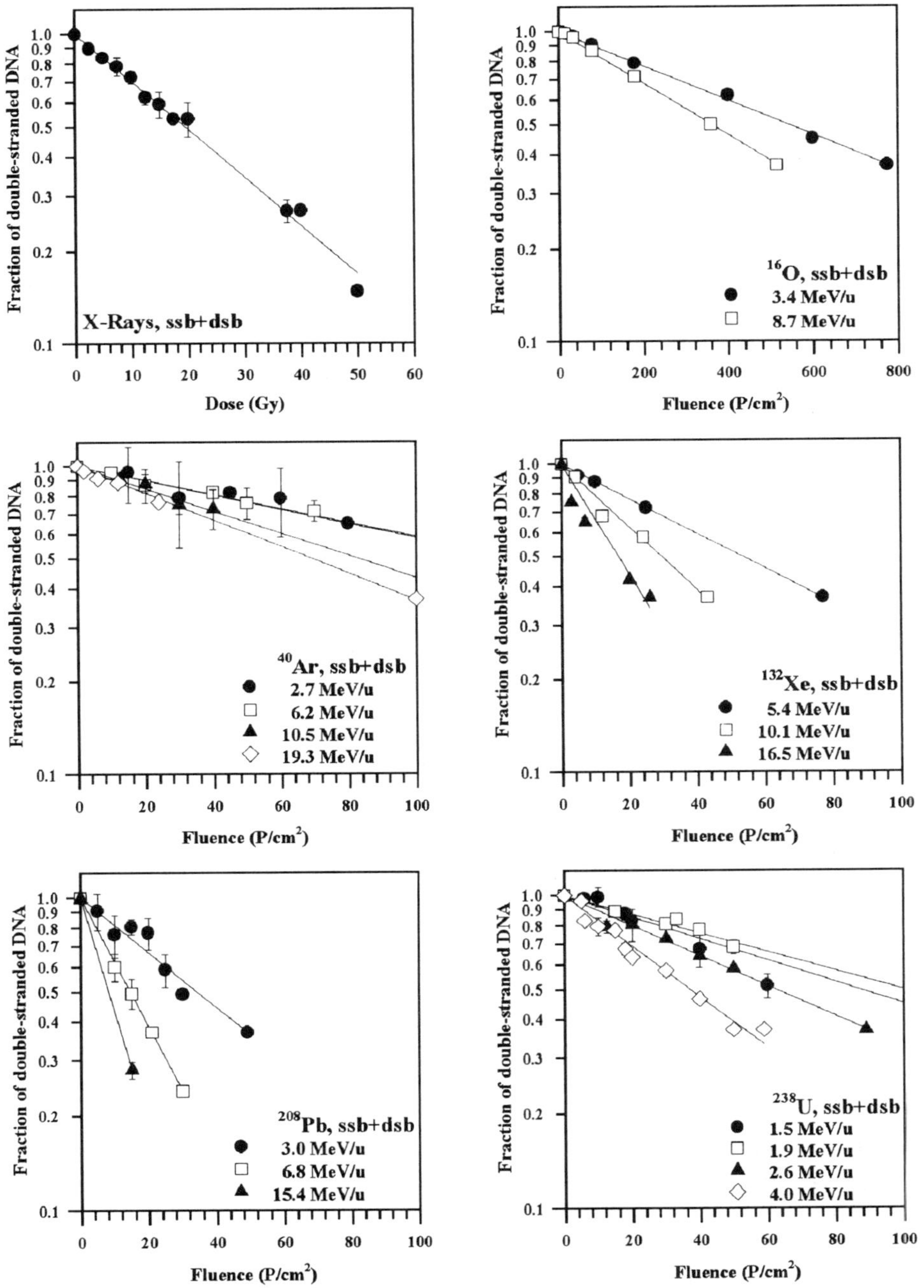

Figure 1. Dose-effect curves for DNA strand break induction measured with the unwinding technique after X-irradiation and exposure with various accelerated heavy ions differing in specific energies and LET.

TABLE 2. Strand break rejoning in lens epithelial cells after irradiation with X-rays and heavy ions

Radiation		Energy kV		Dose Gy	Initial damage	K_t min	RE_∞	Rejoined DNA
X-Rays		300		15	0.5916	9.7	0.4580	1.0496
				50	0.1479	13.6	0.8577	1.0056
Particle	**Z**	**Energy MeV/u**	**LET keV/μm**	**Fluence 10^6 P/cm^2**	**Initial damage**	**K_t min**	**RE_∞**	**Rejoined DNA**
16-O	8	8.7	285	35	0.9600	6.2	0.0279	0.9879
				80	0.8700	20.4	0.1161	0.9861
				180	0.7180	18.6	0.2536	0.9716
				360	0.5000	19.2	0.4577	0.9577
40-Ar	18	2.7	2,200	80	0.6500	38.2	0.3285	0.9785
		19.3	790	6	0.9133	21.8	0.0867	1.0000
				24	0.7650	16.4	0.2203	0.9853
48-Ti	22	14.3	1,440	80	0.3900	120	0.3032	0.6932
84-Kr	36	18.0	3,050	9	0.7900	12.7	0.1813	0.9713
				21	0.6233	7.1	0.2710	0.8943
132-Xe	54	5.4	8,800	5	0.9200	16.2	0.0450	0.9650
				10	0.8800	71.6	0.0916	0.9716
		16.5	6,200	3	0.8000	5.5	0.1799	0.9799
				9	0.6700	17.1	0.3088	0.9788
				21	0.4200	27.1	0.4461	0.8661
139-La	57	10.1	8,400	15	0.5560	38.1	0.1875	0.7435
208-Pb	82	6.8	14,300	30	0.2400	36.1	0.0621	0.3021
		15.4	14,100	15	0.2800	44.0	-0.1001	0.1799
238-U	92	2.6	15,700	40	0.6400	36.2	0.2292	0.8692
		4.0	16,300	5	0.9600	56.0	0.0602	1.0202
				10	0.7960	102.0	-0.0311	0.7649
				18	0.6733	72.0	-0.1808	0.4925
				40	0.4656	6.1	0.0218	0.4874

cell line. For heavy ion irradiation it could be demonstrated, that rejoining of broken DNA pieces slowed down to a great extend. For ions with an LET of less than 10,000 keV/μm more than 90% of the induced strand breaks are repaired within 24 hours. At higher fluences, especially for low energetic particles with a very high local density of energy deposition within the particle track, a higher proportion of (non-rejoined) residual damage is detectable, even after prolonged periods of incubation. At the highest LET value (16,300 keV/μm) no rejoining is seen (Figure 2., TABLE 2.).

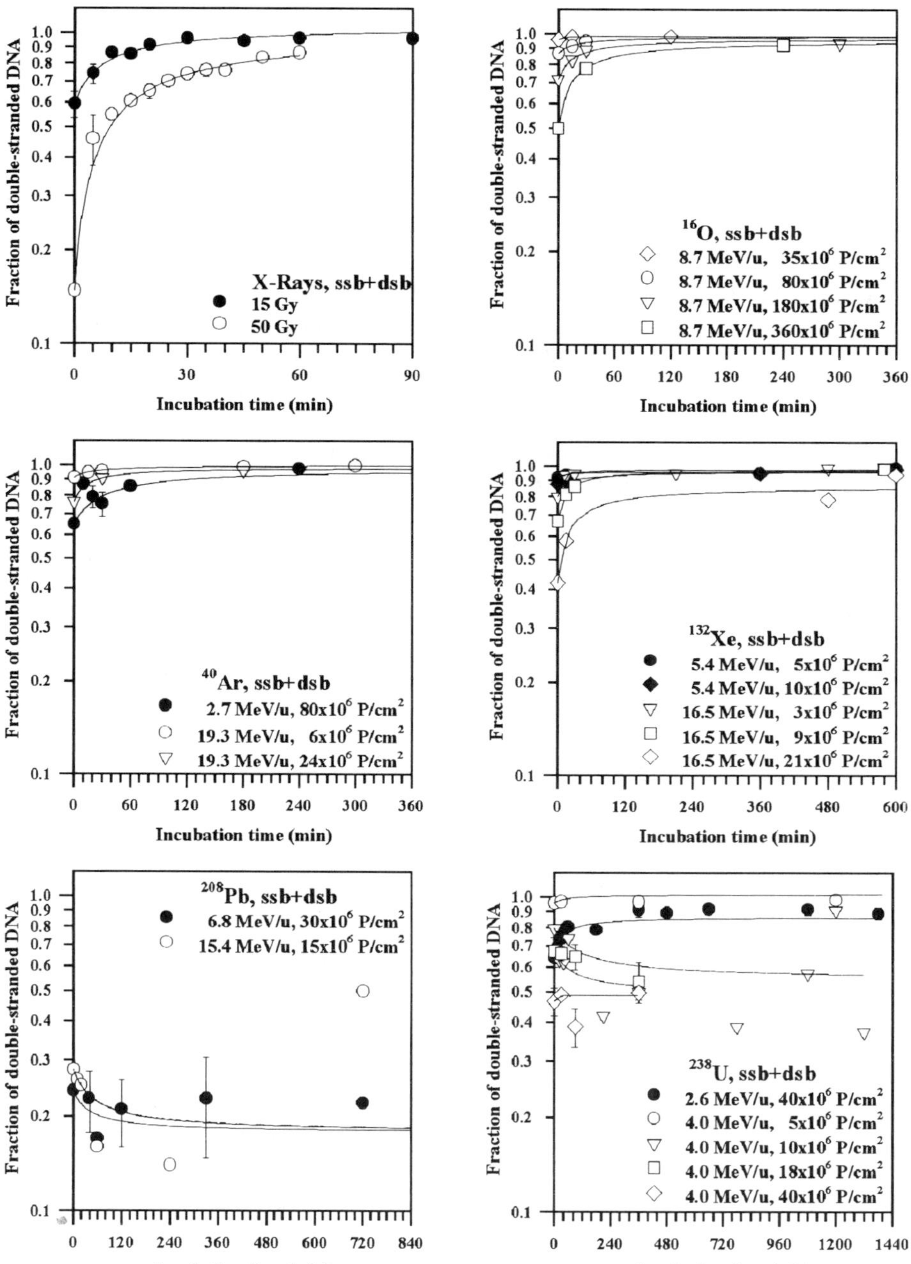

Figure 2. Rejoining curves for DNA strand break repair measured with the unwinding technique after X-irradiation and exposure with various fluences of distinct accelerated heavy ions differing in specific energies and LET

4. Discussion

In view of the irregular spatial distribution of energy generated by particle irradiation, radiation effects should not be expressed per average dose (Gy). Instead, cross sections (μm^2), which represent the probability of a particle to affect a certain target area, are given. For intracellular strand breaks, the critical size is the chromosome. Figure 3. shows standardized cross sections σ for the induction of total strand breaks. For data in the high-LET region so-called hook-structures can be seen (Pb, U). In all cases the cross sections for DNA strand breaks correspond to RBE values smaller than one. Data in the range up to 300 keV/µm are from Kampf [7], obtained for V79 cells with the ions H, He and C. These measurements were performed using the alkaline sucrose sedimentation technique. Our results continue the data from Kampf.

Cross sections of the intracellular induction of DNA strand breaks in lens epithelial cells show the same dependencies from LET as it is reported for other biological endpoints. The low efficiencies (RBE 0.008-0.2) are in good agreement with data for ions with $Z<18$ [8]. In the LET range 800-16,000 keV/µm the efficiency of DNA strand break induction increases with increasing particle energy. With increasing LET and decreasing energy of the ion, the density of energy deposition increases. This increases the probability of recombination of radiolytic products, which then do not affect the DNA. This may account for the low strand breaking efficiencies in general (RBE values well below 1), as well as for the continuous decrease of this efficiency with increasing LET values and decreasing energies.

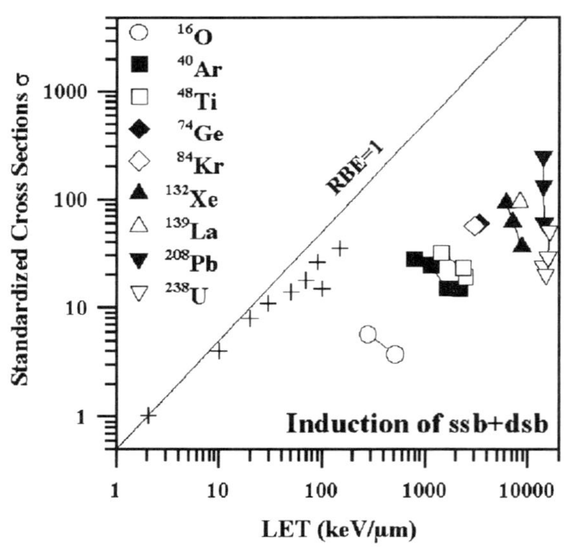

Figure 3. Standardized efficiencies for the induction of DNA strand breaks as a function of LET. V79 cell data from Kampf [7] are included for comparison (crosses). In the high LET range, individual curves exist for the different particles. The solid line corresponds to RBE=1

Three major differences between the repair of DNA strand breaks in lens epithelial cells after low and high LET irradiation have become obvious: (i) The repair after heavy ion radiation is rather slow (K_t >15min), compared to X-irradiation (K_t <15min). This may be due to a higher proportion of DNA dsb [9]. (ii) The rate and extent of repair decreases with increasing radiation dose or particle fluence. Changes in the damage structure could be one explanation. (iii) The proportion of unrejoined breaks in heavy ion irradiated samples is high, even after long periods of repair incubation.

In the experiments using lead and uranium ions at LET values >10,000 keV/μm no significant DNA strand break repair could be determined (Fig. 4). If the dose profile inside the particle track is considered [10], the dose in the track center can be as high as 1.6 MGy for uranium (LET 16,000 keV/μm), while the oxygen ion (LET 524 keV/μm) exhibits only 50 kGy in the track center. As doses of 1,000 Gy have been reported largely to inhibit repair [11], it is possible that DNA damage induced by lead or uranium is irrepairable.

In conclusion, the results show that, after heavy ion irradiation (especially for the very heavy ions Pb and U), rejoining of DNA strand breaks is less complete than after exposure to X-rays. These observations are consistent with the current theory of mechanism of radiation induced cataractogenesis which posts that genomic damage to the surviving epithelial cells the exposure is responsible for lens opacification.

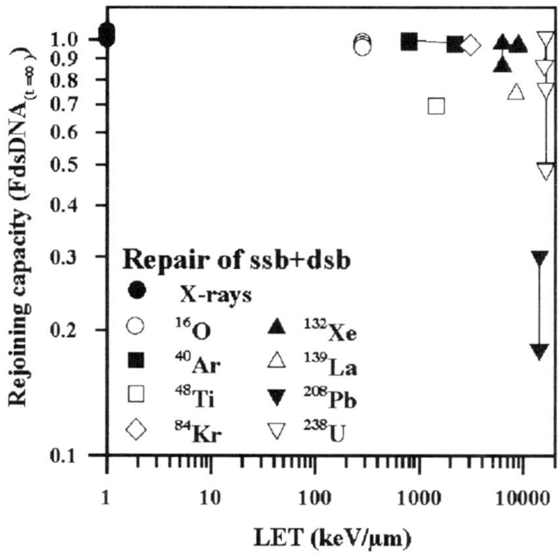

Figure 4. Rejoining capacity for the repair of DNA strand breaks as a function of LET. In the lower LET range (LET<10,000), cells are capable of nearly complete rejoining, irrespectively of particle energy and fluences. In the high LET range (LET>10,000), rejoining capacity strictly depends on the initial amount of DNA damage and thus on particle fluence

5. References

1. Frankenberg-Schwager, M., Frankenberg, D., Blöcher, D., Adamczyk, C. (1980), Repair of DNA double-strand breaks in irradiated yeast cells under nongrowth conditions. Radiat. Res. 82, 498-510
2. Baumstark-Khan, C. (1998), Estimation of environmental burdens by radiation. Radiologic units: From gray to Sievert. in: B.V. Worgul (Ed.), Ocular Radiation Risk Assessment in Populations exposed to Environmental Radiation Contamination, Kluwer, Dordrecht, The Netherlands
3. Rydberg, B., (1975), The rate of strand separation in alkali of DNA of irradiated mammalian cells. Radiat. Res. 61, 274-287
4. Wulf, H., Kraft-Weyrather, W., Miltenburger, H.G., Blakely, E.A., Tobias, C.A., Kraft, G. (1985), Heavy-ion effects on mammalian cells: inactivation measurements with different cell lines. Radiat. Res. Suppl. 8, S122-S134
5. Baumstark-Khan, C., Halbe, E., Rink, H. (1998), X-Ray sensitivity and DNA damage in bovine lens epithelial cells in vitro. in: B.V. Worgul (Ed.), Ocular Radiation Risk Assessment in Populations exposed to Environmental Radiation Contamination, Kluwer, Dordrecht, The Netherlands
6. Catena, C., Mattoni, A. (1985). DNA strand break rejoining in human lymphocytes during the S phase. Int. J. Radiat. Biol. 47, 489-496
7. Kampf, G.(1983), Die Erzeugung von DNS strangbrüchen durch ionisierende Strahlen unterschiedlicher Qualität und ihre Bedeutung für die Zellinaktivierung. Techn. Rep., Zentralinstitut für Kernforschung Rossendorf, KfR 504
8. Ritter, M.A., Cleaver, J.E., Tobias, C.A. (1977), High-LET radiations induce a large proportion of non-rejoining DNA breaks. Nature 266, 653-655
9. Heilmann, J., Rink, H., Taucher-Scholz, G., Kraft, G. (1993), DNA strand break induction and rejoining and cellular recovery in mammalian cells after heavy-ion irradiation. Radiat. Res. 135, 46-55
10. Kellerer, A.M.(1977), Microdosimetric concepts relevant to HZE-particles. Proceedings of the European Symposium on Life Sciences in Space Research, European Space Agency (ESA), Paris, pp 271-277
11. Blöcher, D., Pohlit, W. (1982), DNA double strand breaks in Ehrlich ascites tumour cells at low doses of x-rays. II. Can cell death be attributed to double strand breaks? Int. J. Radiat. Biol. 42, 329-338, 1982

LASER SCANNING FOCAL LENGTH VARIABILITY IS A MEASURE OF DAMAGE IN RAT LENS IN MODEL ASTRONAUT CATARACTS TREATED WITH VITAMIN E (VE) OR R-α-LIPOIC ACID (RLA).

V. BANTSEEV, K. HERBERT*, J.G. SIVAK*, and J.R. TREVITHICK,

*Department of Biochemistry, Faculty of Medicine, University of Western Ontario, London, Canada, N6A 5C1, *School of Optometry, University of Waterloo, Waterloo, Canada.*

1. Abstract

Lenses of rats, selected by clarity and/or low protein leakage during preincubation, were incubated in medium 199 (M199). ^{60}Co-γ-irradiation simulated radiation encountered in space, although γ-irradiation causes less damage than cosmic rays. At the termination of incubation, lenses were scanned by a Scanning Lens Monitor. Protein leakage was positively correlated with variability in focal length ($p<0.04$). Irradiated lenses had a slight, not significant increase in variability. Lenses incubated with dimethyl sulfoxide (DMSO) after irradiation had significantly lower variability, consistent with protective effects of both DMSO and the protective agents vitamin E and R-α-lipoic acid.

2. Introduction

Cataract of the eye lens is a well-known late effect of radiation (1). Recent experiments by Worgul's group (2,3) have indicated that even low doses of more damaging radiation (450 MeV $_{56}$Fe, 600 MeV $_{40}$Ar, and 435 keV neutrons) can induce cataracts in rats irradiated chronically, modelling astronauts in space shuttle flights and to a lesser extent, jet crews in flights over 10,000 meters altitude. Armed forces personnel cleaning up after nuclear accidents could also be at risk of exposure to radiation levels higher than normal background.

Damage caused by radiation is usually mediated by free radicals created either as single radicals or as tracks, if heavy nuclei are involved as the causative agent. Because of this, a model using ^{60}Co-γ-radiation (which is less damaging than neutrons or heavy ions, but more easily available as a radiation source) would be useful for modelling radiation damage and its prophylaxis.

In our experiments (4-6), we have shown that oxidative damage to the lens results in

A. K. Junk et al. (eds.),
Ocular Radiation Risk Assessment in Populations Exposed to Environmental Radiation Contamination, 173–182.

opacity and release of proteins and the intracellular enzyme lactate dehydrogenase (LDH). Both radiation, and elevated glucose in diabetes can result in oxidative stress to the lens. Radiation can directly produce free radicals, and diabetes can result in free radicals as a result of nonenzymic glycation during the Maillard reaction (7,8). Antioxidants acting as free radical scavengers can reduce damage in both model cataracts in the rat lens *in vitro* (9-12).

Another parameter which is associated with cataract is the variability in the lens focal length, which increases significantly in lenses exposed to toxic agents (13). This parameter is measured by a scanning lens monitor developed by Sivak's group (14). The focal length is estimated using a laser beam at 0.2 mm intervals along two perpendicular lines, and the standard errors of the average focal length are determined.

The experiments reported here were designed to ask the questions:
(1) does radiation damage result in increased focal length variability?
(2) is the variability correlated to protein leakage?
(3) can antioxidants reduce the focal length variability?

3. Materials and Methods

Rat lens dissection and incubation in 1.5 ml M199/rat lens were performed as described previously (11). As previously reported, ^{60}Co-γ-radiation (up to 200cGy) and treatments with vitamin E or R-α-lipoate (1 mM) were commenced after an initial 24 hours preincubation at the end of which lenses showing protein leakage ($>$ 30 μg/ml) were discarded. Medium was changed at daily intervals and stored frozen prior to estimation of protein leakage using the Bradford method (15), with an Elisa reader equipped with a computer program (MRX microplate reader with Biolinx 2.0 assay management software, Dynatech, Chantilly, VA).

At intervals, lenses were removed, from the 24 well trays to 13 x 130 mm culture tubes, and transported in an insulated container, in which the temperature was maintained by gel-packs (35.5 °C initially, 30 °C after 2 hr), to the School of Optometry at the University of Waterloo and placed in an incubator at 37°C prior to measuring the focal length variability with the scanning lens monitor.

Protein release and focal length variability were examined for correlation by using the linear regression analysis program of the SPSSPC statistical program (16). Standard errors for each set of focal length measurements for individual lenses were tested for statistically significant differences between sets of lenses.

4. Results

TABLE 1: The parameters of the linear relation between protein leakage and variability (standard error (SE)) of the lens focal length, for groups of treated lenses, either sham controls or irradiated.

Shams Irradiated (I) (200 cGy)	DMSO (D) (1μl/ml)	VE* RLA (1 mM)	Focal Length (mm)	± SE	Variability	± SE	Significance of Variability different from unirradiated sham
S		-	6.00	± 0.13	0.12	± 0.02	N.A
S		-	5.89	± 0.26	0.16	± 0.06	$p<0.071$
S	D	RLA	4.70	± 0.54	0.62	± 0.05	$p<0.00037$
S	D	VE	5.62	± 0.53	0.39	± 0.17	$p<0.069$
I, 200 cGy	-	-	6.09	± 0.31	0.14	± 0.07	$p<0.085$
I, 200 cGy	D	-	6.27	± 0.31	0.11	± 0.08	$p<0.066$
I, 200 cGy	D	RLA	5.00	± 0.85	0.53	± 0.15	$p<0.0077$
I, 200 cGy	D	VE	5.89	± 0.18	0.06	± 0.02	$p<0.090$

*Abbreviations VE (Vitamin E, d-α-tocopherol) RLA (R-α-lipoic acid), SE (standard error).
The following pairs were not significant: DMSO sham vs DMSO irradiated ($p<0.63$), RLA sham vs RLA irradiated ($p<0.11$), VE sham vs VE irradiated ($p<0.10$).

Fig. 1 shows ray diagrams for typical lenses: the top set shows sham controls with no additions and a control with added DMSO, which was used as a vehicle to solubilize additives shown in the second set: (R-α-lipoate, 1 mM) and VE (1 mM); the third set shows a lens irradiated with 200 cGy ^{60}Co-γ-radiation, and an irradiated lens treated with DMSO (1.0 μl/ml medium): the fourth set shows an irradiated lens treated with DMSO containing R-α-lipoate (1 mM) and an irradiated lens treated with DMSO containing VE (1 mM).

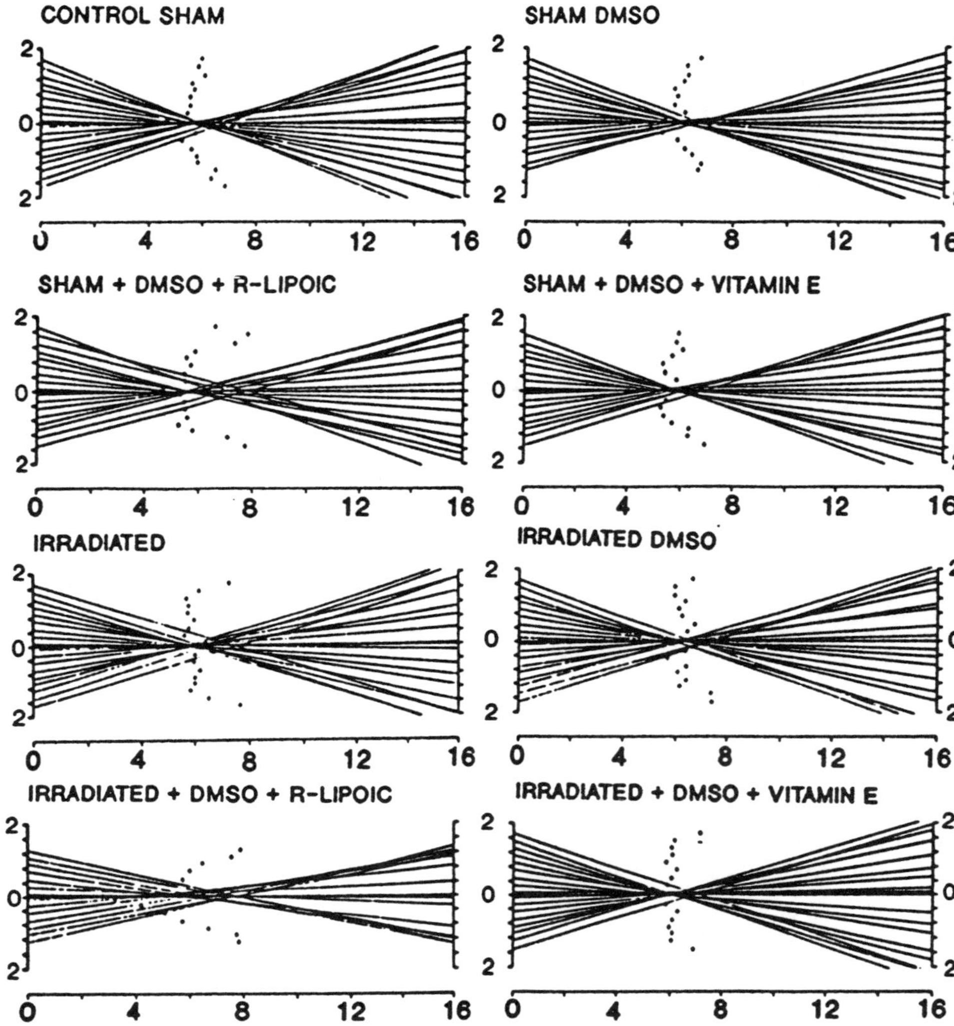

FIG. 1. Typical focal profiles of rat lenses sham-irradiated or irradiated and cultured under a number of different conditions as described in the text. Equivalent focal length (mm) is shown on the horizontal axis. Eccentricity (mm) of laser beam position from optic axis (0.0) is shown on the vertical axis. The points at the position of intersection of the lines indicate where the beams crossed the axis at each eccentric position. Note the smaller spherical abberations indicated by the more vertical alignment of the crossover points for control and irradiated shams, DMSO sham and DMSO irradiated lenses, and DMSO and vitamin E sham and irradiated lenses as compared to the lipoic plus DMSO which show much more concave (to the right) profiles.

The ray diagram focal lengths are used to determine the standard errors for each lens, and each group (usually 6 lenses/group) is tested against every other group. These tests revealed (Table 1) that variability in control lenses was uniformly lower than irradiated or model lenses. Irradiated lenses showed no significant differences in variability after 3 days of incubation. After 8 days and 10 days the irradiated lenses showed a significantly elevated variability when compared to the sham controls. This was decreased by treatment with DMSO or VE (1 mM final added in 1.5 μl DMSO to each 1.5 ml incubation, but RLA (1 mM final, added in 1.5 μl DMSO) increased the variability in either sham controls or lenses irradiated with 200 cGy ^{60}Co-γ-radiation (Table 1). The reason for this was investigated in a more extensive set including lenses treated with DMSO, vitamin E and lipoate.

In one experiment, protein leakage showed a linear dependence on both dose of irradiation and duration of incubation (Table 2). It was correlated with focal length variability (coefficient of correlation, 0.365, $p<0.04$, Table 3).

TABLE 2. Linear regression analysis of plot of protein leakage time course and dose rate.

Variable in Equation	Slope	± SE	Units	Significance
Duration of Incubation	5.11	± 0.57	ng protein /ml/day	p<0.00001
Dose cGy	0.0324	± 0.004	ng protein /ml/cGy	p<0.00001
"Constant"	-8.27	± 3.20	ng protein /ml	p<0.07

TABLE 3. Correlation of variability of lens focal length (mm) with protein leakage (ng/ml), at day 8 of post-irradiation incubation.

Coefficient of correlation	Significance
0.3646	p<0.04

Protein leakage was linearly related to focal length variability (Table 4).

TABLE 4. Regression analysis of variability of lens focal length dependence on protein leakage: parameters of equation.

Parameter in Equation	± SE	Units	Significance
Slope 0.044	± 0.011	mm/ng	$p<0.0003$
Constant 0.312	± 0.044	mm	$p<0.00001$

TABLE 5. Regression analysis of variability of lens focal length dependence on DMSO, vitamin E, lipoate and radiation dose.

Variable	Parameter in Equation	± SE	Units	Significance
DMSO	Slope 0.068	± 0.116	mm /μl(DMSO)	$p<0.57$
Vitamin E	Slope 0.0641	± 0.10	mm /mmol(VE)	$p<0.55$
Lipoate	Slope 0.40	± 0.11	mm /mmol (LIPOATE)	$P<0.0006$
Radiation	Slope 0.279×10^{-4}	$\pm 3.98 \times 10^{-4}$	mm/ cGy	$p<0.49$
	Constant .19	± 0.09	mm	$p<0.05$

Logistic regression analysis of the effect of different variables on focal length variability only demonstrated statistical significance for the effect of lipoate (Table 5). The dependence of protein leakage on these variables was statistically significant for lipoate and radiation dose (Table 6).

5. Discussion

The technique of scanning lens monitor focal length determination has been used in several previous investigations of lens damage - UV, toxic substances, etc. The variation in focal length has been shown to increase in response to cataractous damage (13, 14). Compared to sham-irradiated lenses, irradiated lenses showed increased focal length variability. These experiments indicate a parallel response for both parameters used to monitor lens damage: protein leakage (used previously) and focal length variability, as determined using a scanning laser lens monitor.

TABLE 6. Regression analysis of protein leakage dependence on DMSO, vitamin E, lipoate and radiation dose.

Variable	Parameter in Equation	± SE	Units	Significance
DMSO	Slope - 1.43	± 1.27	ng protein/ml/μL DMSO/ml	$p<0.27$
Vitamin E	Slope - 1.16	± 1.14	ng protein/ml/VE (mM)	$p<0.32$
Lipoate	Slope 4.04	± 1.16	ng protein/ml/Lipoate (mM)	$p<0.0013$
Radiation	Slope 0.017	± 0.004	ng protein/cGy radiation	$p<0.0003$
	Constant 0.45	± 1.04	ng protein	$p<0.67$

The antioxidant VE reduced the variability to normal, but lipoate increased variability in both sham-irradiated and irradiated lenses. Fragmentation of mitochondria in lipoate-treated lenses has been observed by vital mitochondrial staining using confocal laser scanning microscopy in both control and irradiated lenses (17). Such fragmentation could result in the observed increased focal length variability (18). This may be accounted for by light scattering and loss of correlation function reinforcement (18) as the light passes through equatorial lens cells containing the fragmented but functional mitochondria:

The dimensions of the mitochondrial fragments (0.5 x 0.5 μm) are similar to those of globules reported by our group in light scattering opaque regions of human and model rat cortical cataracts (19,20). Srivastava's group (21, 22) has reported globule formation from intact lens fiber cells, but the globules they observed were formed from fiber cells. In their experiments, fiber cells were initially isolated in low calcium, and formed globules immediately when calcium was increased to 1 mM. The potential involvement of calcium in this process was suggested by the observation that elevated glucose potentiates opacification and mitochondrial fragmentation. One of the earliest observed changes in the process of cataract formation is elevation of lens calcium, which vitamin C prevents. Whether VE or lipoate can prevent or reduce calcium uptake has not yet been investigated. It is also possible that during fragmentation of mitochondria, release of Ca^{2+} occurs, leading to calpain activation and globule formation. This could explain in part the protection by vitamin E and lipoate, compared to glucose: vitamin E is a known scavenger of free radicals, and dihydrolipoate, formed from LA, is a powerful antioxidant which could help to protect lens cells against oxidative stress and reduce calcium influx from the medium.

To examine this possibility, the profile of focal length across the lens was examined (Figure 1).

In lipoate-treated lenses, both control and irradiated (groups of 6 lenses for each condition) vs. sham-irradiated untreated or DMSO controls, (6 lenses /group) there was much greater focal length variability in the lipoate-treated lenses. Although in some lenses only half of the lens could be scanned, a pattern of increased focal length in peripheral lens regions (as compared to central regions) was consistently found. The peripheral focal length increased to approximately 8 mm in both controls and radiation groups as compared to the central region in which the focal length was consistently minimal in a range from 3.8 to 5.8 mm, resulting in slopes of focal length vs. distance from the optical axis. Examination of focal length against distances from the central lens optical axis showed small slopes for shams, irradiated controls, and vitamin E-treated lenses, but larger slopes between central region and periphery for RLA-incubated lenses, both sham controls and irradiated lenses.

TABLE 7. Linear regression analysis of plots of normalized focal length vs distance from lens optical centre: effects of radiation, risk reducing agents vitamin E (VE) and R-α-lipoic acid (RLA) and solvent for agents (DMSO): * Not Significant; ** Value of constant in equation 0.661 ± 0.159 units/mm. ($p<0.0001$)

Variable**	Slope of line (units/mm from optical axis)	± SE	SIGNIFICANCE
Vitamin E	0.338	± 0.158	$p<0.036$
R-α-Lipoic Acid	0.554	± 0.158	$p<0.0008$
Irradiation 200 cGy	-0.237	± 0.112	$p<0.038$
Distance from optical centre	0.586	± 0.108	$p<0.00001$
DMSO 1 μl/ml final	0.076	± 0.158	$p<0.632$*

Focal length changes were analysed further: Each data set was normalized by dividing each focal length on the positive side of the optical axis by the average of the data obtained at 0.3, 0.1, -0.1 and -0.3 mm of the visual axis. For each set of lenses the average normalized focal length dependence on distance from the optical axis was analysed at each positive distance from the optical axis, using as variables, the distance, exposure conditions (sham or irradiated), and treatment (DMSO, vitamin E or lipoate). Regression analyses were performed on the data obtained from the lenses incubated after sham or actual irradiation, and treatment using parameters as follows: (1) control, no additives, (2) DMSO, (3) Vitamin E (1 mM) in DMSO, (4) Lipoic acid (1 mM) in DMSO (Table 7).

The results of the regression analysis showed the largest increase in focal length with distance from the optical axis for lipoic acid, about double that for Vitamin E, and no significant effect for DMSO, the solvent used for Vitamin E (Table 7). Radiation with 200 cGy resulted in a decreased slope, indicating a smaller increase of focal length with increasing distance from the optical axis. These results are consistent with the changes induced by lipoate influencing the focal length. Since increased focal length is related inversely to refractive index, this implies a lower refractive index in the lens cortex. Such a lower refractive index could be a result of lower protein concentration or uptake of water into the cortex, swelling the cells.

6. Acknowledgement

The authors gratefully acknowledge financial support from Henkel Chemical Co. Fine Chemicals Division, Eastman Chemical Co., the Natural Sciences and Engineering Research Council of Canada, and the Defence Research Establishment Ottawa (DREO) of the Department of National Defence Canada. Special thanks are due to Dr. W.M. Ross of DREO for helpful discussions, and Drs. K.K. Carroll and E.M. Kurowska for assistance in using the ELISA reader.

7. References

1. Augusteyn R.C., and Collin, H.B. (1980) Chap.13, in *The Eye*, vol.2, Horrobin, D.F. (ed.), Eden Press, Westmount, Quebec, Canada, pp. 250-253.
2. Worgul, B.V. (1988) Accelerated heavy particles and the lens. V. Theoretical basis of cataract enhancement by dose fractionation. *Ophthalmic Res* **20**: 143-148.
3. Worgul, B.V., Medvedovsky, C., Huang, Y., Marino S.A., Randers-Pehrson, G., Brenner, D.J. (1996). Quantitative assessment of the cataractogenic potential of very low doses of neutrons. *Radiation Res.* **145**, 343-349.
4. Ross WM, Creighton MO, Trevithick JR, Stewart-DeHaan PJ, Sanwal M. (1983) Radiation cataract formation diminished by vitamin E in rat lenses in vitro. *Exp. Eye Res.* **36**, 645-653.
5. Ross WM, Creighton MO, Trevithick JR (1990). Radiation Cataractogenesis induced by neutron or gamma irradiation in the rat lens is reduced by vitamin E. *Scanning Microscopy* **4**, 641-650.
6. Bantseev, V., Bhardwaj, R., Rathbun, W.*, Nagasawa, H.,**, and Trevithick, J.R. (1997). Antioxidants and cataract: (cataract induction in space environment and application to terrestrial aging cataract) *Biochem. Molec. Biol. Internat.* **42**, 1189-1197.
7. Wolff, S.P. and Dean, R.T. (1987). "Glucose autoxidation and protein modification. The potential role of 'autoxidative glycosylation' in diabetes." *Biochem.J.* **245**, 243-250.
8. Wolff S.P., Jiang Z.Y., Hunt J.V. (1991) Protein Glycation and Oxidative Stress in Diabetes Mellitus and Ageing. *Free Rad. Biol. Med.* **10**, 339-352.
9. Kilic, F., Mitton, K.P., Dzialoszynski, T., Sanford, S.E., and Trevithick, J.R. (1994). "Modelling cortical cataractogenesis 14: Reduction of lens damage in diabetic rats by a dietary regimen combining vitamins C and E and B-carotene." In Hockin, O., and Sasaki, K. (eds.). *Dev. Ophthalmol.* **26**, 63-72.
10. Kilic, F., and Trevithick, J.R. (1993). "LDH activity as an indication of lens membrane damage during diabetic cataractogenesis." *Proceeding: Mol.Biol.Cell*, **4**, 86a-499.
11. Kilic, F., and Trevithick, J.R. (1995). "Modelling cortical cataractogenesis 16: Reduction of Lens damage". *Biochem. Molec. Biol.Internat.* **35**, 1143-1152.

12. Kilic, F., Handelman, G., Serbinova, E., Packer, L., and Trevithick, J.R. (1995). "Modelling cortical cataractogenesis 17: in vitro effect of α-lipoic acid on glucose-induced lens membrane damage, a model of diabetic cataractogenesis". *Biochem. Molec. Biol. Internat.* **37**, 361-370.
13. Sivak. J.G., Herbert, K.L., and Segal, L. (1994) Ocular lens organ culture as a measure of ocular irritancy: the effect of surfactants. *Toxicol. Meth.* **4**, 56-65.
14. Weerheim, J.A., and Sivak, J.G. (1992) Scanning laser measure of the optical quality of the cultured crystalline lens. *Ophthalmic Physiol. Opt.* **12**, 72-79.
15. Bradford, M., (1976) A rapid and sensitive method for the quantitation of microgram quantities of protein utilizing the principle of protein dye-binding. *Anal. Biochem.* **72**, 248-254.
16. Norusis, M.J./SPSS Inc. (1988) *SPSS/PC+ V2.0 Base Manual.* SPSS Inc., Chicago, IL.
17. Bantseev, V. (1997) *personal communication.*
18. Benedek G.B. (1971) Theory of transparency of the eye. *Appl. Optics* **10**:459-473.
19. Creighton, M.O., Trevithick, J.R. (1979). Cortical cataract formation prevented by vitamin E and glutathione. *Exp. Eye Res.* **29**, 689-693.
20. Creighton MO, Trevithick JR, Mousa GY, Percy DH, McKinna AJ, Dyson C, Maisel H, (1978) Globular bodies: A primary cause of the opacity in senile and diabetic posterior cortical subcapsular cataracts? *Can. J. Ophthalmol.* **13**, 166-181.
21. Srivastava, S.K., Bhatnagar, A., Ansari, N.H. (1994). Isolation of rat lens single fiber cells and morphological studies. *Invest. Ophthalmol.Vis.Sci.* **35,** 1810 (2584).
22. Bhatnagar, A., Ansari, N.H., Wang, L., Khanna, P., Wang, C., and Srivastava, S.K.(1995) Calcium-mediated disintegrative globulization of isolated lens fibers mimics cataractogenesis. *Exp.Eye Res.* **61**, 303-310.

OVERVIEW OF THE EPIDEMIOLOGY OF RADIATION CATARACTS

R.E. SHORE [1], B.V. WORGUL [2]
[1]*Department of Environmental Medicine*
New York University Medical School, New York, NY, USA,
[2] *Eye Radiation and Environmental Research Laboratory*
Columbia University, New York, NY, USA

Abstract

There is currently uncertainty about the parameters of the dose-response curve for radiation-induced lens opacities in humans. Various studies have suggested a dose threshold at >2 Sv, at about 1.5 Sv, or no threshold. The principal human dose-response data are summarized, including several studies that suggest a non-threshold, linear-quadratic curve. The magnitude of a "sparing" effect due to dose fractionation or protraction is also uncertain, although the limited data available suggest there is a sparing effect, at least at higher total doses. The available data suggest that the time for induction of cataracts may be inversely related to the dose to the lens. There are insufficient data on lens opacities vs. age-at-irradiation to determine whether younger persons are more radiosensitive or not. A large, well-designed prospective study of persons with both a wide range of radiation exposures and periodic uniform assessments of lens opacities could make a valuable contribution to our knowledge.

1. Introduction

Although cataracts were among the earliest chronic health effects observed among the Japanese atomic bomb survivors, key epidemiologic features of radiogenic lens opacities in humans are still rather poorly defined, owing to the fact that they have been studied in relatively few irradiated populations. The paucity of studies is due, in part, to the difficulty and cost of making objective, quantifiable assessments of lens opacities. It is generally agreed that posterior subcapsular (PSC) opacities are a hallmark of radiation exposure, rather than cortical or nuclear opacities. The status of our knowledge about several issues regarding ocular radiation effects will be summarized in this review.

A. K. Junk et al. (eds.),
Ocular Radiation Risk Assessment in Populations Exposed to Environmental Radiation Contamination, 183–189.

2. Dose Threshold

It has traditionally been believed that cataract represents a deterministic effect of radiation, i.e., only when sufficient damage is done to the lens tissue is a cataract likely, which implies a dose threshold. This may be true if one limits one's consideration to cataracts serious enough to cause demonstrable visual impairment. For example, Table 1 shows results from the classical study by Merriam and Focht [1] in which they observed no cataracts below 2 Gy of x-irradiation. This study conducted during the 1950's served as the principal basis for conclusions about the low-LET dose threshold for cataracts until recently [2, 3]. However, note in Table 1 the sparse number of subjects with doses below 2 Gy (if those administered radiation for >3 months were also included in the table, then the total would be 33 persons). This small number is hardly sufficient to yield definitive evidence on a threshold dose. In addition, the study probably did not include the smaller opacities one is more likely to see at lower doses.

Table 1. Classical Data on a Dose Threshold from X-irradiation

Dose Range	Percent (# Cataracts / # Examined)
<2 Gy	0% (0/27)
2 - 5.99 Gy	50% (14/28)
6 - 11.99 Gy	71% (34/48)
12 - >30 Gy	100% (19/19)

From: Merriam and Focht [1]. Based on patients with <3 mo. total radiation treatment time.

Otake and Schull [4] reanalyzed the data originally summarized by Miller et al [5] on posterior subcapsular opacities in the Japanese atomic-bomb study. The Miller data were a collation of the results from several early ocular examination programs, which appear to have varied in their criteria for scoring opacities and in the ophthalmologic instruments and degree of mydriasis used. Thus they are not very systematic data, though they were the best available at the time. Otake and Schull applied the new (DS86) dosimetry to those data. A summary of their statistical results regarding dose thresholds is shown in Table 2. When they tried to fit a model that was linear for both gamma and neutron dose (L-L) with no threshold, there was a significant lack of fit, so this model can be rejected. However, a model that included both a linear and a quadratic term for gamma dose and a linear term for neutron dose (LQ-L) provided an adequate fit, as did models that added thresholds. The best-fitting L-L threshold model indicated a gamma threshold of about 0.7 Gy and a neutron threshold of 0.06 Gy, which together indicate a threshold of about 1.5 Sv; however, the confidence intervals on both of the threshold values included zero dose, i.e., they could not reject the possibility of no threshold.

A more recent re-analysis [6] of the Miller et al data examined whether the putative dose threshold and the slope of the dose-response curves differed between those who developed epilation from the bomb exposure and those who did not, where epilation was taken as an indicator of radiosensitivity. They found that, after correcting for dose uncertainties, the slopes and thresholds for the two groups did not differ significantly and that the dose thresholds were in the range of 1.2-1.4 Sv, although, again, the threshold confidence intervals included zero dose.

Table 2. Fit of Statistical Models to Japanese A-bomb Cataract Data Using DS86 Eye Organ Doses

Model	P-value for lack of fit
Lγ-Ln, no threshold	0.03
LQγ-Ln, no threshold	0.15
Lγ-Ln, thresholds a	0.37
LQγ-Ln, thresholds	0.23

[a] γ-dose threshold of 0.73 Gy (95% CI= 0.0-1.4 Gy) & neutron threshold of 0.06 Gy (95% CI= 0.0-0.16 Gy) for L-L model. From: Otake and Schull [4]

In 1983 Choshi et al [7] reported on the results of an ocular screening program in the Adult Health Study sample of the Japanese atomic-bomb survivors. Otake et al [8] attempted a fuller analysis of the dose-response curve for these data and reported that a non-threshold model fit the data better than did a model with a threshold at 1.5 Gy. The model that best fit the data was a linear-quadratic non-threshold model. Part of the reason these data showed no threshold, whereas the earlier data reported by Miller et al [5] were best fit by a threshold model, may be that these data included early indications of ocular changes (posterior lenticular plaque and polychromatic sheen) as well as more advanced lesions.

In our study of children given x-ray treatment vs. medications for ringworm of the scalp in the 1940-50's, Albert et al [9] examined 234 irradiated and 232 unirradiated subjects at ages 10-34 years (a median of 10 years post-irradiation). They reported an excess of posterior subcapsular opacities in the x-irradiated group, based on finding 13 irradiated and 2 unirradiated cases when they were given a blinded examination with a slit lamp. The estimated odds ratio (OR) was 5.9 (95% confidence interval of 1.4-24). The dose to the lens was about 50 cGy [10].

Recently, a large cross-sectional study of risk factors for lens opacities obtained self-reports of prior diagnostic x-ray exposures. The authors reported that a history of CAT scans of the head was associated with posterior subcapsular opacity and nuclear sclerosis [11]. The results are shown in Table 3. However, in the table it is notable that the highest odds ratio (OR) is associated with chest x rays and that ORs nominally greater than unity are seen for each type of x ray, including those where the eye dose would be negligible. This raises the issue of whether response bias may account for some or all of the putative radiation effect in this study.

Table 3. Diagnostic X-ray Exposure and PSC Opacities: Odds ratios adjusted for sex and age

X-ray Type	Odds Ratio (95% CI)
CAT scan, head	1.45 (1.1-2.0)
Head x-ray	1.27 (1.0-1.7)
Chest x-ray	1.74 (0.7-4.1)
Abdomen x-ray	1.18 (0.9-1.6)
Other x-ray	1.20 (0.9-1.6)

From: Klein et al [11].

3. Dose Fractionation and Dose Rate

Another question pertains to whether there are dose-fractionation or dose-rate effects. There is very little systematic data on this issue. Merriam and Focht [1] reported on the minimal x-ray dose at which they found a clinical cataract, broken down according to the length of time over which the dose fractions were administered. They found a minimal cataractogenic dose of 2 Gy to the eye among those who received a single dose, and minimal cumulative cataractogenic doses of 4 Gy and 5.5 Gy for those whose dose fractions were spread over 3 weeks to 3 months or over >3 months respectively. These data suggest a 2- to 3-fold sparing effect for fractionated doses. However, the number of patients with doses less than the minimum cataract doses was very small; it is likely that the observed "threshold" doses would have been somewhat different if there had been more patients with lower cumulative doses.

A recent study by Belkacemi et al [12] compared cataract formation in cancer patients who received total body irradiation prior to bone marrow transplant. The radiation was administered either as a single dose of 10 Gy (to the midplane at the level of L4) or of 6 dose fractions totaling 12 Gy over 3 consecutive days. They found 5-year cataract incidences of 34% and 11% in the unfractionated and fractionated-dose groups respectively. They also found a dose-rate effect, as shown in Table 4. X-radiation administered at a dose rate of over 5 cGy per minute was more cataractogenic than irradiation at a lower dose rate; an analogous result was found when considering just the unfractionated dose group, indicating that the result was not due to confounding of dose-rate by degree of fractionation.

Table 4. Radiation Dose Rate and Cataracts (Bone Marrow Transplant Patients)

Dose-rate Group	Cataracts, Percent (# cataracts / # patients)
< 48 mGy/min.	1% (2/157)
48-89 mGy/min	11% (33/301)
≥ 90 mGy/min	19% (7/36)

From: Belkacemi et al [12].

4. Cataract Latency

The time of appearance of cataracts after lens irradiation is of interest. Merriam and Focht [1] reported a range of 6 months to 35 years after irradiation. They also reported shorter latencies at higher doses (mean latency of 4.3 y for those who received lens doses >6.5 Gy) than at lower doses (mean latency of 8.6 y for those with 2-6.5 Gy). (However, their temporal data should be interpreted cautiously since they have a case series rather than a systematic follow-up of a defined population.) Other clinical reports seem consistent with this interpretation, although there do not appear to be systematic epidemiologic data available to confirm it.

5. Effect of Age

Another question is whether radiation cataract induction differs by age at irradiation. Early reports suggested that young children were more highly susceptible to cataract induction by irradiation than older persons were [13]. Choshi et al [7] also reported this in their cataract screening program among atomic bomb survivors. However, when Otake et al [8] re-analyzed the PSC opacity data in a more systematic way, they found no difference between the dose-response slopes for younger or older atomic bomb survivors. Toda et al [14] reported no difference in cataract risk between atomic bomb survivors exposed in infancy and those exposed later in life. Kawamoto et al [15] reported that those irradiated *in utero* had a small excess of cataracts and Nefzger et al [16] reported that the subgroup with high doses had some loss of visual acuity; however, neither result was statistically significant. Experimental data have also shown mixed results regarding the effect of age at irradiation on cataract induction [17]. A recent study suggested a high incidence of cataracts among 100 children who received 10-12 Gy in 3-6 fractions prior to bone marrow transplantation. After 4.2 years of follow-up on average, 17% had developed bilateral posterior subcapsular cataracts [18]. In contrast, the total cataract incidence was 4.4% among adults who received similar doses in 6 fractions in another bone marrow transplant study with average follow-up of 42 months [12]. This suggests that children may be more susceptible to radiation cataractogenesis.

Age at ocular assessment is clearly an important variable to control, as the background prevalence of lens opacities varies greatly by age. Based on a composite of information from two studies [19, 20], the prevalence of posterior subcapsular cataracts is about 1.6% at ages 40-54, 4.1% at ages 55-64, 10.5% at 65-74, and 14-20% at ages 75-84. On the other hand, neither the background prevalence of PSC cataracts nor the magnitude of radiation effects seems to differ appreciably by sex.

6. Implications of the historical data for new radiation studies of lens opacities

The BEIR V report of the U.S. National Academy of Sciences concluded, based primarily on the Japanese atomic-bomb data, that there is a dose threshold for opacities somewhere between 60 and 150 cGy [3]. The findings by Albert et al [9] suggest that any possible threshold is likely to be below 50 cGy – but it is uncertain whether there is a dose threshold rather than a linear-quadratic non-threshold curve. The latter would be compatible with the more recent Japanese atomic-bomb examination program [8], the scalp ringworm patients and the findings concerning CAT scans. Clearly new studies with systematic ocular assessments are needed that examine the dose-response relationship in the range below 1 Gy. The available data on the effects of dose fractionation or dose protraction are also very limited, so studies that have variation in the degree of fractionation or protraction would be valuable.

The data on the time of appearance of cataracts after irradiation suggest that the latency may be longer at lower doses. On the other hand, if one wishes to observe early lens changes, one should obviously begin ocular surveillance within a few years after exposure. The age-related data on radiation effects are not that well analyzed or compared, so a strategy for choosing a study cohort according to age is rather unclear. However, it is often the case for chronic diseases that it is easier to see environmental effects at relatively young ages, before the "spontaneous" rates of the disease become too high. With this in mind, one would certainly not want to concentrate primarily on the older members of the population.

Acknowledgement: Supported by grants DE-FG01-95EH89658 from the U.S. Department of Energy and ES-00260 from the U.S. National Institute of Environmental Health Sciences.

References

1. Merriam, G.R. and Focht, E. (1957): A clinical study of radiation cataracts and the relationship to dose. Am. J. Roentgenol. Radium Ther. Nucl. Med. 77, 759-785.

2. ICRP (1984): Nonstochastic effects of ionizing radiation. In: Annals of the ICRP, ed. International Commission on Radiological Protection (Report No. 41), pp. 1-33. Oxford: Pergamon Press.

3. NAS/NRC (1990): Health Effects of Exposure to Low Levels of Ionizing Radiation (BEIR V), National Academy Press
421 pp. Washington, DC: National Academy of Sciences - National Research Council.

4. Otake, M. and Schull, W. (1990): Radiation-related posterior lenticular opacities in Hiroshima and Nagasaki atomic bomb survivors based on the DS86 dosimetry system. Radiat. Res. 121, 3-13.

5. Miller, R.J., Funijo, T. and Nefzger, M. (1967): Lens findings in atomic bomb survivors: A review of major ophthalmic surveys at the Atomic Bomb Casualty Commission (1949-1962). Arch. Ophthalmol. 78, 697-704.

6. Otake, M., Neriishi, K. and Schull, W.J. (1996): Cataract in atomic bomb survivors based on a threshold model and the occurrence of severe epilation. Radiat. Res. 146, 339-348.

7. Choshi, K., Takaku, I., Mishima, H., et al. (1983): Ophthalmologic changes related to radiation exposure and age in Adult Health Study sample, Hiroshima and Nagasaki. Radiat. Res. 96, 560-579.

8. Otake, M., Finch, S., Choshi, K., et al. (1992): Radiation-related ophthalmological changes and aging among Hiroshima and Nagasaki A-bomb survivors: a reanalysis. Radiat. Res. 131, 315-324.

9. Albert, R., Omran, A., Brauer, E., et al. (1968): Follow-up study of patients treated by x-ray epilation for tinea capitis. II. Results of clinical and laboratory examinations. Arch. Environ. Health 17, 919-934.

10. Schulz, R. and Albert, R. (1968): Dose to organs of the head from the x-ray treatment of tinea capitis. Arch. Environ. Health 17, 935-950.

11. Klein, B.E., Klein, R., Linton, K. and Franke, T. (1993): Diagnostic x-ray exposure and lens opacities: The Beaver Dam Eye Study. Am. J. Pub. Health 83, 588-590.

12. Belkacemi, Y., Ozsahin, M., Pene, F., et al. (1996): Cataractogenesis after total body irradiation. Int. J. Radiat. Oncol. Biol. Phys. 35, 53-60.

13. UNSCEAR (1962): Report of the United Nations Scientific Committee on the Effects of Atomic Radiation. New York: United Nations.

14. Toda, S., Hosokawa, Y., Choshi, K., Nakano, A. and Takahashi, M. (1964): Ocular changes in A-bomb survivors exposed during infancy. Folia Ophthalmol. Jap. 15, 96-103.

15. Kawamoto, S., Fujino, T. and Fujisawa, H. (1964): Ophthalmological status in children exposed in utero. ABCC Technical Report # 23-64. Hiroshima, Japan: Atomic Bomb Casualty Commission.

16. Nefzger, M.D., Miller, R.J. and Fujino, T. (1969): Eye findings in atomic bomb survivors of Hiroshima and Nagasaki: 1963-1964. Am. J. Epidemiol. 89, 129-138.

17. Merriam, G.R. and Szechter, A. (1975): The relative radiosensitivity of rat lenses as a function of age. Radiat. Res. 62, 488-497.

18. De Marco, R., Dassio, D.A. and Vittone, P. (1996): A retrospective study of ocular side effects in children undergoing bone marrow transplantation. Europ. J. Ophthal. 6, 436-439.

19. Sperduto, R.D. and Hiller, R. (1984): The prevalence of nuclear, cortical, and posterior subcapsular lens opacities in a general population sample. Ophthalmol. 91, 815-818.

20. Klein, B.E., Klein, R. and Linton, K. (1992): Prevalence of age-related lens opacities in a population. The Beaver Dam Eye Study. Opthalmol. 99, 546-552.

PREVALENCE OF LENS OPACITY IN POPULATION WITH CHRONIC LOW-DOSE GAMMA-RADIATION EXPOSURE FROM RADIOACTIVE APARTMENTS IN TAIWAN

T.Y. WANG[1], J.C.CHEN,[2] G.L. GUO,[2] S.F. WU[3], B.F. HWANG,[2] J.Y. D. CHEN,[2] Y.M. A. LEE,[2] W.P. CHANG[2,3]*

*[1]Department of Ophthalmology, [2]Department of Family Medicine, Taipei Municipal Jan-Ai Hospital; [3]Institute of Public Health, National Yang Ming University, Taipei, Taiwan. 155 Section 2, Lih-non Street, Taipei, Taiwan; Email: wpc94@mailsrv.ym.edu.tw; *: corresponding author.*

1. Abstract

In order to evaluate the changes in lens opacity in a population with chronic low-dose γ-radiation exposure in their daily living or school environment from Co-60 contaminated steel in Taiwan, 503 subjects with excess relatively low exposure (RLE) and 95 subjects with excess relatively high exposure (RHE) were examined simultaneously in the Taipei Municipal Jan-Ai Hospital in 1995-1996 in Taiwan. Post detailed slit-lamp biomicroscopy examination by ophthalmology specialists, the frequency of lens with various shapes or sizes of apparent opacity in single or both eyes for the RLE or RHE population were 7/503 (1.4%) and 17/95 (17.9%), respectively. The frequency of either of the lens with any significant opaque change in male and female subjects were 5/237 (2.1%) and 2/266 (0.9%) for the RLE, and 9/46 (19.6%) and 8/49 (16.3%) for the RHE, respectively. The frequency of either of the lens with any opaque changes in those with intrauterine exposure was 3/17 (17.6%). Moreover, various lens changes in shape and morphology were observed, as those with acute high dose radiation exposure. Based on these observations, chronic low-dose radiation exposure was suggested associated with various lens changes and deserved further study on its causal relationship.

2. Introduction

More than twenty thousand tons of Co-60 contaminated steel were accidentally employed as construction steel in 1983 to 1984 and were only identified till 1992 [1]. More than 130 building complexes, 1,200 apartments or families, or up to 6,500

A. K. Junk et al. (eds.),
Ocular Radiation Risk Assessment in Populations Exposed to Environmental Radiation Contamination, 191–196.

people were demonstrated with chronic daily low-dose γ-radiation exposure [1-3]. The exposed cohort, exposure person-year, and the cumulative doses (mSv) received in this unique population in Taiwan could be categorized as school (Yun-Tsun Elementary School, "YES" and Hsin-Hsin Kindergarten, "HHK") and residential exposure, as well as relatively high exposed ("RHE") and relatively low exposed ("RLE"; Table 1). While early biological effects of significant concerns have been evaluated on this unique exposed population [4], more interest has been on clinical effects potentially involved.

TABLE 1. The numbers of total population with chronic low-dose radiation exposure, numbers of person-year of exposure, and the cumulative doses of exposure in 4 different categories of exposure. Average person-year exposure, the mean dose of exposure in one individual and the annul per capital exposure are also illustrated.

Exposure Category	numbers of exposed subjects	Exposure person-year	Cumulative exposure (mSv)
School			
YES	2,900	2,900 X 1= 2,900	2,900 X 3 mSv/person = 8,700 mSv
HHK	1,300	1,300 X 1= 1,300	1,300 X 10 mSv/person = 13,000 mSv
Residential			
RHE	1,100	1,100 X 5 = 5,500	1,100 X 100 mSv/person = 110,000 mSv
RLH	1,200	1,200 X 5 = 6,000	1,200 X 3 mSv/person = 3,600 mSv
Total	6,500	15,700 person-year	135,300 mSv = 135.3 Sv
Average		2.4 year exposure/person	20.8 mSv/person, 8.7 mSv/person.year

In 1995, a comprehensive epidemiological study was launched by the National Health Research institute (NHRI) in Taiwan to follow-up and evaluate this specific exposed subjects. The dose of exposure in the RHE subjects were conducted, under the NHRI study program, by a series of dose reconstruction efforts, including dose estimation of the "Taipei Cumulative Dose of 1996". The TCD96 program was based on information of past living history and a systemic dose rate measurements on living environments of the subjects [5]. As compared with those of personal thermo-luminescence dosimeters (TLDs), the exposure doses reconstructed would be within 20 to 30 % of variance and mostly representing whole body dose (dose of body trunk) [6-7]. The RLH were registered as they were estimated to received less than 5 mSv in any previous year since moved in post 1984. Based on further detailed evaluation on the living and study history and environmental dose estimation, the cumulative doses received by the RLE ranged from 0.2 to 1.2 mSv in excess of background radioactivity received by general public in Taiwan. A comparison between the prevalence of various lens opacity in both groups was conducted in this study.

3. Materials and methods

In order to evaluate the lens change on these subjects with chronic low dose γ-radiation exposure, a free medical examination was arranged in 1995-1996 by the

Ministry of Health to 14 designed hospital country-wide. All these exposed subjects visited the designed hospitals on a voluntary basis. Since the JAH is a regional community hospital, those subjects visited the JAH was not specific than the other exposed population. For those less than 40 years old, 503 subjects of RLE cohort containing 237 male and 266 female subjects and 95 with RHE cohort including 46 male and 49 female subjects were examined in the JAH. All the ophthalmological examinations were conducted by ophthalmologist specialists of the Department of Ophthalmology by biomicroscopy slit-lamp examination post satisfactory pupil dilatation, up to more than 6 mm in diameter. The physicians were single-blinded to the dose of exposure in the examined subjects. Any specific lens opacity change was further taken by photographs immediately and confirmed by an independent ophthalmologist. The location, morphology, and the size of any opacity in the lens in both eyes were read and designed by one single senior ophthalmologist specialist in the JAH. The total cumulative doses for those RHE subjects with specific lens opacity in an of both eyes equal to 4,120 mSv in 17 persons. This is equivalent to 242.4 mSv/person of 122.3 years of exposure, or an average of 1.98 mSv/person-year exposure (Table 2, and 3). Moreover, there were 17 subjects with intrauterine exposure within the RHE population. A detailed history of intrauterine exposure were assessed by trained interviewers, further by interactive and systemic questionnaires.

4. Results

For those with relatively low exposed, 7 in 503 (1.4%) were shown with various changes of lens opacity. The percentage of lens change in male and female subjects were 5/237 (2.1%) and 2/266 (0.9%), respectively. The male subjects were shown with apparently increased frequencies of lens changes than the female subjects. However, no age or dose factor was adjusted. Those with relatively high exposed, the percentage of lens changes was 17/95 (17.9%), while the proportions in male and female subjects were 9/46 (19.6%) and 8/49 (16.3%), respectively. The frequency of lens change in those with intrauterine exposure was 3/17 (17.6%), and was not significantly different from those of the other RHE population. Significant increase in the prevalence rate of lens opacity was observed in the RHE population than the RLE population.

The patterns of lens change observed in our study included (Table 2); (i) mild spoke opacity; (ii) isolated and scattered patchy opacity (0.5-2 mm); (iii) scattered and isolated or in chains of dot opacity (< 0.5 mm); (iv) predominant cortical axial lesions in dots in chains; (v) various sites of lens opacity (posterior capsular, nuclear, and cortex); (vi) non-specific patterns of intrauterine exposure than non-intrauterine exposure; (vii) no apparent difference in patterns between RHE and RLE populations; (viii) no apparent difference in male vs. female in high exposed, but male subjects were shown with increase in frequencies of various lens changes than the female subjects in the RLE population.

TABLE 2. Characteristics of the exposed subjects, including age, sex, lens changes in both eyes, the cumulative doses of exposure, and the age duration of individual's exposure.

Code	age	sex	lens change(OS)	lens (OD)	exposure	exposed age
Relatively low exposed						
#1	15	M	PSC opacity	nil	3	(10-11)
#2	13	M	nuclear opacity	nuclear opacities	3	(9-10)
#3	18	M	multiple dots	nuclear multiple dots	3	(9-10)
#4	15	M	cortical opacity, spoke	multi-dots, patch/plaque	2	(12-13)
#5	12	M	PSC multi-dots, spoke	PSC multi-dots, spoke	3	(10-11)
#6	16	F	multi-dots, multi-patches	multi-dots, multi-patches	2	(11-12)
#7	12	F	multi-dots, scattered, mild spoke	multi-dots in string, ant. cortex, mild spoke	3	(6-7)
Relatively high exposed, intrauterine exposure						
#8	10	M	multiple dots	multiple dots	72	(0-10)
#9	7	M	PSC opacity	PSC opacity	207	(0-3)
#10	6	F	PSC opacity, spoke	PSC opacity, spoke	103	(0-4 months)
Relatively high exposed, non-intrauterine						
#11	37	F	snow-flake opacity	nil	107	(27-35)
#12	12	M	nil	lens opacity	418	(2-10)
#13	31	M	cortical opacity	cortical opacity	395	(17-27)
#14	32	F	cortical opacity multiple dots	cortical opacity multiple dots	37	(27-30)
#15	36	M	nuclear opacity	nuclear opacity	104	(26-34)
#16	39	F	cortical opacity	cortical opacity	240	(24-31)
#17	35	M	multiple dots	PSC multiple dots	29	(28-30)
#18	27	F	multiple dots	multiple dots	240	(12-25)
#19	36	M	cortical opacity	cortical opacity	240	(21-34)
#20	16	M	PSC dots and plaque	PSC dots and plaque	101	(6-14)
#21	13	F	PSC plaque, multi-dots anterior cortex multi-dots	PSC plaque, multi-dots anterior cortex multi-dots	305	(4-7)
#22	14	F	vitreous opacity	vitreous opacity	748	(1-10)
#23	40	M	multi-dots	multi-dots	533	(27-36)
#24	35	F	ant./post. cortical opacity	ant./post. cortical opacity	241	(20-33)

TCD96: Taipei Cumulative Dose 1996, results of a dose reconstruction program in Taipei in 1996.

TABLE 3. Doses of intrauterine exposure in various periods and the total doses of exposure (mSv).

Code	Pregnancy to term	term to relocation (age)	Total dose
#8	18.5	53.9/10 years old	72.4
#9	30.5	176.4/3 years old	206.9
#10	91.6	11.0/4 months old	102.6

5. Discussion

The dose of exposure in these subjects were derived from the Dose Reconstruction Program, TCD96 for the whole body [5, 7]. However, the eye lens dose has not been included in the TCD96 program and should be adjusted during further dose evaluation and risk assessment. Several models of this directions have been employed [8, 9] and would be referred to our future investigation. The locations of these opacities in the lens was primarily described. However, more detailed description for all these changes, including the three-dimensional locations of these changes [10, 11], should allow for more quantitative evaluation and further understanding on the temporal opacity development in these subjects. This would also facilitate future follow-up on the exposed subjects to help understand the evolution of the lens change in the same individual.

It is of great interest that the dose of exposure in these subjects were significantly lower than the threshold levels of 0.5 Gy suggested by the ICRP No. 60 [12]. Particularly in the intrauterine exposure, the mean exposure for those with apparent lens opacity changes were 117 mSv (or equivalent to 0.12 Gy) and far less than 0.5 Gy. For those with any specific lens opacity in the RHE exposure, the mean exposure was around 242 mSv (or equivalent to 0.24 Gy). Both observations suggest that the threshold of radiation-associated lens opacity, if existing, might be far less than that suggested by current level of understanding. It is reasonable that the exposure sufficient to induce lens changes incurred in those with intrauterine exposure was less than those RHE subjects without intrauterine exposure. The latency periods of cataract formation was assumed 3-9 years [13] or 6 months to 3 years [14] post acute high dose of radiation exposure. Since the duration between the exposure and the examination was variable in our study population and limited by the cross-sectional study design, it is difficult to estimate the latency periods of these lens change. However, it was assumed less than the duration described in Tables 2 and 3.

It is also of significant importance to evaluate the causal relationship between chronic low-doe radiation exposure and the lens changes. Most of the studies have been focused on human population and the relative risks derived by comparing with control, non-exposed population. It is suggested that more biological evidences should be collected. As observed in irradiated frog [8], the proliferation activity in the lens epithelium is required for cataract to develop. The targeted lens epithelial cells in different locations of the lens or in subjects with different ages shall be considered in predicting the location or morphology of lens changes in later period. It is valuable to further evaluate the correlation between dose/dose rate of exposure, the initial period and age of exposure, and specific locations of lens opacity evolved. Further investigation in this cohort shall be directed to this direction.

6. Acknowledgments

Special thanks to Professors M.S. Chen, J.D. Wang, Drs. W.L. Chen and Y.C. Li of the National Taiwan University Hospital for technical support and excellent advice.

This study has been part of the Program Project of the National Health Research Institute (NHRI), Taiwan and supported by the Board and Funds of the Education and Development in the Bureau of Health, Taipei City Government for traveling support for author to attend the NATO ARW meeting in Kiev in 1997.

7. References

1. Chang, W.P. and Kau, J. (1993) Taiwan: Exposure to high doses of radiation, The *Lancet* **341**, 750.
2. Chang, W.P. (1993) Spread of Taiwan's radiation panic, The *Lancet* **342**, 1544.
3. Chang, W.P., Chan, C.C., Wang, J.D. (1997) Massive radioactive contamination in recycled scrap steels resulting in massive civilian overexposure, *Health Physics* **73**, 465-472.
4. Chang, W.P., Hwang, B.F., Wang, D., Wang, JD (1997) Chronic low-dose, low-dose rate γ-radiation exposure induced an increased frequency of micronuclei in lymphocytes from residents of radioactive buildings in Taiwan, the *Lancet* **350**, 330-333.
5. Cardarelli, J.C., Hornung, R., Robert, H., Chang, W.P. (1997) Proposed Model for Estimating Dose to Inhabitants of Co-60 Contaminated Buildings, *Health Physics* **72**, 351-360.
6. Lee, J.S., Dong, S.L., Chang, W.P., Chan, C.C. (1997) Determination of external dose with thermoluminescent dosimeter from residents living in the radiation contaminated buildings, *Applied Radiation and Isotopes* **48**, 1237-1248.
7. Hwang, J.S., Chan, C.C., Wang, J.D., Chang, W.P. (1998) Modeling for radiation exposure in living spaces of apartments with multiple radioactive sources, *Health Physics* **74**, 379-386.
8. Holsclaw, D.S., Merriam, G.R., Medvedovsky, C., Rothstein, H., Worgul, B.V. (1989) Stationary radiation cataract: an animal model. *Exp Eye Res* **48**, 385-398.
9. Holsclaw, D.S., Rothstein, H., Medvedovsky, C., Worgul, B.V. (1994) Modulating radiation cataractogenesis by hormonally manipulating lenticular growth kinetics. *Exp Eye Res* **59**, 291-296.
10. Koretz, J.F., Cook, C.A., Kuszak, J.R. (1994) The zones of discontinuity in the human lens: development and distribution with age. *Vision Res* **34**,2955-2962.
11. Graziosi, P., Rosmini, F., Bonacini, M, Ferrigno, L., Sperduto, R.D., Milton, R.C., Maraini, G. (1996) Location and severity of cortical opacities in different regions of the lens in age-related cataract. *Invest Ophthalmol Vis Sci.* **37**, 1698-1703.
12. International Commission on Radiological Protection (1991) Recommendations of the International Commission on Radiological Protection, ICRP Publication 60, Annuals of the ICRP 21 (1-3). Elmsford, New York: Pergamon Press.
13. Henk, J.M., Whitelocke. R.A., Warrington. A.P., Bessell. E.M. (1997) Radiation dose to the lens and cataract formation. *Int J Radiat Oncol Biol Physics* **15**, 815-820.
14. Hempel, M., Hinkelbein, W. (1993) Eye sequeale following external radiation. *Recent Results Cancer Res* **130**, 231-236.

THE EXPERIENCES OF SURVEYS FOR AN EPIDEMIOLOGICAL DATABASE OF DIFFERENT OCCUPATIONAL GROUPS OF RURAL WORKERS IN UKRAINE

P. VITTE, Y. KUNDIEV
Department of Epidemiology, Institute of the Occupational Health Academy of Medical Sciences of Ukraine, Kiev,
75 Saksagansky St., Kiev, 252033, Ukraine

1. Abstract

The epidemiological study of cardiovascular diseases (CVD) consists of 3727 individuals before and an additional 1670 subjects that were included after the Chernobyl accident, living in the contaminated Polessky region. 17 occupations are represented . In general, the database had 270 fields and located in 18 files for each person involved in the study. Under the leadership of the Ministry of Public Health of Ukraine (MPH), the Institute for Occupational Health, the Ukrainian Institute of Cardiology MPH and the Ukrainian Health Education Center MPH and 5 local hospitals cooperated closely in monitoring, survey and data collection. For cardiovascular diseases (CHD), mental and neurological disorders, respiratory diseases, endocrine and labor complications the relative risk for a combination of factors, considered a consequence of the Chernobyl accident rose from 7.0 (confidence limit ± 27%) to 17.3 (± 12%). Due to active intervention over a period of 3 years CHD morbidity decreased.

2. Introduction

Eleven years have passed since the accident at the Chernobyl nuclear power station - the largest man-made disaster in the world. One of the main consequences of the accident appear to be health disorders in clean-up workers (so called Liquidators) and in populations living in contaminated areas [1].

National Institutes of Ukraine, Belarus and Russia as well as experts from Western European countries, USA, Japan and international organizations explored the state of health of affected populations systematically [2]. However, a wide-scale epidemiological investigation aiming to reveal factors of non-radiation nature in combination with radiation exposures has not yet been carried out [3].

A. K. Junk et al. (eds.),
Ocular Radiation Risk Assessment in Populations Exposed to Environmental Radiation Contamination, 197–201.

In order to meet this lack of information in the presented study it was necessary, first, to develop reliable tools for such investigations, a correctly designed questionnaire, an adequate data base and data base management [4].
The following issues were considered most important features for the planned questionnaire:

a) revelation and assessment of tentative levels of radiation exposure;
b) assessment of health shifts and comparison of probable future changes with an adequate control group including exposure to occupational factors, standard risk factors and dietary patterns;
c) confirmation of reliability of the data received by other contributing specialties (dosimetric assessment, chemical analysis, etc.).

Our approach to assess the health effects after the Chernobyl accident in differentiation with various occupational and environmental risks is presented in the following.

3. Methods

Our epidemiological cohort study on cardiovascular diseases (CVD) consists of 3727 individuals before and an additional 1670 included after the Chernobyl accident in the Polessky region. This is one of the areas with the highest radionucleid contamination following the Chernobyl accident and is located very close to the reactor site. The majority of Liquidators recruited immediately after the accident (first generation clean-up workers) came from this area.

In general, the data base had 270 fields and located in 18 files for each person involved in the study. 17 occupations were included in the sample.The data base is closely integrated into the overall structure of the involved organizations. The study is overseen by the Ministry of Public Health of Ukraine (MPH). The Institute of Occupational Health, Academy of Medical Sciences of Ukraine (IOH), the Ukrainian Institute of Cardiology MPH, the Ukrainian Health Education Center MPH and 5 local Ukrainian hospitals are monitoring the surveys and the data collection. Special attention was paid to develop a questionnaire for cardiovascular diseases (including myocardial infarction and stroke), cancer and diabetes mellitus.

4. Results and Discussion

A cross-sectional analysis of the health status in populations near the Chernobyl power station (Polessky region) showed significantly higher morbidity rates in comparison with morbidity data prior to the accident and with the control group. For cardiovascular diseases (CVD), mental and neurological disorders, respiratory diseases, endocrine and labor complications the relative risk (RR) of combination of factors which we consider as consequence of Chernobyl accident rose from 7.0 (confidence limits $\pm 27\%$) to 17.3 ($\pm 12\%$).

Further analysis showed that even 10 years after contact with agrochemicals, the prevalence of coronary heart diseases (CHD) is twofold, and the prevalence of arterial hypertension four times that of workers having had negligible exposure (Table 1). This might not only be due to occupational factors, but represent a bias from better diagnosis of hypertension and CHD during standardized examinations by specialists. The highest risk of CHD was found when subjects were exposed to a combination of occupational factors, for example operators of agricultural machines such as milking machines. The highest relative risk of arterial hypertension was found in swine-breeders, workers in mechanical workshops, plumbers at water-purification plants, and masons.

TABLE 1. Relative risk of cardio-vascular diseases associated with smoking and occupational factors.

Occupation	Occupational RR	Occupational RR & smoking
Tractor drivers	1.19*	3.2*
Workers in mechanical workshops and water-purifying plants	4,9*	11.3*
Field workers not exposed to chemicals	1.2	1.87*
Field workers exposed to chemicals	3,3*	7.0*
Cattle breeders	2.3*	8.8*
Bricklayers	5.2*	6.7*

* Statistically significant ($p < 0,05$)

These results in mind an active intervention program for the studied occupational groups was designed. This program included all subjects and individual schemes for primary and secondary prevention of cardiovascular diseases. Primary prevention focused on therapeutic and hygienic measures. Essential principles of hygienic measures in the preventive intervention design were:

a) optimal labor conditions
b) repeated training in preventive hygienic measures at work and at home for
c) design of optimum work and rest routines
d) decrease of occupational and domestic psychoemotional strain by explanation of actual risks and health advice in order to eliminate bad habits.

These main preventive measures have already been implemented at local, state and country levels. As a result of this active intervention over a period of 3 years CHD morbidity decreased in Ukraine. This effect was higher in the areas of investigation and active implementation of hygienic measures. Preliminary data on the efficiency of the hygienic and therapeutic measures among the investigated individuals is shown in Table 2. A group subjected to therapeutic measures only served as control.

TABLE 2. Efficiency of preventive measures.

	Study group	Control group
Decrease in morbidity level	17.0% *	8.0%
Decrease in mortality level	9.0%	6.0%
Decrease in primary disability	13.0%	7.0%
Shortening of temporary disability of 100 workers	9.2%	2.6%

*- a liability indicator

This favorable tendency in health indices supports the orientation of our investigations and preventive measures.

To provide a model for a population survey in the selected cohorts, weighting coefficients for various factors were established. Multiple regression analysis was applied to determine the portion of all involved factors and their contribution to the occurrence of diseases in the exposed populations. The assessment of weighting coefficients for each factor is given below:

1. relative risk (RR) coefficients;
2. RR trends:
   - in relation to exposure levels;
   - in relations to time intervals;
3. etiological fraction (EF) of each factor and/or their combination;
4. matrix design using health indices of the studied populations (end-points) under consideration of combined exposures;
5. design of a correlation-regression model on the basis of this matrix;
6. tabulate the contribution of weighting coefficients to risk factors
7. determination of RR in consideration of weighting coefficients to develop end-points (in %);
8. prediction of end-points using the obtained data.

5. Conclusion

Sample size is very important in planning epidemiological surveys in order to achieve significance levels. If the sample size is not sufficient even reliable indices should not be considered. This investigation is a subset of wide-scale studies carried out by our institute (IOH), aimed at studying the effects of work-related factors and radiation on human health. After the Chernobyl accident, the clean-up workers, so called “Liquidators” gained our particular consideration.

The described experience in data base management supported the creation of the organization structure of the Ukrainian-American Chernobyl Ocular Study Protocol (UACOS) .

The authors have gained certain experience in development of questionnaires and surveys on epidemiological data bases including long time support and management of follow-up studies since 1976. The questionnaires and studies were directed to reveal the impact of work related and environmental factors on the development of cardio-vascular diseases.

6. References

1. Romanenko, A. Y., The Health Care of the Suffered Populations in Conditions of the Nuclear Power Station Wide Scale Accident (Theoretical and Practical aspects) (1988) *Medizinskie aspekty avariyi na chernobylskoy atomnoy elektrostanziyi.* Scientific Conference publications. Kiev, Zdorobie. - 42-52.
2. Nakadzima,. H. (1995).Preface. *In Medical consequences of the Chernobyl accident (IPHICA Results of Pilot Projects and National Programs). Scientific Report. International Program of the Medical consequences of the Chernobyl accident. World Health Organization.* Sushkevich G. N., Zyib, A. F., (eds.), «*Vidar*» *Ltd.*, 15-16.
3. Dobrovolsky, L. A., Vitte, P. N. EFFECTS OF OCCUPATIONAL AND OTHER RISK FACTORS ON THE HEALTH OF AGRICULTURAL WORKERS (1991). The first Finnish-Soviet Symposium on Occupational Health and Safety in Agriculture. Finland. Ed. V. Notkola, P. Susitaival, M. Kotimaa, Helsinki. Institute of Occupational Health., 28-36.
4. Kundiev Y., Vitte P., Smirnova I., Guslitser L. (1996) COMBINED EFFECTS OF OCCUPATIONAL FACTORS AND RADIATION ON LATE HEALTH EFFECTS AFTER THE CHERNOBYL INCIDENT. *Publication of Armed Forced Radiobiology Research Institute AFRRI, Defense Nuclear Agency, US Department of Defense.* 86.

FINAL RECOMMENDATIONS OF THE NATO ADVANCED RESEARCH WORKSHOP ON "OCULAR RADIATION RISK ASSESSMENT IN POPULATIONS EXPOSED TO ENVIRONMENTAL RADIATION CONTAMINATION", KIEV 1997

Introduction

These proceedings are concluded by the recommendations which were unanimously approved by the participants in the workshop. The recommendations are the result of intense break-out sessions held for each of the three disciplines represented; ophthalmology, dosimetry and epidemiology. The collective goal was to find agreement on the criteria which are considered essential in current and future studies of ocular damage to populations at risk.

The participants, scientists from thirteen nations engaged in a merging of perspectives and approaches allowing consensus on a broad range of issues. Speakers addressed the topics in review fashion or in the detail required to assess specific questions which historically have proven problematic. The break-out discussions resulted in the formulation of criteria for the standardized assessment of populations at risk. Each discipline's views appear in the reports that follow. Together they represent the first true effort to offer a guide to the design and implementation of an ocular follow-up of a population exposed to greater-than-background doses of ionizing radiation.

1. The Ophthalmology Discussion Group

The Ophthalmology Discussion Group met to discuss the minimum requirements for the conduct of eye follow-ups in populations exposed to environmental radiation contamination. A secondary goal was to discuss more robust or maximal requirements for such a study. The overall aim was to offer consensus recommendations for the design and implementation of a radiation effects study on the eyes of individuals in populations at risk.

The Ophthalmology Discussion Group was co-chaired by C. Medvedovsky, N. Sergienko and T. Kodama. Participating members of the group were: A. Aparin, M. Avakian, M. Bausz, N. Bushueva, M. Charles, S. Denyer, A. Deyev, J. Gladun, M. Froemel, A. K. Junk, N. Kovalenko, T. Kovalchuk, V. Lishchenko, A. Madekin, T. Makarenko, S. Maximenko, S. Mikhaylovsky, G. Parkhomenko, V. Serduchenko, V. Serduk, A. Smirnova, S. Sosnovsky, L. Sushina, M. Vinogradova, E. Voice, V. Vit, L. Zlatopolskaya, N. Zlenko. Some portions of the deliberations included both Y. Kundiev and B. Worgul.

A. K. Junk et al. (eds.),
Ocular Radiation Risk Assessment in Populations Exposed to Environmental Radiation Contamination, 203–219.

Because of its relative non-ambiguity and the fact that agencies historically have conditioned their risk assessments on the induction of cataract, study design necessarily focused on cataract onset. There were readily agreed upon basic points which should be considered in the design and conduct of an eye study:

- Cataract progression while not readily amenable to unequivocal subjective assessment, would be noted and, at a minimum, semi-quantitatively assessed.
- Careful coordination with the epidemiological component must be implemented from the outset, to agree on such things as the best way to handle confounders and/or one and two-eyed data acquisition.
- Qualified ophthalmologists must be used as primary examiners and if a site employs more than one examiner, the most qualified or senior member should be given oversight authority and be assigned responsibility for overall compliance.
- Examiners must receive program-specific training.
- Mydriatrics should always be used to maximize posterior lens visualization. A study should not even be considered if the subjects eyes cannot be dilated.
- Examiners must utilize, at a minimum, a slit-lamp biomicroscope. Ophthalmoscopy can be employed as part of the overall eye examination but the lens status must be assessed using a slit-lamp.
- Standardized forms and the training to properly use them are critical.

1.1. OPHTHALMIC ASSESSMENT

1.1.1. Eye Examination

Although the goal of most eye follow-up studies will be cataract assessment, a relatively thorough eye examination should accompany the lens evaluation. Not only would it help to reveal undiagnosed potential confounders but would assure the ophthalmic health of the subject for continued longitudinal study. The examination should be reported on dedicated forms (figure 1) not only to assure their having been done but to allow a retrospective analysis if unexpected pathologies occur. An example of this is the observations of fundus changes in irradiated populations. Because the previous radiation follow-ups did not do detailed fundus examinations little is known about changes in the back of the eye at cataractogenic dose levels.

1.1.2. Evaluation of Potential Confounders

Working closely with the epidemiological investigators, the ophthalmology component must aware of and alert to the problem of confounders which might affect the transparency of the lens and the interpretation of the radiation effect on it.

Careful assessment will be made to exclude from enrollment those who suffer from one of a number of potent risk factors for cataracts which could complicate radiation cataract assessment. They fall under several categories:

Intraocular diseases

Aniridia, anterior segment necrosis, Fuchs' syndrome, glaucoma, Harada's syndrome, high myopia, Jacobsen-Brodwall syndrome, Laurence-Moon-Bardet-Biedl syndrome, Leber's congenital amaurosis, microphthalmia, Norrie's, persistent hyperplastic primary vitreous, O'Donnell-Pappas' syndrome, Peter's anomaly, retinal detachment, retinal degenerations (retinitis pigmentosa, gyrate atrophy), sclerocornea, retinoblastoma, retrolental fibroplasia, retinal anoxia (Buerger's disease, Takayasu's pulseless disease), trauma (Glassblowers cataract, ocular contusion syndrome), uveitis/inflammations (anterior and posterior).

Systemic diseases

a. Metabolic disorders: Albright's disease, Bassen-Kornzweig syndrome, Diabetes mellitus, Fabry's disease, galactosemia, Hand-Schüller-Christian syndrome, hemochromatosis, Heerfordt's syndrome, homocystinuria, hypertension, hypoparathyroidism / hypocalcemia, Kussmaul's disease, Lowe's syndrome, Oculo-oto-ororenoerythropoietic disease, Refsum's disease, Sjögren's syndrome, Wilson's disease.

b. Skin diseases: Acrodermatitis chronica atrophicans, atopic dermatitis, Bloch-Sulzberger syndrome, congenital ectodermal dysplasia, Kyrle's disease, neurodermatitis, Pemphigus foliaceus, Rothmund-Thomson syndrome, Werner's syndrome.

c. Connective tissue/skeletal disorders: Abefeld's syndrome, bone dysplasias (Engelmann's syndrome, Paget's syndrome), Conradi's disease, dislocated lenses (Marfan's syndrome, Ehlers-Danlos syndrome), Leri's syndrome, myotonic dystrophy, Pierre-Robin syndrome, Stickler's syndrome, Still's disease.

d. Renal diseases: Alport's syndrome, Lowe's syndrome.

e. Central nervous system: bilateral acoustic neuroma (neurofibromatosis 2), Hagberg-Santavuori syndrome, Marinesco-Sjögren syndrome, Meckel's syndrome, von Recklinghausen's syndrome (neurofibromatosis 1).

Drugs

Alcoholism, allopurinol, chlorpromazine, dinitrophenol, busulfan (Myleran), DMSO, ergot, indapamide, miotics, naphthalene, ouabain, paradichlorobenzene, phenothiazine, psoralen, selenium, smoking (Roy's syndrome), steroids, thallium, trinitrotoluidine, triparanol.

If, one of these factors come into play during the course of the study, for example if a subject develops diabetes, that individual can be carried along in the study, but should be flagged and may have to be analyzed as a separate stratum or deleted from selected analyses. Those with some presenile or congenital lens changes which are not located in the PSC area or which do not interfere with visualization of that region, need not be disqualified from enrollment.

F O R M 1 - L E N S 1

ОСМОТР ХРУСТАЛИКА 1

(Биомикроскопия с расширенным зрачкои > 5 мм)

ВИЗИТ	ДАТА	ИССЛЕДОВАТЕЛЬ	ФАМИЛИЯ БОЛЬНОГО	КОД

ИЗМЕНЕНИЯ ХРУСТАЛИКА	ПРАВЫЙ ГЛАЗ		ЛЕВЫЙ ГЛАЗ	
ПРОЗРАЧНЫЙ	НЕТ ▭	ДА ▭	НЕТ ▭	ДА ▭
ПРЕКАТАРАКТАЛЬНЫЕ ИЭМЕНЕНИЯ	НЕТ ▭	ДА ▭	НЕТ ▭	ДА ▭
1. Полихромн. переливч. в плоскости задней капсулы	НЕТ ▭	ДА ▭	НЕТ ▭	ДА ▭
2. Единичные "точки" <10	НЕТ ▭	ДА ▭	НЕТ ▭	ДА ▭
под передней капсулой	НЕТ ▭	ДА ▭	НЕТ ▭	ДА ▭
в передней коре	НЕТ ▭	ДА ▭	НЕТ ▭	ДА ▭
под задней капсулой	НЕТ ▭	ДА ▭	НЕТ ▭	ДА ▭
в задней коре	НЕТ ▭	ДА ▭	НЕТ ▭	ДА ▭
в экваториальн.области	НЕТ ▭	ДА ▭	НЕТ ▭	ДА ▭
вокруг ядра	НЕТ ▭	ДА ▭	НЕТ ▭	ДА ▭
3. Единичные вакуоли <5	НЕТ ▭	ДА ▭	НЕТ ▭	ДА ▭
под передней капсулой	НЕТ ▭	ДА ▭	НЕТ ▭	ДА ▭
в передней коре	НЕТ ▭	ДА ▭	НЕТ ▭	ДА ▭
под задней капсулой	НЕТ ▭	ДА ▭	НЕТ ▭	ДА ▭
в задней коре	НЕТ ▭	ДА ▭	НЕТ ▭	ДА ▭
в экваториальн.области	НЕТ ▭	ДА ▭	НЕТ ▭	ДА ▭
вокруг ядра	НЕТ ▭	ДА ▭	НЕТ ▭	ДА ▭

1

Figure 1. Lens examination form, a part of the 9 page eye examination form used in the UACOS effort. The entire packet is available in Russian and English translation upon request. Contact Prof. B. V. Worgul, Eye Radiation and Environmental Research Laboratory, Columbia University, 630 W 168th St., New York, NY 10032, USA, Tel.: +1-212-305-6748, Fax.: +1-212-305-6749, email: "bvw1@columbia.edu"

1.2. LENS ASSESSMENT

It is critical that the population is examined at intervals not exceeding 24 months. Longer intervals reduce resolution and consequently the value of the study. If precataractous changes are noted a re-examination at 6 months is recommended.

After a standard ophthalmological work-up, a mydriatic must be used to obtain maximum pupil dilatation (>5 mm) for lens examination. If the pupil cannot be dilated the data should not be included in the study. Because onset is the primary criterion for the assessment, reliable identification of early lens changes in the posterior subcapsular (PSC) region of the lens is essential. The emphasis is on detection rather than quantification of cataract. This strategy recognizes that at relatively low dose ranges the cataracts which develop are not likely to become severe and in many cases may not be progressive. Therefore clear and unambiguous criteria which define the endpoint, cataract, are essential.

1.2.1.Early (precataractous) lens changes

Typically one of the earliest clinical expressions of radiation exposure of the lens is the appearance of a "polychromatic sheen" or "beaten brass" look to the posterior capsule. A study design should acknowledge its presence by scoring it as one of three possible early, or precataractous, lens changes. Equally common transient dots or vacuoles appear in the PSC area or posterior superficial cortex. As has been the general experience with radiation cataract development, typically when more than 10 dots or 5 vacuoles are present they are not likely to be transient.

Therefore the proposed Lens Examination Forms provide for three possibilities in scoring early or precataractous lens changes:

- A polychromatic sheen associated with the posterior capsule.
- Individual (non-aggregated) dots which number fewer than 10.
- Individual vacuoles numbering fewer than 5.

Although the radiogenic changes will occur in the PSC region there is always the possibility of dots or vacuoles occurring elsewhere in an otherwise unremarkable lens. Therefore for completeness the scorer should be asked to localize the observed changes as; anterior, posterior, equatorial and/or supranuclear. The forms used by the practitioner should have provision for binary responses to each.

1.2.2. Cataract Scoring

While not pathognomonic, radiation cataracts develop in a characteristic, sequential fashion. The sequela is so predictable it can serve as a semi-quantitative scoring technique as was been done by Merriam and Focht in 1962. Because it was specifically designed for gauging radiation cataract and its inherently unambiguous nature, a myriad of modified versions of the method have employed by a number of laboratories.

The method is as follows:

- **Stage 1+** Discrete opacity which can take the form of a small spot readily discernible with retroilluminated light; aggregates of dots (>10) or vacuoles (>5), cortical spokes, waterclefts, or granulated opacities. The scorer must record the location as described above.
- **Stage 2+** More extensive cortical changes collectively occupying approximately 25% of the noted area of the lens. If markedly less or more than 25% is involved a **Stage 1.5+ or 2.5+**, respectively, is scored. For the "x.5" stages the lens forms provide "comment" space but are not sensitive to that staging for binary recording.
- **Stage 3+** Advanced changes. Light does not reach vitreous.
- **Stage 4+** Premature cataract. Near-total lens opacification. In some areas it is possible to see the nucleus or posterior cortex of the lens.
- **Stage 5+** Mature cataract. Total lens opacification.

The scoring method used to stage the cataracts incorporates the localizations as described for the early lens changes. Because of the low-dose nature of many studies radiogenic cataracts beyond the 1-2+ stage generally will not be encountered. Nonetheless, the later stages may appear. The study is designed so that cataract onset is defined by the 1+ stage which will be the common endpoint used to determine risk. Although that juncture will be the critical cataract data point as regards risk analyses, the patient will remain in the cohort and continue to be followed for the remainder of the study. The more advanced staging criteria for evaluation should be employed, optimally in concert with the application of advanced imaging techniques to immortalize the raw data and reduce the subject analytical components.

The examining ophthalmologist should also determine the location of the changes observed i.e., central, medial, superior / inferior medial, lateral, superior / inferior lateral. The importance of this lies in the possibility of significant beta exposure which might result in a sidedness to the opacity particularly in an acute exposure situation. This could help in dose estimations and accounting for a potentially significant beta dose. The beta contribution could vary as a function of lens depth so that age at time of exposure is an important parameter to consider. For the same reason whether the individual is myopic, hypermetropic, eutropic or emmetropic should be noted and considered in data analysis.

2. The Dosimetry Discussion Group

The Dosimetry Discussion Group addressed the minimum requirements for the conduct of dosimetry to support an epidemiologic study of radiation cataracts in populations exposed to environmental radiation contamination. A secondary goal was to discuss the optimum requirements (or maximum support) for such a study. Most of the considerations were rather specific for the population of Chernobyl Liquidators;

thus, while many requirements might be generalized, many concerns and needs are specific to the considered problem.

The Dosimetry Discussion Group was co-chaired by V. V. Chumak and L. Anspaugh. Additional members of the group were H. Bakhanova, C. Baumstark-Khan, W. Chang, M. Charles, V. Krujchkov, and V. Shevchenko. Brief consultations were made with R. Shore and B. Worgul during the course of the discussions.

2.1. SOME GENERAL NEEDS AND GOALS FOR DOSIMETRIC SUPPORT OF EPIDEMIOLOGIC STUDIES ARE

- Dosimetrists and epidemiologists should be involved early in joint discussions of possible studies so that even approximate estimates of dose can be used to examine whether a postulated epidemiologic study would have enough power to detect, in a statistically significant way, the effect to be studied.
- Central estimates of dose and estimates of uncertainty should be provided for absorbed dose for each type of radiation of significantly different linear energy transfer (LET), such as alpha particles, beta-gamma radiation, and neutrons; information as specific as possible should be provided on the nature of the irradiation experienced by the studied population. The use of radiation-protection concepts, such as weighting factors, equivalent dose, and effective dose, should be avoided in a scientific study on the derivation of risk. The use of the International System of units is strongly encouraged; that is, dose should be expressed in Gy or mGy and activity should be expressed in Bq.
- For case-control or cohort studies, doses and associated uncertainties should be determined for each individual in the study.
- Significant dosimetric support should continue over the life of any epidemiologic study of potentially significant value (or investment). Opportunities should be pursued that might increase the accuracy of or reduce the uncertainty in estimates of dose. Such opportunities may well arise from new developments that occur during the life of an epidemiologic study.
- The results of the discussions are summarized as follows for the two charges to the Discussion Group. The Ukrainian-American Chernobyl Ocular Study (UACOS) is used and was discussed as a concrete example of the conduct of an epidemiologic study of ocular risk. Other studies of ocular risk are either ongoing or can be envisaged. These populations of interest include the workers at the Mayak Complex, the population exposed through contamination of the Techa River, the general population exposed by the Chernobyl accident, and several others.

2.2. MINIMUM PROGRAM FOR DOSIMETRY

Adequate dosimetry support for the proposed UACOS is a challenge for the dosimetry community, as dosimetry support for this study will necessitate the solution of many difficult problems. Adequate dosimetry support is understood to have the following requirements:

- Assistance in the cohort-selection phase to ensure that proposed members of the cohort have a reasonable probability of having a 'knowable" dose with as little uncertainty as possible.
- Ultimate provision of a dose to the eye lens that includes both beta and gamma components with as small an amount of uncertainty as possible. The uncertainty requirements are not specified, but a goal should be to have individual doses with an uncertainty factor of three or less. An uncertainty factor of two or less would be highly desirable.

The steps required for the minimum dosimetry program are as follows:

2.2.1 Assemble the cohort

For several reasons the dosimetrists will have major responsibility for the assembly of the cohort for the UACOS. First, adequate power for the study requires that as large a number as possible of Liquidators with doses over 1 Gy be included in the cohort. Second, it is important that those included in the study have a high probability of having a 'knowable" dose, at least in the future. Third, it may be possible to select some members of the cohort who will have more certain doses than others. For example, some prospective members of the cohort can be presumed to have had no external beta dose due to the conditions of their exposure; as external gamma dose is presumed to be more knowable, such persons might be given priority for selection (unless they all might have low doses). Although this task or requirement of assembling the cohort is listed first, its success depends on the successful completion of some of the steps outlined below.

2.2.2. Verification of existing dose records available in the State Chernobyl Registry and other databases

Dosimetric data concerning about 90,000 early Liquidators from Ukraine are maintained in several databases. Many persons have questioned the quality of such data and there are persistent concerns that some data may have been falsified. In reality it is likely that some subsegments of this database contain quite reliable data, and the reliability may be determined by the organization responsible for the dosimetry records. The potential value of such records is very great, and it is critical to examine them carefully and to filter such data to select those segments that have a high probability of being reliable. It is presumed at this time that such dose records would pertain to gamma doses only. However, some data from dosimeters sensitive to beta radiation might have been recorded in the databases.

2.2.3. Assemble all monitoring and research data on external beta dosimetry

Measurements of external beta dose and of beta dose as a function of depth in tissue equivalent material were made by investigators, especially those from the Institute of Biophysics. Information collected simultaneously on external gamma dose provides data on the ratio of beta-to-gamma dose for the eye lens. This information is extremely valuable for this study, and special efforts will be made to collect all such data.

2.2.4. Validation of dose records by means of retrospective dosimetry

After the dose records in item 2.2.2. are filtered to select those deemed to be most reliable, it will be necessary to perform a validation study for some subset of such doses. It is assumed that such presumed reliable doses will be external gamma doses. Validation of such doses will be examined by the measurement by electron paramagnetic resonance of external gamma doses in a selected number of tooth samples to be collected as the opportunity arises due to dental health requirements for extraction.

2.2.5. Evaluation of individual doses by analytical and expert assessment methods

Most individual members of the proposed cohort will not have reliable (or any) dosimetry records. For these individuals it will be necessary to perform an analytical reconstruction of doses; this analytical method will rely upon calculational procedures to deduce both beta and gamma doses based upon rather complex calculations of the mixture of radionuclides present at times following the accident (and therefore the energies of the emitted betas and gammas) and geometry of the presumed sources for each individual. If possible, detailed interview data will be used to assist in the analytical procedures. Information will be sought on location and times in location during the course of liquidation work, but such interview data will not be helpful for many of the cohort members due to the lack of specific memory of where the interviewed individuals were. Information from interviews will also be sought on whether goggles or glasses were worn during the course of any major exposure period. Where necessary, the "analytical" doses will be derived on the basis of "expert judgment" of qualified individuals. One important outcome will be the best possible estimate of the ratio of beta-to-gamma dose to the eye lens.

2.2.6. Reconstruction of doses using electron paramagnetic resonance (EPR) of tooth enamel

A tooth-collection system has already been implemented among prospective members of the cohort. The acquisition of a tooth will be one of the primary selection criteria for inclusion in the cohort. The acquisition process will continue during the life of the study for all members selected for the cohort. As many teeth as possible from the cohort members will be analyzed by EPR to determine the external gamma dose.

2.2.7. Derive the best possible estimate of external gamma dose and estimate its uncertainty

Information from steps 2.2.2, 2.2.4, 2.2.5, and 2.2.6 above will be used to derive the best possible estimate of external gamma dose for each member of the cohort; and the uncertainty in the estimated gamma dose will be estimated.

2.2.8. Derive the best possible estimate of eye-lens external beta dose and estimate its uncertainty

The results of steps 2.2.2, 2.2.3, 2.2.4, and 2.2.5 above will be used to estimate beta-to-gamma-dose conversion factors for each member of the cohort and this estimate will be multiplied by the estimated gamma dose determined in step 2.2.7 above to determine the best estimate of beta dose to the eye lens. The uncertainty in the beta dose will also be estimated.

2.2.9 Develop a method to validate the estimated beta dose to the eye lens

Members of the discussion group agreed that it is essential to have a method of validating the calculated beta dose to the eye lens. No such method now exists. A possible solution to this problem was presented by Prof. Worgul during a plenary session of the workshop. This is the development of the eye-lens micronuclei dosimetry system, which if successful, could be used to assay the beta plus gamma doses to the eye lens. It is believed that this proposed research and development program would be extremely valuable, and this activity is supported strongly by the Dosimetry Discussion Group.

2.3. OPTIMUM (OR MAXIMUM) PROGRAM FOR DOSIMETRY

The goals and requirements for the optimum program are the same as for the minimum program. However, the probability for success of the dosimetry support can be enhanced by using some additional methods available for retrospective dosimetry and by performing directed, but limited, research and development for validation of total dose to the eye lens.

The steps required for the optimum dosimetry program are indicated below. Additions to the minimum program are in "hyphenations".

2.3.1. Assemble the cohort

For several reasons the dosimetrists will have major responsibility for the assembly of the cohort for the UACOS. First, adequate power for the study requires that as large a number as possible of Liquidators with doses over 1 Gy be included in the cohort. Second, it is important that those included in the study have a high probability of having a 'knowable" dose, at least in the future. Third, it may be possible to select some members of the cohort who will have more certain doses than others. For example, some prospective members of the cohort can be presumed to have had no external beta dose due to the conditions of their exposure; as external gamma dose is presumed to be more knowable, such persons might be given priority for selection (unless they all might have low doses). Although this task or requirement of assembling the cohort is listed first, its success depends on the successful completion of some of the steps outlined below.

2.3.2. Verification of existing dose records available in the State Chernobyl Registry and other databases

Dosimetric data concerning about 90,000 early Liquidators from Ukraine are maintained in several databases. Many persons have questioned the quality of such data and there are persistent concerns that some data may have been falsified. In reality it is likely that some subsegments of this database contain quite reliable data, and the reliability may be determined by the organization responsible for the dosimetry records. The potential value of such records is very great, and it is critical to examine them carefully and to filter such data to select those segments that have a high probability of being reliable. It is presumed at this time that such dose records would pertain to gamma doses only. However, some data from dosimeters sensitive to beta radiation might have been recorded in the databases.

2.3.3. Assemble all monitoring and research data on external beta dosimetry
Measurements of external beta dose and of beta dose as a function of depth in tissue equivalent material were made by investigators, especially those from the Institute of Biophysics. Information collected simultaneously on external gamma dose provides data on the ratio of beta-to-gamma dose for the eye lens. This information is extremely valuable for this study, and special efforts will be made to collect all such data.

2.3.4. Validation of dose records by means of retrospective dosimetry
After the dose records in item 2 are filtered to select those deemed to be most reliable, it will be necessary to perform a validation study for some subset of such doses. It is assumed that such presumed reliable doses will be external gamma doses. Validation of such doses will be examined by the measurement by electron paramagnetic resonance of external gamma doses in a selected number of tooth samples to be collected as the opportunity arises due to dental health requirements for extraction. "Additional validation studies will be made by the collection of small amounts of blood for the derivation of dose by fluorescent in situ hybridization (FISH) analysis of stable chromosomal translocations in lymphocytes."

2.3.5. Evaluation of individual doses by analytical and expert assessment methods
Most individual members of the proposed cohort will not have reliable (or any) dosimetry records. For these individuals it will be necessary to perform an analytical reconstruction of doses; this analytical method will rely upon calculational procedures to deduce both beta and gamma doses based upon rather complex calculations of the mixture of radionuclides present at times following the accident (and therefore the energies of the emitted betas and gammas) and geometry of the presumed sources for each individual. If possible, detailed interview data will be used to assist in the analytical procedures. Information will be sought on location and times in location during the course of liquidation work, but such interview data will not be helpful for many of the cohort members due to the lack of specific memory of where the interviewed individuals were. Information from interviews will also be sought on whether goggles or glasses were worn during the course of any major exposure period. Where necessary, the 'analytical' doses will be derived on the basis of 'expert judgment' of qualified individuals. One important outcome will be the best possible estimate of the ratio of beta-to-gamma dose to the eye lens.

2.3.6. Reconstruction of doses using electron paramagnetic resonance (EPR) of tooth enamel and fluorescent in situ hybridization (FISH) analysis of circulating lymphocytes
A tooth-collection system has already been implemented among prospective members of the cohort. The acquisition of a tooth will be one of the primary selection criteria for

inclusion in the cohort. The acquisition process will continue during the life of the study for all members selected for the cohort. As many teeth as possible from the cohort members will be analyzed by EPR to determine the external gamma dose. "In addition, blood samples will be collected from a selected sample of individuals for analysis of external gamma dose by FISH analysis of stable chromosomal translocations."

2.3.7. Derive the best possible estimate of external gamma dose and estimate its uncertainty

Information from steps 2.3.2, 2.3.4, 2.3.5, and 2.3.6 above will be used to derive the best possible estimate of external gamma dose for each member of the cohort; and the uncertainty in the estimated gamma dose will be estimated.

2.3.8. Derive the best possible estimate of eye-lens external beta dose and estimate its uncertainty

The results of steps 2.3.2, 2.3.3, 2.3.4, and 2.3.5 above will be used to estimate beta-to-gamma-dose conversion factors for each member of the cohort and this estimate will be multiplied by the estimated gamma dose determined in step 7 above to determine the best estimate of beta dose to the eye lens. The uncertainty in the beta dose will also be estimated.

2.3.9. *Develop a method to validate the estimated beta dose to the eye lens*

Members of the discussion group agreed that it is essential to have a method of validating the calculated beta dose to the eye lens. No such method now exists. A possible solution to this problem was presented by Prof. Worgul during a plenary session of the workshop. This is the development of the eye-lens micronuclei dosimetry system, which if successful, could be used to assay the beta plus gamma doses to the eye lens. It is believed that this proposed research and development program would be extremely valuable, and this activity is supported strongly by the Dosimetry Discussion Group. Research and development should also be directed toward a second candidate system. One system judged to have a reasonable probability of success is to an assay using FISH applied to cells cultured from skin taken very close to the eye. It may be possible to culture cells taken from hair follicles from eyelashes as well.

3. The Epidemiology Discussion Group

The Epidemiology Discussion Group met to discuss both the minimum "essential" epidemiologic standards for studies of ocular radiation risk and additional "recommended, but optional" criteria for such studies. Although the core of the discussion concerned studies of Chernobyl Liquidators, an attempt was made to generalize the criteria to other studies of ocular radiation effects or even to other hazardous exposures.

The Epidemiology Discussion Group was co-chaired by P. Vitte and R. Shore. Additional members of the group were Y. Kundiev, A. Abdullina, V.F. Danilichev, L. Dobrovolsky, A. Eglite, B. Fountos, I. Galstyan, L. Guslitser, I. Masnyk, T. Mikhailina, G. Ozola and O. Tsvetkova.

The criteria below which are regarded as minimum, essential criteria for an adequate study are designated as "(ESSENTIAL)" at the end of their description and are prefaced with a "**". Other criteria that are desirable but are not essential are designated as "(Recommended)". In addition, for completeness, two items are included that describe methods that have been used by some investigators but are not recommended for anything but preliminary, exploratory studies; these are designated as "(NOT recommended)".

3.1. STUDY DESIGN CONSIDERATIONS

3.1.1. Geographic study

A geographic study, which correlates compiled rates of some ocular disorder in various geographic areas with an index of average exposure levels in those areas, is occasionally useful as a "hypothesis generating," preliminary study, but it is potentially subject to serious biases. A geographic study is intrinsically incapable of establishing a causal relationship, and its estimates of the magnitude of risks are apt to be seriously biased. (NOT recommended)

3.1.2 Cross-sectional study

A cross-sectional study is one in which a random or representative "cross-section" of a population is given ocular examinations. The results may then be correlated with exposure or other characteristics. The exposure characteristics are usually inferred from either geographic location or subjects' recall. This is a useful type of descriptive study and can be used for hypothesis generation, but the weak nature of the exposure data limit their usefulness in inferring a causal relationship. (NOT recommended for studying disease causation, but may be useful as a descriptive study)

3.1.3. Case-control study

In a case-control study the exposure history of a series of cases of ocular disease/disorder is compared to the exposure history of a matching group ("controls") who do not have disease. This can be a useful type of study if it is carefully designed and carried out. However, it is very difficult to select proper controls in this type of study, so there may be "selection biases". In addition, such studies usually rely on personal recall of exposures in the past. Such information is subject to "recall bias," i.e., where cases and controls have a different degree of under-reporting or over-reporting of past exposures. When possible, a cohort study is therefore preferable (or possibly a case-control study in which objective records of past exposures are obtained rather than relying on personal recall). Case-control studies are useful primarily for rare diseases or disorders. If the disorder is fairly common (as cataracts are), then a cohort study is the preferred study design. (Recommended in some circumstances, but not preferred)

3.1.4. Cohort study

A cohort study is the preferred study type whenever it is feasible. In a typical cohort study, a group of persons who have had an exposure is systematically identified and another group without that exposure, but who are comparable to the exposed group in other characteristics, serves as a comparison ("control") group. For a dose-response type cohort study in which the doses range from high to quite low, it may be possible to dispense with a purely unexposed group and rely on the dose-response curve, i.e., compare subgroups with various dose levels. When possible, it is desirable to define a study cohort with a substantial range of radiation doses, so that dose-response analyses can be conducted, as these are potentially more informative than simple exposed/unexposed comparisons. (Recommended, preferred)

3.2. STATISTICAL POWER **

In planning a study it is vital to determine the sample size required to yield adequate statistical power; otherwise the study is unlikely to produce meaningful results. It is recommended that the investigator consult with a statistician regarding this, as statistical methods are available to determine statistical power but they require some statistical expertise to implement and interpret them properly. The statistical power of a study is a function of several factors: the sample size, the baseline frequency of the disease endpoint, the range of doses (or how large the average dose is), and uncertainties in the dose estimates and in disease ascertainment. (ESSENTIAL)

For a planned dose-response analysis, it is important to have a wide range of doses, because the dose range strongly affects the statistical power of the study. It follows that, in determining the likely statistical power of a planned study, one should be realistic about the likely results. To be realistic, one can estimate the expected magnitude of the relative risk in the projected study based on the estimated average dose multiplied by an average risk coefficient (per unit dose) from the best available studies. (For example, for a low-dose study one might expect a relative risk of only 1.2, in which case a statistical power calculation based on a relative risk of, say, 3.0 would be unrealistic and therefore meaningless.)

3.3. DEFINED "SAMPLING FRAME" **

Design the study so that the sample of subjects will be systematically drawn from a defined population, not just a "convenience sample" or whoever volunteers. (ESSENTIAL)

3.4. PARTICIPATION RATES **

The rates of subject participation and follow-up in the study must be kept high. Non-participants and study dropouts tend to be a nonrandom (i.e., biased) subset of the study sample; if they become too numerous they potentially can introduce bias into the study results. Maintaining a high rate of participation in a study usually requires the allocation of considerable resources and should be planned for in advance. (ESSENTIAL)

3.5. MULTIPLE ASSESSMENTS OF DISEASE INCIDENCE

It is advantageous to design a cohort study so that there are periodic re-examinations of study subjects. This allows one to study the changes in ocular status over time, and permits the study subject to serve as his/her own control. Having multiple measurements increases the precision of the investigation and reduces the amount of error variance, which will increase the statistical power of the study. (Recommended)

3.6. DATA COLLECTION PROCEDURES

3.6.1 Comparable intensity of screening **

It is essential that a cohort study be designed so that subjects at all dose levels receive ocular examinations with the same frequency and thoroughness. If this is not done (e.g., if the high dose subjects get more frequent or more detailed examinations) it will introduce bias into the data. Similarly, in a case-control study it is essential that any questionnaires or other procedures be administered in an identical way to the cases and controls. (ESSENTIAL)

3.6.2. Objective data **

Whenever possible, objective data (i.e., those obtained by measurement) are preferable. For those data which necessarily have a subjective element to them (e.g., the ophthalmologist's examination findings), it is important to specify, in advance and as completely as possible, the criteria for various categories or designations. Similarly, in a case-control study it is essential that the interview be standardized, including the specific wording of the questions and of any follow-up probes that will be used to clarify or amplify answers persons might give to questions. (ESSENTIAL)

3.6.3. Blinded data collection **

In a cohort study, to help assure the validity of the data and prevent unconscious biases from creeping in, it is essential to keep those who collect the data from knowing the exposure status of the study subject being examined (i.e., whether the subject is in the exposed or unexposed group or what his/her dose was). Those who collect interview/questionnaire data from subjects should be kept from knowing either the exposure status or the ocular status of the subject. (ESSENTIAL)

Any laboratory procedures which are performed should be done in a blinded fashion, i.e., the laboratory personnel should be given samples with only identifiers that do not reveal the exposure status or ocular status of the subject. (ESSENTIAL)

Similarly, in a case-control study interviewers should be kept unaware of whether the person they are interviewing is a case or a control; if the interviewee himself tells the interviewer this information, that fact should be noted and coded in the database, so that subsequent analyses can evaluate whether the unblinding introduced any bias into the study data. (ESSENTIAL)

3.6.4. Intermixed data **

In order for "blinding" to be effective, subjects with various amounts of exposure should be intermixed in the data collection process, so that the examiners or data collectors are kept thoroughly ignorant of exposure status. The analogous principle for a case-control study is that interviewing of cases and controls should be intermixed (rather than interviewing the controls at separate locations or separate time periods from the cases). The same principle applies to laboratory assays; a given batch or run with a laboratory procedure should contain samples from persons at various dose levels. This will reduce the possible biases that could be introduced by inadvertent variations in laboratory procedures, reagents or calibration from batch to batch. (ESSENTIAL)

3.6.5. Quality assurance monitoring **

An integral part of an epidemiologic ocular study is the quality control/quality assurance (QA/QC). For a major study, a quality assurance committee should be formed that **1)** includes expertise in the dosimetric, ophthalmologic, epidemiologic and data management aspects of the study, and **2)** is given authority to see that suitable changes or corrections are implemented when necessary. This will help assure that the quality and integrity of the data are maintained at the highest level. The QA/QC committee would define a plan to monitor the data collection procedures on a regular ongoing basis and to periodically review samples of the data for accuracy, completeness and validity. The QA/QC committee should make data and procedures fully available for inspection. The QA/QC committee would normally report directly to the study director(s). They would submit written reports that note any irregularities or weaknesses found in the data or procedures, and the responsible data-collection groups should be required submit written responses documenting how they have corrected these problems. (ESSENTIAL)

3.6.6. Inter-scorer reliability

A useful technique is to have a fraction of study subjects re-examined by a second, independent ophthalmologist (where "independent" means that the second examiner does not know the findings of the first examiner). The independent scorings by the two examiners should be recorded and preserved; this will permit calculations of inter-examiner reliability, which is a valuable statistic to report. (Once the examiners have made their independent scorings, if there is a discrepancy the two examiners can discuss the case and arrive at a consensus scoring.) A second function of this re-examination process is that it allows ongoing monitoring of when an examiner is scoring differently from other examiners, so that timely re-training of the examiner in the use of the scoring criteria can be performed. (Recommended)

Periodic re-calibration of examiners: It is valuable to bring all the ophthalmologic examiners together periodically (perhaps yearly or biennially) and have a re-calibration session in the use of the scoring/diagnostic criteria. Part of the re-calibration should be to have each examiner independently examine and score a small series of persons and then have a group discussion about the scoring with the chief ophthalmologists (who represent the "gold standard" for scoring). It is preferable to choose persons to be examined in this session who represent a range of scoring categories and who are somewhat difficult to score, as these will help train for the maximum standardization in scoring. These procedures will increase the uniformity of ocular scoring/diagnosis among individual examiners and, in a multi-institutional study, will also help minimize differences in scoring between the examining centers. Differences in scoring between various examining centers can be of special concern if the average dose levels of the Liquidators seen at the various centers happen to differ systematically. (Recommended)

3.6.7. Data Analyses

The fundamental concept in the analysis is to estimate the relative risk in the exposed group, or to assess the trend in relative risk according to dose levels if there is a range of radiation doses. When a range of doses is available and the data set is reasonably large, it also becomes possible to evaluate whether the dose-response trend best fits a linear non-threshold function, a linear-quadratic function, a linear with threshold function, or other plausible dose-response functions. These analyses will be of value in that they address questions pertinent to the radiobiology of cataracts. Questions about the variation in risk over elapsed time since exposure can also be addressed. (Recommended)

3.6.8. Control for confounders **

The data analyses will need to control for confounders, preferably using modern multivariate statistical methods. (A "confounder" is a variable which is correlated with both the disease/disorder and the exposure in the data set; because of these joint correlations, the confounder variable can introduce bias into the analysis if not controlled for.) Therefore, preliminary analyses should be conducted to determine whether sociodemographic factors or other disease risk factors are acting as confounders; if so, they would be included as covariates in the analysis, either by stratification or by modeling. Since age is such a strong risk factor for ocular disorders, it should routinely be controlled for in analyses. (ESSENTIAL)

If there are multiple ocular examinations of each study subject over time (i.e., a longitudinal study), then a statistical method that takes into account the intra-individual correlation over time is needed, unless only a summary measure over time is being analyzed. Methods based on "generalized estimating equations" (Liang & Zeger, 1986) can be used to appropriately account for intra-individual correlation. (Recommended, if appropriate).

SUBJECT INDEX

AUTHOR'S INDEX